ENCYCLOPAEDIA OF EMBRYOLOGY

ENCYCLOPAEDIA OF EMBRYOLOGY

(Vol. 1)

Dr. A. Tyagi

ANMOL PUBLICATIONS PVT. LTD.

NEW DELHI - 110 002 (INDIA)

ANMOL PUBLICATIONS PVT. LTD.
H.O.: 4374/4B, Ansari Road, Darya Ganj,
New Delhi-110 002 (India)
Ph.: 23261597, 23278000

B.O.: No. 1015, Ist Main Road, BSK IIIrd Stage
IIIrd Phase, IIIrd Block,
Bangalore - 560 085 (India)
Visit us at: www.anmolpublications.com

Encyclopaedia of Embryology

First Published, 2006

ISBN 81-261-2676-0 (Set)

PRINTED IN INDIA

Published by J.L. Kumar for Anmol Publications Pvt. Ltd., New Delhi - 110 002 and Printed at **Arora** Offset Press, Delhi.

Contents

Preface

Literally, embryology is the study of embryos, where embryo denotes the juvenile stage, either within the egg-shell, egg membranes or in the mother's womb. In the development stage, the embryo undergoes a number of changes. The changes occur not only in the body of the larva but also in habit or behaviour also. It is due to these dramatic changes that embryology has now been termed 'Developmental Biology' preferably.

Metamorphosis, embryonic induction, embryonic nutrition, regeneration, cleavage, parthenogenesis (development of egg without fertilization), gametogenesis and fertilization are few of numerous other points of study under embryology.

Though a number of books on every subject are available in the market, there is being felt a dearth of such an encyclopaedia as may answer any queries regarding any of the points which come under embryology.

Present encyclopaedia may prove to be an appreciable step in this direction. Hopefully, this would cater to the maximum requirements of the bio-enthusiasts.

Editor

Preface

Literally, embryology is the study of embryos, where embryo denotes the juvenile stage, either within the egg-shell, egg membranes or in the mother's womb. In the development stage, the embryo undergoes a number of changes. These changes occur not only in the body of the larva but also in habit or behaviour also. It is due to these changes, mainly that embryology has now been termed developmental biology preferably.

Metamorphosis, embryonic induction, embryonic differentiation, regeneration, cleavage, parthenogenesis (development of egg without fertilisation), gametogenesis and fertilization are few of numerous other points of study under embryology.

Though a number of books on every subject are available in the market, there is being felt a dearth of such an encyclopaedia as may answer any queries regarding any of the points which come under embryology.

Hence, this endeavour may prove to be a pioneering step in this direction. Hopefully, this would cater to the maximum requirements of the bio-enthusiasts.

Editor

1

Metamorphosis

Definition : Metamorphosis (Gr. *metamorphoun :* to transform) is an important phenomenon during development in a number of animals which involves dramatic changes in habit, habitat, morphology, physiology and behaviour of larva so that it is transformed into the adult having entirely different habit and structure. For example:

(i) the change from a planktonic to a benthic existence in sea urchin,

(ii) from an aquatic to a terrestrial existence in frogs and toads and

(iii) from non-flying to a flying existence in insects.

Occurrence of Metamorphosis

Larval forms and accompanying metamorphosis occur in many phyla of invertebrates from sponges to echinoderms and in several chordates including amphibians. Based upon the presence or absence of metamorphosis, two type of embryonic developments are recognized-

1. Direct development in which the fertilized egg develops directly into the young one and there is no larval stage. The young one that comes out of the egg is a miniature adult as in reptiles, birds and mammals.
2. Indirect development in which the fertilized egg hatches into larva, entirely different from adult both in structure and habit. It leads an independent existence for a brief period and then gradually changes into the adult. The larvae found in different groups have different structure and are known by special names.

The occurrence of larva and metamorphosis depends upon the amount of yolk present in the ovum.

1. In eggs with large amount of yolk (as in reptiles and birds), the development is direct with no larval stage and no metamorphosis because the supply of food is sufficient for complete development.
2. In eggs with very little or no yolk (as in placental mammals), the developing embryo receives food supply from mother through placenta and again the development is direct without larval stage.
3. In eggs with yolk but not sufficient for the complete development (as in *Herd mania, Amphioxus,* frog and insects), the developing embryo diapause at larval stage. The larval stage is free swimming and feeds voraciously to store food material for further development.

Types of Metamorphosis

Depending upon whether larva exhibits advanced characters or the adult, metamorphosis can be of following types —

Retrogressive Metamorphosis : Retrogressive metamorphosis includes degeneration of certain advanced characters of the larva during metamorphosis so that the adult's organization is more simple and primitive. The adult, in such cases, is known as degenerated. This metamorphosis is found among Ascidians. Its details have been discussed in the embryology of an Ascidian.

Progressive Metamorphosis-V : In progressive metamorphosis simple larval organization changes into more complex organization of the adult. Metamorphosis in amphibians and in insects is of progressive type.

Neoteny : In this case larva attains adulthood without undergoing any metamorphic changes. Thus in neoteny larva develops gonads and reproduces its own kind. This phenomenon is called paedogenesis. Axolotl larva of *Ambystoma* exhibits neoteny.

S.No.	*Phylum*	*Larval form*
1.	Porifera	Amphiblastula
2.	Coelenterata	Planula
3.	Platyhelminthes-	
	(a) Turbellaria	Muller's larva
	(b) Trematoda	Miracidium, sporocyst, redia, cercaria and metacercaria, etc.
	(c) Cestoda	Onchosphere
4.	Nemertenea	Pilidium
5.	Annelida	Trochophore
6.	Mollusca	Trochophore and veliger
7.	Arthropoda	
	(a) Crustacea	Nauplius, metanauplius, zoea, megalopa
	(b) Insecta	(i) No larva i.e. insects with no metamorphosis.

Contd...

S.No.	Phylum	Larval form
		(ii) Nymph i.e. insects with incomplete metamorphosis.
		(iii) Caterpillar, grub, etc. i.e. insects with complete metamorphosis.
8.	Bryozoa (Ectoprocta)	Cyphonautes larva
9.	Echinodermata	Bipinnaria, auricularia, doliolaria and pluteus, etc.
10.	Enteropneusta	Tornaria larva
11.	Ascidiacea	Tadpole
12.	Cyclostomata	Ammocoete
13.	Amphibia	Tadpole larva

Metamorphosis in Chordates

Progressive Metamorphosis in Amphibia : Metamorphosis of frog can be studied as an example of progressive type of metamorphosis. The metamorphosis of tadpole larva into adult frog involves changes associated with the transformation of an aquatic, gill-breathing, fish-like and herbivorous larva into a semi-terrestrial lung breathing and carnivorous adult. The changes taking place during this transformation can be studied under following three categories —

1. Ecological changes
2. Morphological changes
3. Physiological changes.

Ecological Changes : These include changes in habitat and feeding habit —

1. Aquatic and fish-like tadpoles change into semi-terrestrial frogs.
2. The herbivorous tadpoles feeding on vegetable matter with the aid of horny teeth (in frog) or plankton feeder (in clawed toad) change into carnivorous adult living on insects, worms, small frogs and small rodents.
3. Change from aquatic mode of respiration (by gills) to terrestrial (by lungs) mode of respiration.

Morphological Changes : The changes in structure of tadpole during metamorphosis are grouped into three categories—

(a) regressive changes,

(b) progressive changes and

(c) remodelling.

Regressive changes during Amphibian Metamorphosis : These changes include the gradual reduction and final disappearance of all those larval structures which were essential in the larva but are no more needed in the adult. These include:

Tail : The long tail with a tail fin, necessary for larva swimming is no more required on land and hence it is gradually absorbed during metamorphosis. Its degenerating tissue provides ourishment to the metamorphosing tadpole.

Gills and Gill-clefts : The larval gill clefts are closed and the operculum and opercular chamber disappear.

Sucker : The larval sucker completely disappears.

Jaws : The horny projection from lips of tadpole and also the horny teeth are shed off. The larval jaws are replaced by true jaws first formed of cartiage and then get ossified into bony structure.

Cloacal tube becomes short and reduced.

Lateral-line sense organs are lost.

Branchial vessels supplying gills also disappear with the disappearance of gills.

Progressive changes during Amphibian Metamorphosis : These changes involve the progressive development and specialization of the larval organs such as—

Limbs : The two pairs of limbs that had just made their appearance in larva gradually increase in size and become functional. The hindlimbs become greatly enlarged and adapted for jumping and for swimming (webbed). The forelimbs also grow out.

Head : The head becomes broad and triangular.

Mouth : The small, rounded mouth gape changes into a broad crescentric aperture without lips and horny projections. Teeth develop in the upper jaw only.

Tongue : Tongue develops from the floor of buccal cavity.

Eyes : The eyes become large, more prominent and bright. They come to occupy highest position on the head.

Nictitating Membrane : Develops in the eyes.

Middle ear or tympanum and tympanic cavity develop in connection with the first branchial pouch.

Hyoid apparatus develops from the branchial (gill) arches.

Lungs : Lungs develop for aerial breathing.

Remodelling of Existing Larval Structures : During amphibian metamorphosis certain larval structures are modified or remodelled to suit the need of adult. These are:

Heart : Heart becomes three-chambered and maintains an isolation of deoxygenated and oxygenated bloods which are pumped together.

Blood Vascular System : In tadpole, the blood vascular system is like that of a fish. During metamorphosis it is modified to supply lungs. Some other changes in portal systems also occur.

Intestine : In herbivorous tadpole, the intestine is very long and coiled like a watch-spring. During metamorphosis it gets greatly shortened due to carnivorous habit of the adult.

Skin : The soft and moist larval skin becomes thick and glandular suited to live on land. Its two-layered epidermis becomes many layered and the surface layers become cornified. Multicellular serous and mucous glands develop and sink into the subcutaneous tissue as pocket. The pigmentation of skin also changes.

Physiological Changes : Alongwith the above-mentioned morphological changes, the following biochemical and physiological changes occur during metamorphosis in the larva:

(i) The islets of Langerhans of pancreas start functioning to produce insulin(endocrine).

(ii) Liver becomes more active. Its enzyme system becomes more elaborate to metabolize more carbohydrates and to synthesize urea from ammonia.

(iii) The ammonotelic larva changes to ureotelic adult and as such the larval kidney are replaced by mesonephric kidney.

(iv) The larval visual pigment-porphyropsin (retinene-2) is replaced by rhodopsin or retinene-1.

(v) The larval haemoglobin is replaced by adult haemoglobin. The serum albumin and serum proteins increase in concentration.

(vi) *Autolysis :* The disappearance of larval tail, gills and other structures is brought about by autolysis. It is facilitated by amoeboid phagocytes (macrophages).

Their lysosomal enzymes like cathepsin, etc. record a steep rise in concentration and utilization. The autolysed or phagocytosised material is reabsorbed and is used in the construction of new organs of the adult.

(vii) *Degrowlh :* During metamorphosis feeding is suspended. Therefore, reserve food is utilized by the larva to produce energy required for the completion of various processes of metamorphosis. Therefore, there is loss of weight. The miniature frog produced, at the end of metamorphosis, is lighter and smaller than the mature tadpole. This reduction of body mass is called 'degrowth'. The reduction of body mass is also caused by the shrinking of some parts of larval body. For example, the head and trunk become smaller during metamorphosis.

(viii) *Enzymes :* There is a remarkable change in the types and amount of enzymes produced during metamorphosis to facilitate the completion of metamorphic processes. Some larval enzymes not required in the adult are synthesized no more, whereas synthesis of some new enzymes begins during the process.

(ix) There are changes in the metabolism of carbohydrate, lipid and nitrogen.

(x) *Water Balance :* The absorption power of kidney tubules increases considerably to avoid loss of water in urine. This is associated with the terrestrial existence of adult and leads to the replacement of less efficient larval mesonephric kidney by the more efficient, elaborate mesonephric kidney of adult.

The study of metamorphosis in frog indicates that all the morphological and physiological changes occurring during metamorphosis have a direct adaptive value relating to the transition from freshwater habitat to terrestrial existence.

Summary of Metamorphic Changes in Anurans

S.N.	*System*	*Larva*	*Adult*
1.	Locomotory	Tail fin	Tail lost; 2 pairs of limbs develop for locomotion on land.
2.	Respiratory	Gills, gill clefts and operculum	All lost; lungs develop for aerial respiration.
3.	Circulatory	(i) Heart two chambered.	(i) Heart becomes three-chambered.
		(ii) Aortic arches and ventral aorta like that of fish.	(ii) Aortic arches modify into carotid, systemic and pulmo-cutaneous arches of the adult.
		(iii) The cardinal veins of venous system are similar to fish.	(iii) Replaced by jugular and caval veins.
4.	Nutrition	(i) Herbivorous.	(i) Carnivorous (insectivorous).
		(ii) Mouth small with horny lips and labial teeth.	(ii) Mouth large cresentric, jaws replaced with bony jaws, horny lips lost.
		(iii) Intestine very long and coiled like a watch-spring.	(iii) Intestine short with just a few coils.
		(iv) More of carbohydrases enzymes	(iv) Enzyme proteases are more abundant.
		(v) Liver less developed	(v) Liver more developed
5.	Excretory	(i) Excretory product largely ammonia (ammonotelic).	(i) Excretory product largely urea (ureotelic).
		(ii) Liver unable to convert ammonia into urea.	(ii) Liver possesses enzymes necessary for changing ammonia into urea (enzymes of ornithine urea cycle).
6.	Nervous System and Sense organs	(i) Corneal reflex absent	(i) Corneal reflex developed due to development of ocular muscles.
		(ii) Nictitating membrane absent.	(ii) Eye with nictitating membrane.
		(iii) Visual pigment porphyropsin or retinene 2.	(iii) Visual pigment is rhodo-psin (retinene 1)
		(iv) Lateral line system and its sense organs are well developed.	(iv) Lateral line system degenerated
		(v) Tympanum, tympanic membrane and columella are absent.	(v) Tympanum, tympanic membrane and the columella well developed.

Hormonal Control of Amphibian Metamorphosis

Metamorphosis in Amphibians is initiated by:

1. Thyroid hormone-thyroxin and tri-iodothyronine
2. Iodine.

Thyroid and Metamorphosis

Experimental Evidence : Metamorphosis is initiated by the functional development of thyroid gland. The thyroid hormone is carried by blood to different parts of the body, where it enhances wide-spread changes. Thyroid is essential for initiating metamorphosis has been proved by the followed experiments-

(i) It was first demonstrate by Gudernatsch (1912) when fed some frog tadpoles on dried and powdered sheep thyroid and found that they metamorphosed precociously.

(ii) Allen (1918) removed thyroid rudiment in frog tadpoles at tail-bud stage. The thyroidless tadpoles showed normal growth and attained a much larger size (123 mm.) than the normal tadpole (60 mm.) but failed to metamorphose. This proves that metamorphosis cannot be initiated without stimulus from thyroid gland.

(iii) When these thyroidless tadpoles were immersed in water containing soluble extracts from thyroid gland, they immediately underwent metamorphosis (Allen 1938).

(iv) Feeding the young tadpole with thyroid gland or injecting thyroid extract or by putting young tadpoles in water containing thyroid extract, the metamorphosis is induced to occur in young larvae.

Similar experiments were carried out on Urodeles by Marx (1935). Axolotl larva of *Ambystoma maxicanum* which under normal conditions does not metamorphose, may be induced to do so by thyroid treatment.

Chemical Composition of Thyroid Hormone **:** The thyroid secretion is a complex protein, thyroglobulin, which has molecular weight of about 675,000. It is in inactive form and is formed of several molecules of low molecular weight compounds. The compounds are tri-iodo-thyronine and thyroxine or tetra-iodo-thyronine. In both these compounds two residues of amino acid tyrosine are joined together. Three atoms of iodine in tri-iodothyronine and four atoms of iodine in thyroxine are attached to the tyrosine molecules. Of the two compounds of thyroid secretion, thyroxine forms the main active substance, but tri-iodothyronine is more effective on tissues.

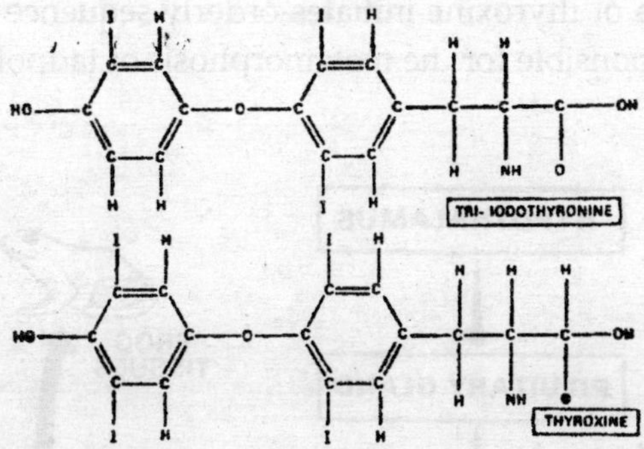

Structural formulae of tri-iodothyronine and thyroxine.

Mechanism of Hormone Action

According to W. Etkin (1968)-

(i) The pace of metamorphic events depends on the concentration of thyroid hormone. Because of this reason, the thyroid hormone concentration in blood and tissues gradually increases during last two-third of larval life upto the phase of metamorphic climax and then drops suddenly.

(ii) The reactivity of different larval tissues to different concentrations of thyroid hormone is inherent in the tissue. It means different tissues have different critical threshold.

(iii) The concentration of thyroid hormone in the blood and tissues at the time of metamorphosis is increased by the thyrotropin releasing factor (TRF) secreted by the hypothalamus.

It is now presumed that at a critical point in the development, some genetic mechanism makes the hypothalamus sensitive to low concentration of thyroid hormone circulating in the larval blood. It, then secretes thyrotropin releasing factor (TRF) which stimulates the anterior pituitary or hypophysis to release thyroid stimulating hormone (TSH). TSH in turn, causes an increase of thyroid hormone. The increase of thyroxine initiates orderly sequence of tissue-changes responsible for the metamorphosis of tadpole into the adult.

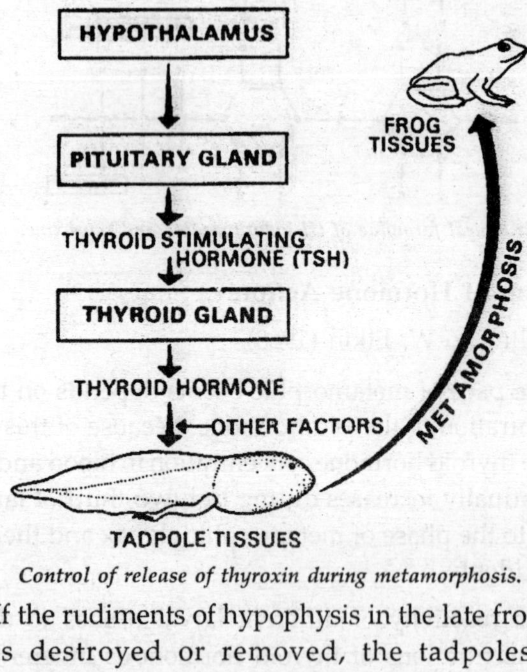

Control of release of thyroxin during metamorphosis.

1. If the rudiments of hypophysis in the late frog embryo is destroyed or removed, the tadpoles do not metamorphose but if piece of hypophysis from metamorphosed or adult frog are implanted the

metamorphosis sets in, provided the thyroid gland is intact.

2. If part of hypothalamus attached to the pituitary is isolated from the latter, the TSH level fails to increase and consequently thyroid gland remains sluggish and tadpole fails to metamorphose.

Another hormone of anterior pituitary, the prolactin acts as an inhibitor. The overall control on metamorphosis is the interaction of TSH and prolactin.

The pituitary thyroid axis is kept at a low level of activity during growth-phase of tadpole, i.e. during premetamorphosis phase. During prometamorphosis period, TRF increases by the action of hypothalamus. TRF induces secretion of thyroxin which reaches climax during metamorphosis. Therefore, prolactin acts as an antagonist to TSH. The metamorphosis is the result of dynamic balance of these two hormones.

Tissue Reactivity in Amphibian Metamorphosis : In amphibian metamorphosis, a single agent, the thyroxin (a low molecular weight compound) evokes multiple responses in diversified tissues. The responses, though diversified, are specific and are both constructive and destructive depending on the target tissue. This depends on two points—

(1) The reactivity of the tissues of the target organ to the thyroid hormone (the competence).

(2) The threshold value of different larval tissues for thyroid hormone concentration.

Competence of Larval Tissues or Multiple Response : The reactivity or responsiveness of different larval tissues to thyroxin is markedly different. For example, tissues of tail and gills become necrotic and undergo degeneration owing to the action of thyroid hormone, while the tissues of limbs increase and undergo differentiation. Thyroxine induces rapid ageing and destruction of R.B.Cs of metamorphosing tadpoles (carrying larval haemoglobin) and simultaneously stimulates the development of cells that synthesize the haemoglobin of adult frog type.

The tri-iodothyronine reduces biosynthesis of nucleic acids in tail but increases their synthesis in liver. Moreover, muscles of the tail show degeneration while those of trunk remain unaffected.

The above examples clearly show that the response and reactivity of larval tissue is very different to the same agent. It can also be demonstrated by experiments that the reactivity of tissues is tissue-specific and is not associated with their location in the body. (i) Parts of a tadpole tail if transplanted to the trunk of a tadpole undergoing metamorphosis undergoes necrosis alongwith the host tail and becomes absorbed. (ii) If an eye of a tadpole is transplanted to the tail of a tadpole before the tail shrinks and degenerates but the eye remains normal and is brought nearer to the trunk and finally comes to lie in the sacral region.

Threshold Value : Kollros (1961) has demonstrated that different larval tissues have different threshold value i.e. are sensitive to different concentrations of thyroid hormone. In general, structures that change early during metamorphosis are more sensitive and have low threshold than those undergoing change at a later stage. Even different parts of one organ may have different threshold. For example, threshold for perforation of operculum is lower than the threshold for gill absorption. A higher dose of thyroid hormone is required for the breakthrough of forelegs and an even greater dose of thyroid hormone is necessary for absorption of tail. In case of hindlimbs long exposure to low concentration of thyroxine promotes differentiation to three-digit stage.

A higher concentration is required for the differentiation of five digits and a still higher one for the formation of interdigital web. Such experiments clearly indicate that:

(i) the parts which have a low threshold responses earlier during metamorphosis than the parts having a high threshold value, i.e. the threshold value is reflected in the order in which the metamorphic changes proceed in the normal development. In urodels, the bulging of eyes reacts to the weakest dose of thyroid hormone (minimum threshold) and is the first event during metamorphosis. Next follows the reduction of fin fold, and shortening and disappearance of external gills, followed by closure of gill-clefts and transformation of skin.

(ii) there is a progressively-increasing threshold at different stages of development of a particular organ and even during the entire process of metamorphosis.

Regulation of Metamorphic Molecular Events by Hormones in Amphibian Metamorphosis : During metamorphosis there is an extensive re-orientation of protein synthesis. Synthesis of some larval proteins diminishes while synthesis of a number of new proteins commences. Tata (1970) has reported in the hepatocytes of metamorphosing tadpoles production of rRNA and mRNA increases leading to the formation of new ribosomes and polysomes and finally an increase in protein synthesis.

Insect Metamorphosis : One of the most characteristic features of insects development is that they almost always hatch in a condition morphologically different from that assumed in the imago. In order to reach the latter instar they pass through changes in form and structure and sometimes in habit which are collectively termed metamorphosis. However, the degree of metamorphosis varies in different groups. Broadly, three types of metamorphosis have been recognised:

No Metamorphosis or Slight Metamorphosis (Ametabolous Development) : In primitive wingless insects (Apterygota) like silver fish, spring tails, etc. and in secondarily apterous exopterygotes the young one that emerges from the egg is essentially similar to the imago, differing from it only in size, immature reproductive organs and external genitalia. It moults several times leading to gradual increase in size accompanied by maturation of sex organs and appearance of external genitalia. The moulting and growth continues even after reproductive maturity. These insects are, therefore, regarded to have no metamorphosis. But, since the changes discussed above are marked, it is now described that these have slight metamorphosis and these insects are called ametabolus.

Egg → Young → Imago

Incomplete Metamorphosis (Hemimetabolous Development) : Insects of Exopterygota exhibit simple metamorphosis. The young ones that hatch out of the eggs resemble the adults or imago in general form and metamorphosis in them includes gradual growth and acquisition of wings, genitalia and gonads. Therefore, a pupal stage is wanting and the young ones are known as nymphs. The degree of metamorphosis varies in hemimetabolous forms but two major types are very distinct: (i) Gradual metamorphosis — In insects like cockroaches, grasshoppers and crickets, etc., the nymph is similar to adult both in structure as well as in habit, but lacks wings, gonads and external genitalia. It moults several times as it grows and develops gonads, genitalia and also the wing pads in the second and third thoracic segments in the later larval period. The transformation of wing pads into functional wings occurs at the last moult. This last nymphal stage with wing pads and genitalia is called imago stage which moults finally into a winged adult, after which the insect does not moult anymore. There is no quiescent stage and no disappearance or remodelling of larval parts.

Egg → Nymph → Imago

Partial Metamorphosis : In insects like dragonflies, Mayflies, damselflies the nymphs differ from adult both in external structure as well as in habits. The nymphs are aquatic and herbivorous. Therefore, they possess tracheal gills for respiration, mandibulate mouthparts for cutting vegetables and some organs for locomotion. These young ones are known as niads. These undergo extensive remodelling to assume adult organization, by shedding gills, modifying mouthparts and developing wings. There may be one or more quiescent or semiquiescent stages (recalling pupa) and disappearance of a few larval parts (gill, etc.) and remodelling of some other parts (mouth parts).

Therefore, this type of metamorphosis is known as partial or incomplete metamorphosis.

$$\text{Egg} \rightarrow \text{Niad} \rightarrow \text{Imago}$$

Complete Metamorphosis or Holometaboly : In all endopterygota insects like butterflies, moths, bees, wasps, beetles and flies, etc. the egg hatches into a worm-like larva, very much different from imago or adult in structure, appearance and habit. The larva has a worm-like body, biting and chewing type of mouthparts, simple eyes and poorly developed walking legs. It has quite a different way of life. For example, the larva of butterfly crawls on the ground, eats leaves, while adult butterfly flies in the air and drinks nectar from flowers. The mosquito larva lives in water and eats algae and protozoa while the adult sucks blood or flower and fruit juices.

The larvae crawl or swim, eat voraciously, grow in size and moult several times and finally change into a quiescent state, called pupa. The pupa neither moves, nor feeds and is enclosed in a pupal case or puparium (cocoon in butterflies and moths) secreted by the labial glands of the larva. Inside the puparium two types of changes occur at a fast speed. These are histolysis and histogenesis.

Histolytic Changes : In histolysis all the larval organs except the central nervous system are broken down by special amoebocytic cells, called phagocytes. The tissue fluid formed by their destruction is utilized as raw material in the construction of adult organs.

Histogenesis : This includes the development of adult organs from group of cells of imaginal buds, or imaginal discs. The imaginal buds are actually the rudiments of future organs of the adult such as wings, walking legs, antennae, mouthparts and internal organs etc. These develop directly from egg and remain quiescent or nonfunctional all through the larval stage. During pupal stage these discs or buds grow in size and differentiate into adult structures which remain collapsed and folded. When reorganization is completed, it undergoes another moult and the young insect or imago emerges out. At its emergence, the blood is pumped into these collapsed structures, which unfold and inflate and chitin is deposited to make them hard.

Egg → Larva → Pupa → Imago

Hormonal Control of Insect Metamorphosis : The process of moulting and metamorphosis in insects is controlled by hormones secreted by

(i) brain (protocerebrum),

(ii) corpora allata and

(iii) prothoracic gland.

The hormonal control of insect metamorphosis was worked out by Wigglesworth in England and Carroll Williams at Harvard. While working on giant Cecropia moth, Williams has demonstrated that neurosecretory cells in the protocerebellum of larva brain are arranged in four groups. These produce prothoracotropic hormone (PTTH) which stimulates prothoracic gland located in the thorax. The prothoracic gland, in turn secretes growth and differentiation hormone which is known as ecdysone. Edysone stimulates epidermis to secrete moulting fluid leading to moulting in larva and initiates metamorphosis i.e. moulting of larva into pupa and that of pupa into the imago or adult.

1. Ecdysone is a steroid with the formula $C_{27}H_{44}O_6$. Karlson and Butenandt in Germany were able to isolate ecdysone in pure form from the silkworm-*Bombyx*. Ecdysone is present in all insects and other arthropods similar to the presence of thyroid hormone in all classes of vertebrates. Ecdysone has two different effects :
   1. Induces growth.
   2. Causes moulting by removing old cuticle and its replacement by the new cuticle. But this hormone does not determine whether the moult will be a larval moult producing next larval stage, or the pupal moult converting the larva into pupa or the imaginal moult, leading to the emergence of imago.
2. Another hormone, the juvenile hormone (JH) secreted by the endocrine gland, corpora allata (located near insect brain), ensures the occurrence of larval moults and inhibits metamorphosis. Therefore, its presence or absence determine whether the larva will moult into a larva or into a pupa.

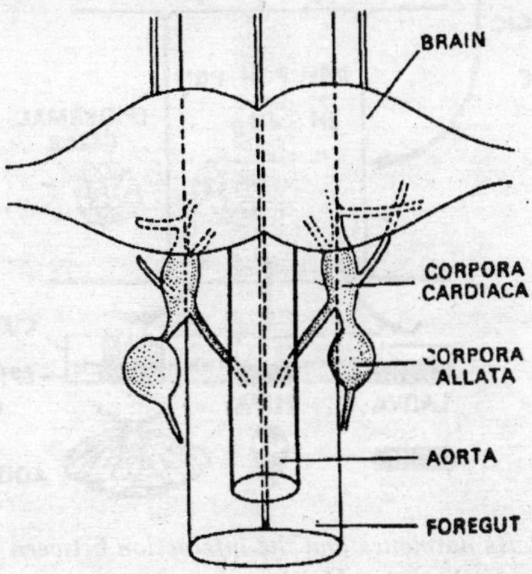

Endocrine glands in inserts associated with metamorphosis.

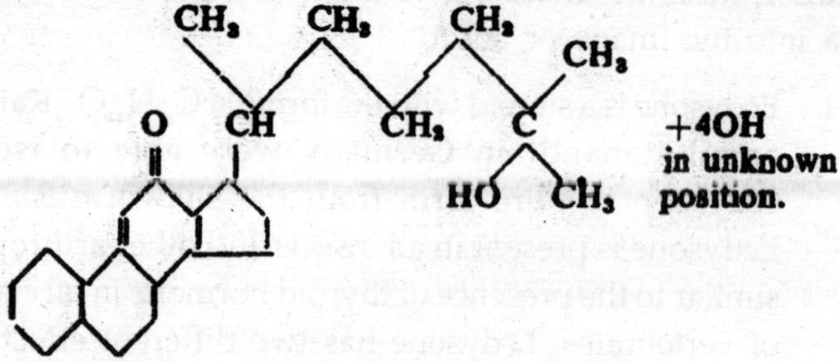

Structural formula of ecdysone.

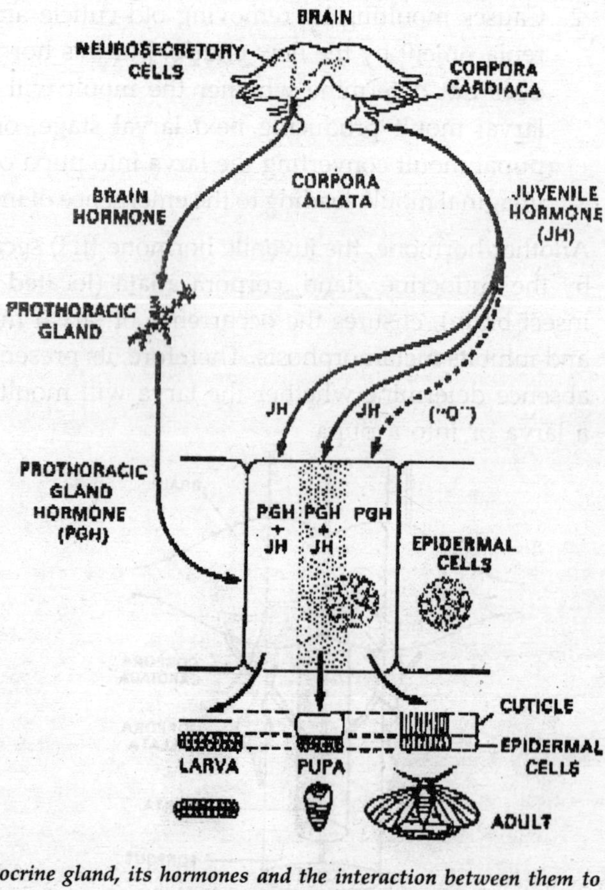

Endocrine gland, its hormones and the interaction between them to induce metamorphic changes in insects.

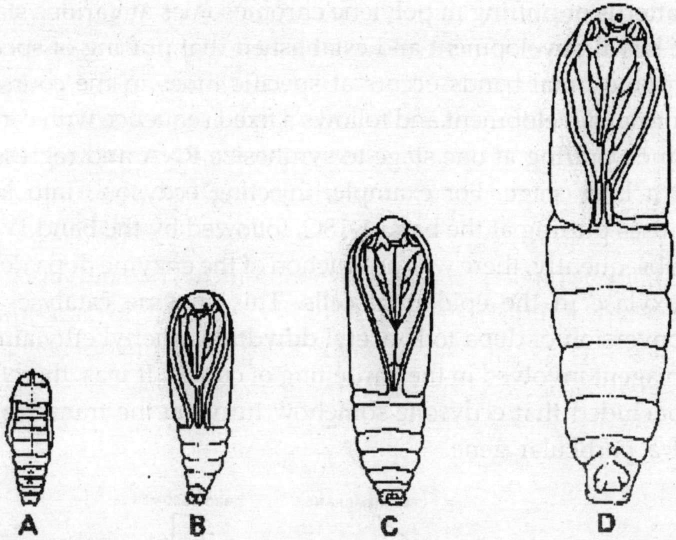

Diagram showing the effect of extra amount of juvenile hormone which produces a giant larva.

In the presence of ecdysone, the juvenile hormone promotes larval development or maintains the *status quo.* It means that presence of JH in an immature insect, whether larva or pupa, ensures that after moulting it retains larval or pupal characters. In other words withdrawal or absence of JH initiates metamorphosis. Conversely, if extrajuvenile hormone-producing gland from second-stage larva is transplanted to a late or fourth-stage larva, it undergoes additional larval moults and grows to a giant size. Removal of corpora allata early in the larval life results in premature metamorphosis.

Mechanism of Hormone Action in Insects : Insect-moulting hormones work at the chromosomal level. These influence the specific gene loci, control their transcription and finally influence cell differentiation. This was first reported by Clever and Karlson (1960) when he injected minute amount of ecdysone into' the larvae of dipteran insect *Chironomus tetanus.* Within fifteen minutes, the hormones induced puffing or swelling of specific region of a particular chromosome. He also studied the patterns of puffing in polytene chromosomes at various stages of larval development and established that puffing of specific chromosomal bands occurs at specific times in the course of normal development and follows a fixed sequence with certain bands puffing at one stage to synthesize RNA and regressing at a later stage. For example, injecting ecdysone into larva causes puffing at the band 1-18C, followed by the band IV-2B. Subsequently, there was production of the enzyme dopa decarboxylase in the epidermal cells. This enzyme catalyses the conversion of dopa to N-acetyl dihydroxy phenyl ethylamine, an agent involved in the hardening of cuticle. It was, therefore, concluded that ecdysone somehow turns on the transcription of a particular gene.

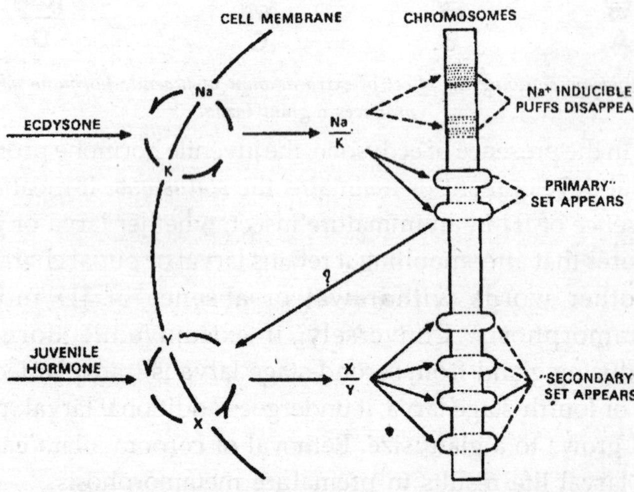

Probable effect of ecdysone on gene puffing by changes in membrane permeability for Na/K ions. (After Berrill, 1971)

There is evidence that ecdysone activates only one or two genes which produce puffs very early after ecdysone injections. This in turn, starts a chain reaction, involving puffing of other genes one after the other ending in moulting or metamorphosis as the case may be (Clever 1961,65).

It is still not well understood whether ecdysone as such

acts on gene or it changes the intra-nuclear milieu and a change in intranuclear milieu then affects the gene. Goodenough and Levine (1974) have suggested that ecdysone might control puffing and transcription of genes by any one of the following methods—

(i) By serving as a regulatory molecule, it might interact with the controlling elements that maintain the polytene DNA quiescent.

(ii) By serving as an effector molecule, it might modify the activity of some regulatory proteins associated with DNA.

(iii) By influencing the uptake of certain ions that stimulate the transcription of genes involved with moulting.

According to Kroeger (1968) ecdysone causes accumulation of K^+ ions by increasing its uptake.

(iv) According to Berrill (1971) the hormone acts at two sites. At cell membrane level, it alters cell permeability and consequently the intracellular and intranuclear electrolyte media. At chromosomal level it causes a differential pattern of mRNA synthesis by influencing the histones bound to DNA.

Comparison of Amphibian and Insect Metamorphosis : The process of metamorphosis in insects and amphibians exhibits marked similarity as follows —

(i) In both cases, the diffusible chemical substances (hormones) influence differentiation of cells and morphogenetic processes during metamorphosis.

(ii) The stimulus for secretion of hormones responsible for initiation of metamorphosis is provided by neurosecretory cells of brain (hypophysis in amphibians and protocerebrum in insects).

(iii) The neurosecretion does not act directly on the larval tissues but stimulates the secretion activity of a second endocrine gland (thyroid in amphibians and prothoracic gland in insects).

(iv) Metamorphosis in both cases involves some destructive activities (histolysis) and some constructive activities (histogenesis).

Metamorphosis in Insects

The changes undergone by an immature larval insect into a sexually mature adult form, the imago, is collectively known as metamorphosis. The imago is often quite different from the immature young in form, structure, habits and habitat. Metamorphosis in these animals is a special form of moulting. It is the periodic shedding of the cuticle of the skin which necessarily accompanies growth.

Types of Metamorphosis : In some insects metamorphosis is more pronounced whereas in other it is less conspicuous. Insects exhibit 4 types of metamorphosis :

Development without Metamorphosis or Ametabolous Development: In certain insects, like the *silver fish* and *spring tails,* metamorphosis does not take place and the newly hatched young resembles the adult in form, structure and mode of life, though it is smaller in size. It grows and after a few moults attains the adult stature without undergoing any transformation. The life history of these insects, therefore, includes three stages :

eggs ⟶ young ⟶ imago (adult).

Gradual Metamorphosis or Paurometabolous Development: In *cockroaches, locusts, grasshoppers, white ants* and bugs, the newly hatched young resembles the adult in general body form, habits and habitat, but lacks wings and external genital appendages. The young gradually grows and develops the rudiments of the wings externally in the form of flat outgrowths of the second and third thoracic segment. These rudiments increase with every subsequent moult, but at the last moult there is an abrupt and very marked increase in the size of the wings, and after this moult the wings become functional.

This type of metamorphosis in which the young undergoes slow but steady change for becoming an adult is known as the gradual metamorphosis. The young of insects with gradual metamorphosis is called a nymph. In these insects too, there are three stages in the life history.

egg ⟶ nymph ⟶ imago (adult).

Incomplete Metamorphosis or Hemimetabolous Development: In *dragonflies, mayflies,* and *damselflies,* the immature stages are called naiads which are aquatic and respire by tracheal gills, whereas the adults are terrestrial or aerial. The young lacks wings but the adult is winged. It respires by tracheae. In these insects again there are three stages in the life history :

egg ⟶ naiad ⟶ imago (adult).

Complete Metamorphosis or Holometabolous Development: This type of metamorphosis includes four development stages :

egg ⟶ larva ⟶ pupa ⟶ imago (adult)

Complete metamorphosis takes place in several insects like *caddisflies, beetles, butterflies, moths, bees, and wasps, mosquitoes* and *flies.* In the type of metamorphosis, the young differs from the adult in shape, structure and mode of life.

The young on hatching, is worm-like in appearance and is called the larva. It varies in structure in different insects and is known by specific names. In the *housefly,* the larva is without legs and is called the maggot. The mature larva is about 12 mm long. It has a small head with a pair of oral lobes and hooks.

The head is followed by 12 segments. *In butterflies and moths,* the larva is called the caterpillar. It has three pairs of jointed true legs on the thorax and several short, thick prolegs on the abdomen. The larvae of *mosquitoes* are known as wrigglers because they exhibit wriggling movements in the water. The larva of *culex* has a large chitinous head, a thorax and an abdomen of nine segments with a respiratory siphon and four tracheal gills.

The intake of food in the larva is very high.

In insects with complete metamorphosis a resting stage, the pupa is intercalated between the larval and the adult condition. In the pupal stage the insects do not take food and are very restricted in their movements, if they move at all. The pupa of *culex* is comma-shaped and is often called a tumbler. It possesses a large cephalothorax with a pair of respiratory trumpets and a ventrally flexed abdomen made up of nine segments.

The terminal segment has a pair of chitinous leaf-like paddles by which the pupa swims, the pupa of *house-fly* is enclosed in a dark brown-coloured barrel-shaped chitinous casing the puparium. Such a pupa is called coarctate. The puparium is segmented externally. It shows traces of larval spiracles and spiny pads which are non-functional. In silk-worm, the covering around a pupa is called the cocoon. It is formed of silk threads.

During metamorphosis, most of the larval organs in the pupa, except the central nervous system and the developing sex organs, are broken down. This process of the disintegration of larval organs is called histolysis which is brought about by phogocytic blood corpuscles. The latter feed upon the tissues of disintegrating organs and products of their digestion are then utilized for constructing new structures.

Groups of formative cells called imaginal discs are set

aside in the pupa. These are the rudiments of the future organs reaching full differentiation in the imago. The process of formation of organs of the adult inside a pupa is called histogenesis. Not only *wings* but also *mouth parts, antennae* and *legs* develop from imaginal discs. During complete metamorphosis of higher insects the larval *muscles* are broken down and their residues are consumed by phagocytes. The adult muscles, particularly the flight muscles, are then developed. The *eyes* of the adult insects are developed from special imaginal discs.

Physiological Control of Metamorphosis : It has been established that the moulting and metamorphosis in insects is controlled by hormones. Three organs of internal secretion are concerned with this process : (1) the brain (protocerebrum) (2) the prothoracic glands and (3) the corpora allata. The glandular cells of all three organs show secretory activity prior to each moult, and the three types of secretion are essential for the normal course of larval moults.

The Brain (protocerebrum): There are four groups of *neurosecretory cells* in the brain. Of these, two groups lie near the midline and one group on each side. The neurosecretory cells secrete a hormone which serves to activate the prothoracic gland as a result of which the moulting is initiated. The secretion of the brain, therefore, cannot act directly but only through the activation of the prothoracic gland.

The Prothoracic Gland: It is an irregular branching mass of glandular cells located in the thorax. The prothoracic gland lies in close association with the tracheal tubes. The hormone produced by the prothoracic gland is called the growth and moulting hormone or ecdysone. It has the following functions :

(i) It initiates the process of moulting in the epidermis as a result of which the epidermal cells undergo growth and proliferation.

(ii) It is responsible for the shedding of the old cuticle and the production of the new one.

Butenandt and Karlson (1951) prepared ecdysone in a chemically pure form from silkworm pupae. 25 mg of the pure substance was isolated from five hundred kilograms of silkworm pupae. It was found that 0.0057 mg of ecdysone thus isolated was enough to cause the pupation of a fly larva. Karlson and Hoffineister (1963) carried out the chemical analysis of the ecdysone and gave the empirical formula as $C_{27}H_{44}O_6$. Chemically, it is a steroid. Its structural formula is as follows:

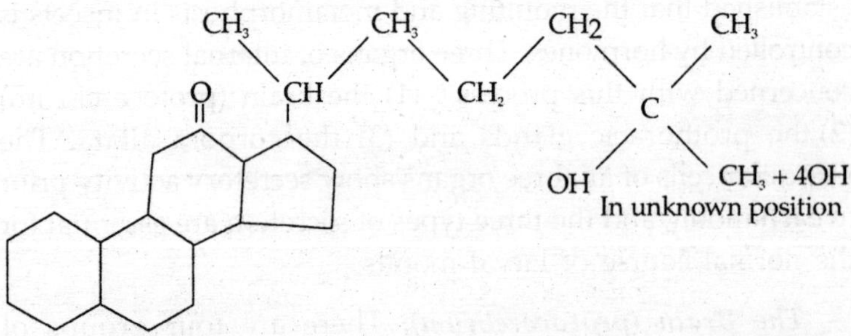

The Corpora Allata: In most insects there are found two pairs of bodies connected by nerve strands to the protocerebrum and lying alongside the dorsal aorta. First of these bodies on each side is the corpora cardiacae which is of the nature of nerve ganglia. Located more posteriorly is the corpora allata which consists of secretory cells.

The secretion of the corpora allata controls the nature of the change that is going to take place at the time of moulting. The hormones secreted by the protocerebral neurosecretory cells and the thoracic gland induce an insect to moult but they do not determine whether it will be a larval moult, the pupal moult, or the imaginal moult. On the other hand, the secretion of the corpora allata controls the qualitative changes in the body of the insect during metamorphosis.

The presence of the corpora allata is necessary to prevent metamorphosis and to keep the insect in the larval state. Therefore, the secretion of the corpora allata has been called the juvenile hormone. At every larval moult the cells of the corpora allata show signs of secretory activity but no such activity is observed during the pupal or imaginal moult. It is inferred, therefore, that at the time metamorphosis takes place, the corpora allata do not produce their hormone or at least are less active. It is actual the absence of the juvenile hormone that is the necessary condition for metamorphosis. The juvenile hormone is chemically related to ecdysone and also a steroid or a substance of the terpene group (Schheiderman and Gilbert, 1964).

2

Nucleocytoplasmic Interactions

All the activities of the cell are governed by an interaction between the nucleus and cytoplasm. Just as the nucleus controls the activity of cytoplasm, the cytoplasm surrounding the nucleus also controls the activity of the nucleus. This fact has been proved in many nuclear transplant experiments. During the whole process of development there is a balanced interplay of the nucleus and the cytoplasm. Though nucleus plays an important role, the role of cytoplasm is also considerable. It shows tremendous influence on the nucleus.

The experiments of Lester Goldstein (1966) have revealed that the exchange of molecules takes place between the nucleus and the cytoplasm. On entering the nucleus from the cytoplasm these molecules cause the selective activation of the nuclear genes. Goldstein cultured *Amoeba proteus* in a medium containing radio-active protein. He also fed Amoeba with labelled radioactive protein. Very soon the radioactive proteins entered the cytoplasm and were incorporated into the nucleus.

He removed this radioactive nucleus and transplanted it to another Amoeba which had a normal nucleus. This amoeba now had two nuclei viz. the transplanted radioactive nucleus and the normal host nucleus. The radioactive proteins from the transplanted nucleus slowly found their way to the host nucleus through the cytoplasm. Both the nuclei reached equilibrium and soon shared the radioactive proteins equally. This was verified by autoradiography or by a Geiger counter. This experiment clearly establishes the two-way traffic that exists between the nucleus and cytoplasm.

Cytoplasmic Influence of Nucleus

Cytoplasmic Stimulation of Nucleus : DNA synthesis ceases in the brain cells of the adult *Xenopus.* In an experiment, the nucleus taken from the adult brain cell was transplanted to a mature unfertilised egg. The nucleus which has already stopped the synthesis of DNA now becomes active and starts synthesising DNA. This is a clear case where the dormant nucleus is made active by the surrounding young cytoplasm of the egg. On the other hand if nucleus from brain cell is transplanted to an immature egg cell, similar activity is not seen in the nucleus. This is because the cytoplasm of the mature egg alone contains certain factors that can initiate protein synthesis

Harris (1965) collected a few human tumour cells and fused with it the nucleus taken from the red blood corpuscle of chicken. Under normal conditions these nuclei do not synthesize DNA or RNA. However when they are fused to the tumour cells they begin to synthesize DNA and RNA. The cytoplasm of the tumour cell has activated the dormant chicken nucleus.

If a mature cap is grafted on to a young *Acetabularia* stem, the nucleus begins to undergo division as though it is already old. This is another interesting case of the cytoplasm stimulating the nucleus to do an act which it normally does not do.

Cytoplasmic Inhibition of Nucleus : If the cap of a mature *Acetabularia* which is ready to undergo nuclear division, is removed, the activities of the nucleus are inhibited and the division and migration stops. The nucleus also shrinks and becomes very small.

Transplant experiments conducted on toad, *Xenopus* provide another interesting example. The synthesis of rRNA is very high during orogenesis but is retarded during maturation. It continues to remain so till gastrulation. In young tadpoles rRNA synthesis takes place vigorously and the nucleolus is prominent. The nucleus taken from a young tadpole is transplanted to a just mature egg where rRNA synthesis has stopped. In about forty minutes nucleolus disappears and rRNA synthesis is inhibited till it reaches the gastrulation stage. This experiment clearly shows that the genes of nucleus are inhibited by the repressors released from egg cytoplasm.

Cytoplasmic Influence on Nuclear Maturation : *Amoeba* grows bigger with an increase in the cytoplasmic volume. There is a relationship between the volume of cytoplasm and the maturation of the nucleus and its ability to divide. Once the cytoplasm reaches a particular size or quantity the nucleus begins to divide. In experiments, *Amoeba* was kept at a constant size by the periodic removal of cytoplasm. This resulted in the nucleus remaining without any division throughout (Hartmann 1924 & Prescott 1956). This clearly shows that the maturation of the nucleus is dependent on the cytoplasm.

The size of the nucleus is related to age in *Acetabularia.* In young *Acetabularia* the nucleus is small while in mature forms the nucleus is large. In an experiment the nucleus from a young *Acetabularia* was transplanted to an enucleated mature *Acetabularia*. Immediately the nucleus undergoes rapid changes and assumes the role of mature form. This proves that the maturation of nucleus is entirely influenced by the cytoplasm.

Hammerling (1953) noticed that in *Acetabularia* the nucleus begins to divide only after the cap formation is completed. In his experiments he removed the cap just before it was completed. This was followed by the formation of a new cap. He again repeated the same act. In this way he was able to keep the nucleus in an immature stage for a long time. He demonstrated by this experiment that cytoplasm controls the maturation of the nucleus.

Cytoplasmic Influence of Chromosomal Elimination

Example 1 : In the early cleavage stages of *Ascaris* the cells that are destined to become the germ cells retain their full quota of genetic factors while others suffer diminution. At the end of second cleavage the chromosomes are thrown into the cytoplasm where they disintegrate. The mid part of the chromosome breaks into many parts. The cell that is situated at the vegetal pole of the egg alone retains the chromosomes in their original shape. This gives rise later to the germ cells. This strange behaviour of the chromosomes is attributed to the influence of the cytoplasm on the nucleus. In experiments where the cytoplasmic contents were disturbed by centrifugation elimination does not take place.

Example 2 : The gall midget *(Mayetiola destructor)* have different number of chromosomes in the somatic and germ cells. The somatic cells have eight chromosomes while the germ cells have nearly forty chromosomes. The cytoplasm of the posterior part of the egg has special properties and this cytoplasm is called the germplasm. During cleavage the zygote nucleus (with forty chromosomes) divides first but not the cytoplasm. After third cleavage there are eight nuclei of which one moves to the posterior part of egg and gets surrounded by the germplasm. In the next cleavage sixteen nuclei are formed of which the posterior two along with germplasm form two cells. These two cells lead to the formation of germ cells, while other become the somatic cells. In somatic cells only eight chromosomes undergo duplication while the rest do not duplicate and get eliminated. In experiments the germplasm of the egg was irradiated with ultra-violet rays just before the nucleus migrated into it. On migration the behaviour of the nucleus was different and it also suffered chromosomal elimination. Though these nuclei lead to the development of reproductive tissue they could not produce sperm or eggs.

Structural variations and differential activities result by the influence of cytoplasm on the nucleus. This particular aspect has been well studied in the case of the polytene chromosomes. The polytene chromosomes have many swellings called puffs. The location of the puffs in the same chromosomes varies during the different stages of the development of the animal. Kroeger (1960) transplanted the salivary gland nucleus of the larval Drosophila into the egg cytoplasm. This resulted in changed puffing pattern in the chromosomes. This change is due to the action of the egg cytoplasm on the transplanted nucleus. Beerman and Clever (1964) proved that the changes in puffing pattern takes place in relation to the developmental stage of the animal.

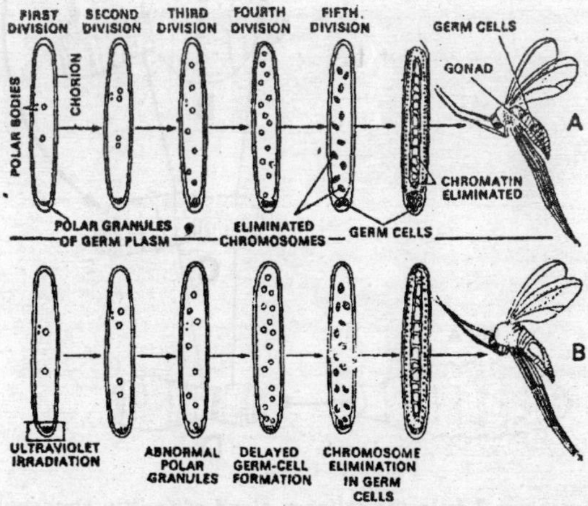

A-Germ cell specialization in gall midget. The germ cells are separated at third and fourth divisions. The somatic nuclei after fourth division show chromosome elimination. Each nucleus loses 32 chromosomes and retain only 8 chromosomes. The germ cells, on the contrary, retain all the 40 chromosomes.

B- The posterior end of egg containing germplasm is (radiated with ultraviolet rays. The nuclei entering this region also show chromosomal elimination).

Cytoplasmic Influence on Chromosomal Activity : Clever and Karlson (1969) injected ecdysone into the larva of *Chironomous.* This hormone normally initiates metamorphosis in insect larva. After injection the larva begins to develop quickly into a pupa. When the nucleus was observed in a microscope the chromosomes showed changes in puffing even within thirty minutes of injection. The experiment proves that the hormone acts first on the cytoplasm and through it on the genes.

Sally Hennen (1963) made inter-specific nuclear transplantation in *Rana.* He transplanted the diploid nucleus of one species into the enucleated egg of the other.

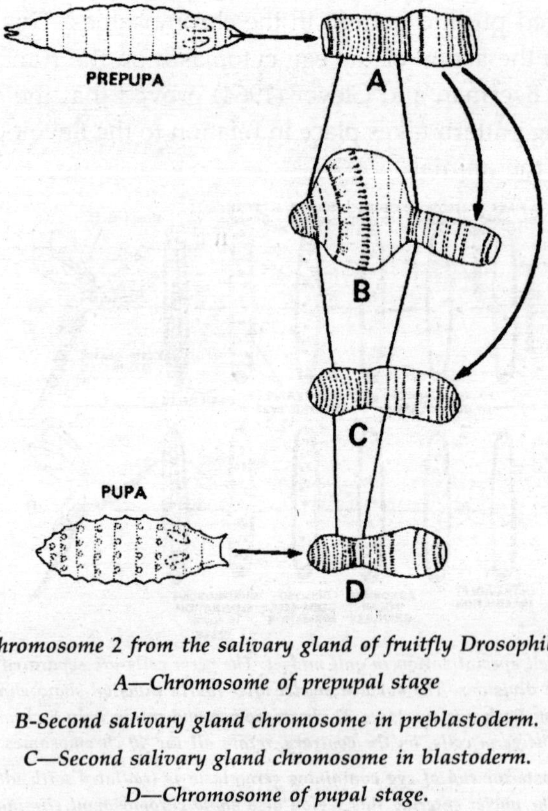

Chromosome 2 from the salivary gland of fruitfly Drosophila.

A—Chromosome of prepupal stage

B-Second salivary gland chromosome in preblastoderm.

C—Second salivary gland chromosome in blastoderm.

D—Chromosome of pupal stage.

This egg develops Upto the gastrula stage but stops without further development, because of the incompatibility between the nucleus of one species and the cytoplasm of another. On microscopic examination the nucleus revealed rings, minute dots and a reduction of one chromosome happen.

Cytoplasmic Influence on Mitosis

Amoeba divides only when the cytoplasmic mass reaches a critical level. In experiments cytoplasmic mass was periodically removed from *Amoeba*. This prevented the nucleus from dividing. In this way nuclear division can be permanently postponed.

Nuclear division in *Acetabularia* takes place only when the cap completes its development. Removal of the cap just before it completes its development results in the stoppage of nuclear division. In this way nuclear division can be postponed indefinitely by continuous removal of the cap. On the other hand, if a mature cap is grafted to the young *Acetabularia* the nucleus begins to divide. Here again it is clear that the nuclear division is controlled by the size and age of cytoplasm.

Moore (1941) transplanted sperm nucleus of *R. paulustris* into the enucleated egg of *R. pipens*. The rate of cleavage was that of *R. pipens* only. In the next experiment he transplanted the sperm nucleus of *R. pipens* into the enucleated egg of *R. paulustris*. This time the rate of cleavage was that of *R. paulustris*. This shows that cytoplasm influences the role of cleavage and in turn the mitotic divisions.

Cytoplasmic Influence of Nuclear Differentiation : Danielli (1955) transplanted nucleus from *Amoeba proteus* into *Amoeba discoides* thus producing a hybrid form. The hybrid (proteus nucleus and discoides cytoplasm) was found to be intermediate in shape but more like discoides in nuclear diameter and division rate. After a number of generations if the transplanted proteus nucleus is transferred back to an enucleated *Amoeba* *proteus*, it was found that due to its long sojourn in discoides cytoplasm, the transplanted nucleus has been modified to resemble that of the discoides nucleus. This experiment proved that the nuclear differentiation is influenced by the cytoplasm.

Cytoplasmic Role in Inactivating "X" Chromosome : Bakr (1949) observed that the two 'X' chromosomes present in the cells of female mammals including human beings differ in appearance. One of them is said to be typical and active while the other heteropycnotic (i.e.) condensed and deeply stained. In the interphase nucleus the typical 'X" chromosome is not clearly visible but the heterophycnotic 'X' chromosome appears as the chromocenter now designated as sex chromatin or Barr body. Thus cytological studies clearly establish that one 'X' chromosome has been inactivated. Auto-radiographic studies also reveal that the heteropycnotic chromosome does not take part in nucleic acid synthesis. Both the 'X' chromosomes are active in the beginning but one is inactivated later. Lyon (1961) has stated that the genetic inactivation of one 'X' chromosome takes place early in development due to the cytoplasmic changes. Thus it is the cytoplasm that controls the inactivation of the 'X' chromosome.

Cytoplasm and Enzyme Synthesis

Spencer and Harris (1964) in their studies on *Acetabularia* found that even enucleated *Acetabularia* can synthesize the enzyme phosphatase. It synthesizes three kinds of phosphatases at the optimum pH of 5,8,5, and 12. The phosphatase synthesized at *pH* 12 is formed only when the cap is being formed. Though it has the ability to produce this enzyme even earlier, cytoplasmic factors inhibit it. Thus cytoplasm plays an important role in controlling the synthesis of enzymes.

Nucleocytoplasmic Interaction in Differentiation : The differential activation of the genes influenced by the cytoplasm result in differentiation. The environment provided by the different early blastomeres is different. If all the blastomeres had the same atmosphere and same genes, differentiation is not possible. Electron microscopic studies also show differences in different areas of the egg cytoplasm. Moreover, the egg cytoplasm itself is a heterogenous mixture of substances that are distributed neither uniformly not at random. The genes find themselves in different environment in the different blastomeres. Thus differentiation is brought about by selective activation or inhibition of the genes by the cytoplasm.

Differentiation can occur at two stages viz at transcription level and 'translation level. Hammerling in his experiments with *Acetabularia* found that differentiation takes place at the translation level. He noticed that *Acetabularia* can regenerate a new cap even a few days after the nucleus has been removed. This shows that the cytoplasm definitely possesses the ability to differentiate. He also noticed the existence of the cap-producing substance present in the cytoplasm in different concentrations at different levels. He called it gradients. The production of a cap in *Acetabularia* is thus an interaction of both nucleus and cytoplasm.

Nucleocytoplasmic Interaction in Protein Synthesis : Protein synthesis involves active interaction of both nucleus and cytoplasm. The main factors that are involved in this process are DNA, RNA and ribosomes. While DNA and RNA have their activities in the nucleus, ribosomes and RNA have their activities in the cytoplasm. The study of genetic code and knowledge of genetics has established that the primary role is played by the nucleus, the cytoplasm also has an equal and important role in the synthesis of proteins.

Danielli (1955) in his experiments (described earlier) has come to the conclusion that while the molecular structure of the protein was controlled by nucleus, cytoplasm influenced the physiological and morphological characters.

Garen (1963) and Lavinthal (1962), who studied the structure of the enzyme alkaline phosphatase in *Escherischia coli* found that it is formed of two polypeptide chains. While one of these chains is determined by the chromosomal gene, the other by the cytoplasmic factors called episomes.

Nucleocytoplasmic Interaction in Regeneration : Hammerling found that if *A. mediterranea* stalk is grafted to the nucleated base of *A. crenulata,* the cup that is regenerated resembles that of mediterranea. After this first cap is removed and the successive caps produced all resemble that of *A. crenulata* only. This is because of the existence of the morphogenetic factors that already exist in the cytoplasm due to the nucleocytoplasmic interaction before the stalk was grafted. After this when the cap is removed the further caps are produced by the cytoplasmic interaction with the new nucleus (that of *A. crenulata).* Thus regeneration also depends on the interaction of nucleus and cytoplasm.

The whole process of life activity of a cell is a constant interaction between nucleus and cytoplasm. This interaction seems to be more pronounced and active during development.

3

Embryonic Induction

Transplantation is a method by which small pieces are cut out of embryos in various stages of development and inserted into suitably prepared incisions of the same or another embryo. The embryo from which a part is taken is referred to as the donor, and the embryo to which the part is transplanted is called the host. The process of transplantation may be of the following types :

Autoplastic: When a piece of the same embryo is transplanted to another place, the transplantation is called autoplastic.

Homoplastic: If the transplantation is from one individual to another of the same species, the transplantation is homoplastic.

Heteroplastic: When a part is transplanted to an individual of another species belonging to the same genus, the transplantation is said to be heteroplastic.

Xenoplastic: A transplantation to an individual more distantly related than species of one genus is known as xenoplastic. For example, tissues of Hydra, insects, fishes, reptiles, birds and mammals can be transplanted in the newt.

Spemann's Experiment and the Embryonic Induction : German embryologist Hans Spemann and his pupil Hilde Mangold (1924) succeeded in cutting out the cells of the dorsal lip of the blastopore of an early gastrula of a newt *Triturus cristatus* (unpigmented, pale variety) before their inward migration. Then they transplanted (heteroplastically) this small bit of tissue near the lateral lip of the blastopore of another newt *Triturus taeniatus* (pigmented, dark variety). They observed that the transplanted piece of dorsal lip invaginated into the interior and developed into a second notochord and the somites. It induced the host ectoderm above the site of the graft to form a neural groove. This neural groove was made up exclusively of host (dark) cells. It underwent normal development, forming a neural tube initially and then a central nervous system. Finally, a two-headed creature was produced.

A microscopic study revealed the presence of a notochord, kidney tubules and an additional lumen in the endoderm which represented gut of the secondary embryo. Most of the neural tube, parts of the somites, the kidney tubules and the ear rudiments of the secondary embryo consisted of host cells. All these parts would not have developed if the transplant had not been present. This led Spemann to conclude that the transplanted cells had altered the normal course of development of the host cells around them. Instead of producing the abdomen of the newt, the host cells above the graft were stimulated to produce a second central nervous system. This influence, causing the development of certain organs of the embryo, is called *embryonic induction* or simply induction. The tissue which is the source of this influence is called the inductor.

Primary Organizer : When Spemann transplanted portions of gastrulas other than the cells of the dorsal lip of the blastopore, no induction was seen. Only grafts taken from the dorsal lip of the blastopore and the adjoining parts of the marginal zone were found to be able to induce. It is the ability of the dorsal lip of the blastopore (future notochord and axial mesoderm) to cause, when transplanted, the fabrication of a total embryo that Spemann called it organizer. Spemann gave the active region the name of organizer, meaning this was the part which *organizes* the process of development. He imagined the organizer as initiating the process of morphogenesis and differentiation by inducing the formation of the neural tube. The latter then might induce the development of still other embryonic structures like eye, ear, etc. The interaction of the grafted dorsal lip of the blastopore (chordo-mesoderm) and the overlying ectoderm is the first stage of interacting system in the induction process. The dorsal lip of the blastopore, therefore, is called the primary organizer. The organizer of the gastrula is that region of the egg that coincides with the gray crescent before the beginning of cleavage.

Secondary, Tertiary and Quaternary Organizers : As gastrulation proceeds, the various organ systems of the embryo are laid down under the influence of the primary organizer and they themselves then acquire the power of inducing later—formed structures to develop. These, in turn, develop organizing properties—and so on. It is thus possible to recognise a series of secondary, tertiary and quaternary organizers, which are arranged in a sort of hierarchy at whose summit is the primary organ zervot follows, therefore, that one embryonic tissue layer interacts with an adjacent one and the latter is thereby induced to develop in a particular way. This developed tissue then interacts with another tissue in turn and induces it to develop. In other words, progressive development takes place by sequential induction. One tissue provides the stimulus for the development of the next.

Eye development provides a classic example of chain of inductive events :

1. The chordo-mesoderm, a primary organizer (inductor) induces the differentiation of the fore-brain and the optic area within it. The development of eye begins with the evagination of a pair of saclike optic vesicles from the lateral walls of the prosencephalon. The optic vesicles push outwards until they reach the epidermis, displacing and intervening mesenchyme.
2. The external surface of the optic vesicle now flattens out and invaginates inward, so that the vesicle is transformed into a double-walled cup-like structure—the optic cup. The invaginated layer, i.e., the inner layer of the optic cup is much thicker than the external wall. The first is to develop into the *sensory layer*, whereas the second develops in *the pigment coat* of the retina. The pigment and sensory layers eventually fuse.
3. The optic cup serves as a secondary organizer inducing the formation of the lens. As the optic vesicle is transforming into an optic cup, the somatic ectoderm immediately overlying the cup undergoes a thickening to form a lens placode. The placode then invaginates inward and finally pinches away from the parent ectoderm to form a lens vesicle lying in the pupil.
4. The lens, acting together with the retina serves as a tertiary organizer of the cornea. The layer of mesenchyme left in front of the anterior chamber of eye combines with the overlying somatic ectoderm to form the cornea.

It becomes evident from the foregoing account that in the induction sequence, one tissue provides the stimulus for the development of the next. As each structure is induced, it can then induce still other structures. Successive waves of induction could thus account for the orderly, properly timed, complete, and organized embryonic development of the animal.

A few other examples of an organizer taking effect after the main embryonic axial structures have been laid down under the influence of the primary organizer, are as follows:

(i) The development of the posterior lobe of the pituitary body depends on the presence of the tip of the notochord.

(ii) The development of the nasal placodes depends on the presence of the fore-brain.

(iii) The development of teeth depends on the pharyngeal endoderm.

(iv) The formation of sympanic membrane requires the presence of the annular cartilage.

(v) The development of dorsal fin in fishes depends on the presence of the mesenchyme derived from trunk neural crests.

Regional Specificity of the Organizer : The induction of chordo-mesoderm are regionally specific i.e., every part of the organizer induces a particular organ or organ system. Accordingly the organizer is divided into two parts : (i) head inductor and (ii) trunk or spinocaudal inductor.

The anterior part of the archenteric roof induces head organs and may be called a head inductor. It may be further differentiated into (i) the *archencephalic inductor,* inducing the forebrain, eyes and nose rudiments ; and (ii) the *deuterencephalic inductor*. The latter induces hindbrain and ear vesicles (Lehmann, 1945). The posterior part of the archenteric roof induces trunk organs and tailbuds. It is known as the *trunk* or *spinocaudal inductor.*

Survey of Organizer in the Chordates : Although the primary organizer was first discovered in urodele amphibians, it was soon found that dorsal lip of the blastopore and the roof of the archenteron of lower chordates *(e.g., Amphioxus)* and other vertebrates has the same function in development.

Amphioxus: Tung, Wu and Tung (1962) grafted pieces of tissue from the inner surface of the dorsal blastopore lip of an early gastrula of *Amphioxus* into the blastocoel of another embryo in the same stage of development. They observed that a secondary embryo developed in the ventral region of the host with a notochord ana mesoderm produced by the transplant. A neural tube, however, was induced from host tissue.

Cyclostomes and Fishes: In lampreys, whose cleavage is holoblastic and whose blastula and gastrula resemble those of amphibians, the dorsal lip of the blastopore, when transplanted into the blastocoel of another young gastrula, induces the development of a secondary embryo.

In bony fishes, induction of secondary embryos were produced by grafting the posterior edge of the blastodisc into the blastocoel of another embryo (B. C. Oppenheimer, 1936, in *Fundulus* and *Perca).* In this case, the posterior edge of the blastodisc corresponds to the dorsal lip of the blastopore. Neural inductions were also obtained by transplanting the chordomesoderm and endoderm (Luther, 1935, in *Salmp).* Ginsburg and Dettlaff (1944) produces neural induction in the *Sturgeon* by grafting the dorsal lip of the blastopore.

Amphibians: In frogs the formation of a secondary embryo can be induced by the transplantation of the dorsal lip of the blastopore into the blastocoel of a young gastrula. This process takes place in very much the same way as in newts and salamanders.

Reptiles: Although no experiments on the primary organizer have been done in reptiles, it is believed that the archenteron has the same inducing activity in this group as in other vertebrates.

Birds: In the birds, the existence of the primary organizer was established by experiments by Waddington and Schmidt (1933). The anterior half of the primitive streak was found to be the inducing part. It was recognized as corresponding to the lips of the blastopore in amphibians.

Mammals: Waddington (1934) successfully carried out neural induction in a rabbit embryo by cultivating the early blastodisc on a plasma clot and implanting the primitive streak of the chick as an inductor. This experiment proved that the tissues of a mammalian gastrula have the ability for neural induction.

Nature of Induction

Soon after Spemann's discovery, it was found that the inducting properties of the organizer (dorsal lip of the blastopore) were retained even if the cells were killed by various means - by boiling, by treating with alcohol or petrol, either, by freezing or by dessication. When implanted into a living embryo, it was found that a killed organizer can still induce (Bautzmann, Spemann and Mangold 1932). It indicated that the vital activity of the organizer is not essential for induction. Probably, the roof of the archanteron produces its effect by liberating some chemical substance which is the immediate cause of induction. It is acceptable that such a substance could be liberated even from dead tissues. Waddington, Needham and Co-workers Concluded that this natural inducing substance is a steroid. Arey (1966) called it an evocator.

Abnormal inductors and induction by substances of known chemical substance. It has been found that not only the chordo-mesoderm but also a wide variety of tissues like liver, kidney, muscles, gut and skin etc. are able to produce inductions. Induction can also be performed by tissues of various animals belonging to different phyla of the animals kingdom. For example, the tissues of *Hydra*, insects, fishes, reptiles, birds and mammals were found to be effective as inductors of newt. Neural inductions may result from such an unlikely agent as methylene blue or a mechanical irritant such as silicious earth.

Some workers have presented evidence that ribonucleoprotein, i.e., a complex of RNA and protein may have inductive properties. Besides, a number of weak organic acids are good inductors. These include *muscle adenylic acid (AMP), thymonucleic acid (DNA), dihydroxystearic acid, linolenic acid* and *stearic acid.*

Competence : During induction, the reacting cells of the host must be in a particular physiological state so as to differentiate into nervous system under the influence of the inductor. This special state of reactivity is called competence. It is restricted to the ectoderm and is present during a short period only. If the perspective ectoderm is not stimulated to differentiate into nervous system during this period, it differentiates as epidermis.

The Competence : Do cells in a growing embryo influence each other? What is that force which determines the pattern of growth and differentiation? Do some cells have a better influence than other cells in the process of development? Experiments conducted by Hans Spemann, Hiwe Mangold and others have answered these questions.

Dependent Differentiation or Embryonic Differentiation : During embryogenesis of multicellular organisms, some cells are induced to differentiate into specific organs or tissues by the presence of other cells. This process of inducement by cells (tissue interaction) is called embryonic induction or dependent differentiation. The *embryonic induction is a morphogenetic effect in which one embryonic tissue transmits a chemical stimulus that influences another embryonic part to produce a structure that otherwise would not come into existence.*

The embryonic tissue that exerts the inductive influence is termed as inductor. The chemical substance given off by the inductor is called evocator. The tissue or cells that react to the stimulus is said to be responsive tissue, or competent.

Thus embryonic induction is a determining mechanism of

development which exerts a control on the pattern of protein synthesis in the responsive tissue. This leads to the formation of new types of cells with a new behaviour.

History of Embryonic Induction.

1. 1924	Hans Spemann and Mangold	Neural induction in amphibians
2. 1930	Schotte	In frogs
1937	Daleq and Pasteels	
3. 1937	Saltz	In Lampreys and Cyclostomes
1938	Yamada	
4. 1935	Luther	In bony fishes
1936	Oppenheimer	
5. 1933 and 1952	Weddington	In brids
6. 1934	Weddington	In rabbit
7. 1960	Reverberi, Ortalani and Furruzza	In ascidian
8. 1962	Tung, Wu and Tung	In *Amphioxus*
9. 1960, 1963	Curtis	In *Xenopus laevis*
10. 1934, 1947 and 1968	Holtfreter	
11. 1966	Nieuwkoop	Provided account of nature of embryonic induction
12. 1968 and l969	Barth and Barth	

Spemann's Experiments on Organizers : Hans Spemann, a German zoologist, while working with newts won Nobel Prize in 1935 for his discovery of 'Organizer effect in embryonic development.' Some of his experiments are being summarized here —

Experiment 1 : In one of his early experiments, Spemann constricted the newts egg lengthwise with a baby hair by making a noose. The noose passed through grey crescent dividing the egg into two equal halves but the two halves still had a narrow cytoplasmic connection. Only one half had the nucleus, the other half was enucleated. The nucleated portion of the egg underwent cleavage. The enucleated half was passive. At 16 cell stage, the nuclear material passed into the enucleated half through the cytoplasmic bridge. Now both halves showed cleavage and further development. With the tightening of the noose the two parts got separated completely and each one developed into a full-fledged larva.

Spemann preferred newt eggs for transplant experiment, because (i) he found newt eggs better than frog's egg for surgery, (ii) In newt eggs the animal half is colourless, vegetal half is dark. The gray crescent area is gray in colour and lies between the two. The elements of each area can easily be followed during development and differentiation and their future can easily be ascertained.

Spemann's most famous experiments were conducted to discover the mechanism of differentiation of nervous system.

Experiment 2 : In another experiment, the newt egg was constricted in such a fashion that the constriction was laid parallel to the gray-crescent and not through it. The normal embryo developed from that half of the egg which had gray crescent. The other half without gray crescent developed into an unorganized cell-mass, it was called 'bauchstuck', which in German means a belly piece. It had materials for liver, lungs, intestine and other abdominal organs, but had no axial skeleton.

The comparison of these two results clearly showed that gray-crescent is essential for the proper development of an embryo.

Experiment 3 : Spemann cut out the ectoderm from the top of the embryo and put it into a separate dish. The embryo healed up and developed into a tadpole which lacked nervous system. The isolated ectodermal piece failed to develop.

Spemann concluded that ectoderm can differentiate into nervous system only when it is attached to the embryo. Also some embryonal part causes its differentiation.

Experiment 4 : Spemann cut a flap of ectoderm from the top of embryo and removed the mesoderm from beneath, the ectoderm fold was placed back or the original position. The ectoderm healed but the embryo failed to develop nervous tissue. From the above experiment Spemann concluded that mesoderm influences the differentiation of nervous system from ectoderm.

Experiment 5 : In another experiment Spemann studied the importance of gray crescent in both blastula and gastrula. He removed dorsal lip of blastopore (Which is represented by gray crescent) from the early gastrula. The early gastrula failed to develop any further. Spemann transplanted this dorsal lip of early gastrula to the ventral portion of another gastrula. The graft invaginated inside the host embryo and developed into a secondary embryo with complete system of all organs such as notochord, nerve cord, somites, kidney tubules, eyes, ears, etc. Here the graft became self differentiated and formed all those structures which it would have given rise to in its normal position. It also induced the adjoining host tissue to participate in the formation of induced embryo.

Conclusion : Spemann arrived on following conclusions based on the series of transplant experiments-

1. Dorsal lip of blastopore induces and organizes the normal gastrulation.
2. Embryonic ectoderm is uncommitted or unspecialised. It may be directed by other tissues to take different paths of differentiation.
3. Neural differentiation is triggered by the activity of underlying tissue, the presumptive notochord and presumptive mesoderm (chorda-mesoderm).
4. Dorsal lip of blastopore has a high capacity for self differentiation. It also serves as an organization centre.
5. The inductor tissue must be in virtual contact with the responsive tissue. The chemical substance (evocator)

passes to the target tissue by diffusion and becomes less effective over a distance.

6. An inductor acquires inductive power for a limited period.
7. The target region of the embryo responds to a particular inductor for a limited period, when the tissue is non-committed.
8. The target tissue has the competence. The inductor tissue induces it to differentiate
9. The organs developed from the graft are usually supplemented by parts from the host tissue.

Spemann called the dorsal lip of blastopore as organizer. Because this tissue was able to organize the whole embryo it was called the primary organizer. Though this reaction is the first to take place in the sequence of embryonic interactions, embryologists, however, prefer to use the term embryonic induction or inductive interaction or dependent differentiation.

Properties of the Organizer : Scientists found that various types of tissues and tissue substances, some alive and some dead and tissues from many animals can act as inductors in amphibibians for neurulation. But the organizing activities of dorsal lip tissue are more comprehensive. It directs the normal gastrulation, determines the entire dorsal axial system of the embryo (i.e. notochord, neural tube and somites). Therefore, the dorsal lip of embryo as an organizer has following important characteristic which make it the most indispensable part of the growing embryo such as:

1. It can induce and influence the surrounding cells to undergo changes to make them from structures like neural tube, etc.
2. It has the capacity for self organization. It behaves as if it carries a particular mission in the development of the embryo and acts as the chief architect.

3. It has the capability of self differentiation i.e. it not only induces the other cells nearby to form certain organs but it also forms a part of that organ.
4. The primary organizer determines the main features of axiation and organization of the embryo. It directs the development of an axiated gastrula from non-axial blastula.
5. Normally the organizer does not interfere with the work of another organizer when two such organizers are present in one embryo as in artificial transplant experiments.

Neural Induction

The primary organizer of Spemann (the chorda-mesodermal tissue or the dorsal lip of blastopore) induces the formation of neural plate and neural tube. Therefore, it is called neural inductor and this type of induction as neural induction.

Role of Gray Crescent in Neural Induction : A. S. G. Curits (1962) in a series of experiments on Xenopus laevis proved that gray crescent gives rise to dorsal lip of blastopore and that gray crescent acts as neural inductor.

1. The gray crescent material was removed from a fertilized egg just before cleavage and was grafted to another egg on the opposite side. Gastrulation produced two neural plates in the embryo with two separate nervous systems at the opposite ends. This clearly shows that gray crescent is the portion of the egg that is primarily concerned with gastrulation, neurulation and other aspects of growth.
2. Curtis removed gray crescent from the fertilized egg. The cleavage continued but gastrulation does not occur. Curtis also conducted similar experiments with embryos of 8 cell stages:-

1. Gray crescent material was removed from the eight-celled embryo, it is able to gastrulate and proceed to develop normally.
2. Gray crescent material was removed from a fertilized egg just before cleavage. This graft was transplanted to the 8-celled embryo on its ventral side, the 8-celled embryo did not show any reaction.
3. Graft from the gray crescent cortex from 8-celled embryo was transplanted to the ventral side of uncleaved fertilized egg. Embryo with two separate nervous systems at the opposite ends was formed. This indicates that 8-celled embryo still possessed the inductive ability especially when grafted to younger stages.

From above experiment Curtis concluded that gray crescent controls gastrulation and the inducting or organizing effect from gray crescent is spread out to the adjacent cortical region during second and third cleavages.

Time of Neural Induction : When exactly does the neural induction take place? Is there any particular time interval when this can occur? These two questions are well answered by the simple experiments conducted by Saxen. L., and S. Toivonen (1962) on the gastrula of newt.

1. In first experiment they removed the presumptive neural plate from an early newt gastrula and transplanted it on to the ventral side of another gastrulae of the same stage. Surprisingly no induction took place and the grafted material began to develop according to its new location.
2. In the second experiment a small piece of the presumptive neural plate was removed from a late gastrula and transplanted to another gastrula. The grafted material caused neural induction and formed

the second nervous system thereby proving its ability to induce according to the original plan irrespective of the new surrounding into which it is grafted.

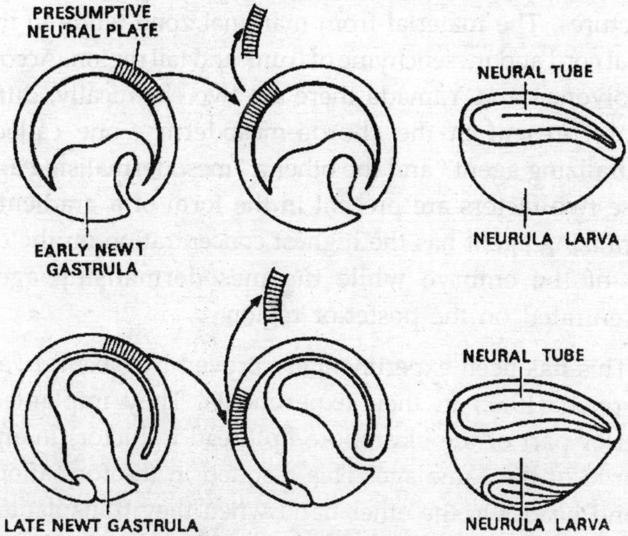

Saxen and Toivonen's experiments on the gastrulae of newt to show the time of neural induction by substituting regions of neural plate at different stages of development

From these experiments it becomes evident that neural induction occurs at the time when the material of chorda-mesoderm moves from the dorsal lip of blastopore inward and forward. The inductive stimuli exhibit a time-gradient which may be crucial with regard to action and reaction events.

Regional Differentiation of Primary Inductor : Though the entire chorda-mesoderm was thought to be the sole cause for inducting the embryo to differentiate, later studies have proved that different regions of the chorda-mesoderm have different types of induction. Most of the dorsal and dorsolateral blastoporal material is necessary for a graft to induce the complete secondary embryo. If only the prospective endo-mesodermal material of dorsal lip is grafted into another early gastrula, it induces a partial secondary embryo containing ectodermal head structures (brain, sense organs, mouth, etc.). Graft of median portion of dorsal lip induces formation of eyes and olfactory pits and its lateral parts induce posterior cephalic structures. The material from marginal zone tends to induce spinal cord and mesenchyme of trunk and tail region. According to Toivonen and Yamada there are two chemically, different factors present in the chorda-mesoderm - one called the "neuralizing agent" and the other a "mesodermalising agent". These two factors are present in the form of a gradient. The neuralizing agent has the highest concentration on the dorsal side of the embryo while the mesodermalising agent is concentrated on the posterior region.

This has been experimentally proved by Saxen. L. and S. Toivonen (1962) in their experiments. They implanted the anterior part of the blastopore lip (head inductor) to another embryo of the same age. This resulted in the formation of a second head. On the other hand when they transplanted the (trunk inductor) posterior region of the late gastrula it induced the formation of trunk and tail only.

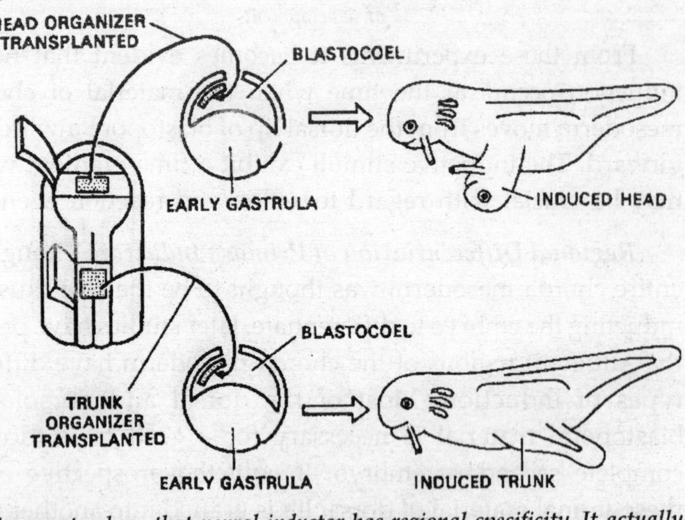

Diagram to show that neural inductor has regional specificity. It actually comprises of neuralizing and mesodermalising regions which induce the formation of head and trunk regions respectively.

During gastrulation the chorda-mesodermal tissue gradually invaginates inside the embryo and finally forms roof of archenteron in the middorsal line. Based on its inducting ability, the different parts of archenteron roof in antero-posterior direction are classified by Lehmann (1945).

These are: (i) Archencephalic inductor induces the formation of forebrain, eyes, and nose rudiments (head inductor). (ii) Deutrencephalic inductor tends to induce formation of hindbrain and ear vesicles. (iii) Spino-caudal inductor induces posterior part of the embryo including tail bud.

Lovtrup (1974) classified embryonic induction into following two categories-

Endogenous Induction : The endogenous inductors are produced within the cells or tissue endogenously and cause self transformation. As a result of self diversification new types of cells and tissues are formed.

Example : (i) Mesenchyme cells of ventral pole of Echinoidea and (ii) Cells of dorsal lip of amphibian blastopore.

Exogenous Induction : In this type of induction the differentiation and diversification of cells or tissue is caused by the influence of neighbouring cells through the process of contact induction. The exogenous induction may be homotypic if the inductor provokes formation of its own kind of tissue or heterotypic if the induced tissue is of different type.

Secondary, Tertiary and Quaternary Organizers : As gastrulation advances, the various organ systems of the embryo begin to differentiate under the influence of primary organizer. These early-differentiated organ systems or their primordia then acquire the power of inducing the differentiation of later formed structures or organs such as eyes, ears, limbs, lungs, etc. These, in turn, develop organizing property and themselves become the source of induction. Thus, there is a series of organizers which can be called as secondary, tertiary and quaternary organizers.

During embryonic development, one embryonic tissue interacts with the adjacent one and induces it to develop in a particular direction. This developed tissue then interacts with another neighbouring tissue and induce it to develop in a specific direction, which in turn may induce the successive tissue. In other words progressive development of embryonic organs is dependent on sequential induction.

Development of Eye as an Example of Sequential Induction

1. The chorda-mesoderm—the primary organizer induces the formation of forebrain and optic area within it in the anterior part of the embryo. The optic area evaginates forming optic vesicle. By invagination it changes into a double-walled cup-like optic cup.
2. The optic cup acts as a secondary organizer. It induces the formation of lens from the ectoderm overlying the optic cup.
3. The lens acts as a tertiary organizer and induces the formation of cornea. The layer of mesenchyme left in front of the anterior chamber of eye combines with the overlying somatic ectoderm (epidermis) and forms cornea.

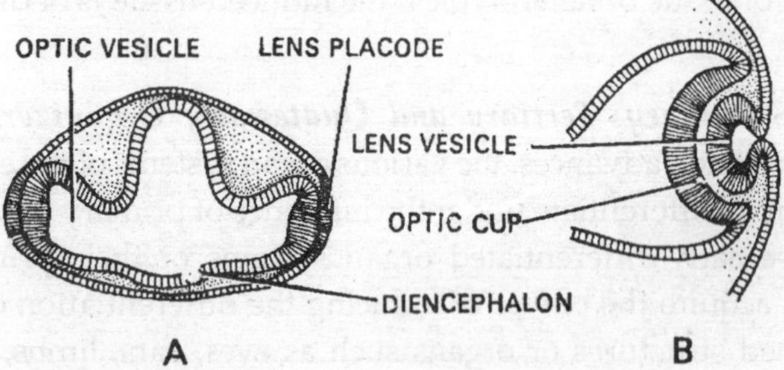

Diagrammatic representation of development of eye in frog embryo. List of Inductors and the Organs Induced by them.

S.No.	Inductor	Type of Induction	Organ Induced
1.	Roof of archenteron (chorda-mesoderm)	Primary organizer	1. Neural tube, its differentiation into fore, mid and hindbrain and optic placode.
2.	Optic cup	Secondary organizer	Formation of lens
3.	Lens	Tertiary organizer	Formation of cornea
4.	Forebrain	Secondary organizer	Nasal placodes
5.	Hindbrain	Secondary organizer	Posterior lobe of pituitary
6.	Annular cartilage	"	Ear vesicles optic capsule and ear placodes
7.	Notochord	Tertiary inductor quaternary organizer	Tympanic membrane
8.	Pharyngeal endoderm	"	Dev. of teeth
9.	Neural crest in trunk region	Secondary organizer	Mesenchyme
10.	Mesenchyme	Tertiary inductor	Development of dorsal fin.

Chemistry of Inducing Substances or Chemical Basis of Induction

1. Experiments of Bautzmann, Holtfreter, Spemann and Mangold have shown that the organizer material whether living or dead is capable of induction. The dorsal lip of blastopore induced the differentiation even when it was boiled or treated with alcohol or ether and transplanted into another embryo. Sometimes the inductor tissue has a better effect after being killed. In some cases, the tissues that do not normally induce, were found to have inductive effect after being killed Holtfreter (1934) demonstrated that presumptive ectoderm and endoderm when killed and transplanted into the blastocoel-induced neural plate formation.
2. Inductor can induce growth and differentiation even in distantly related or unrelated animals. The organizer

tissue from insects, birds, mouse, guinea pigs was found to induce development of frog.

3. Inorganic substances like iodine or kaolin, exposure to high or low ph or saline solution, a variety of weak organic acids, adenosine monophosphates. Thymonucleic acid, linoleic acid and even local mechanical injury also cause induction. Dye like methylene blue are also chemical inductors.

The inductors release the inducing substances into the medium in which they are found. Niu and Twitty (1953) found that the inductor tissue when kept suspended over a coverslip in a nutrient medium begins releasing the inducing substances into the medium, the maximum concentration in the medium is attained in about ten days. This medium which contains the inductor substances is now called the "conditioned medium". The conditioned medium is capable of inducing differentiation on any tissue. This clearly shows that the inductive effect can be brought about even without direct contact (Niu, 1956).

To identify the substances responsible for neural induction, molecules were separated from gray crescent or dorsal lip or blastopore having chorda-mesoderm elements by various biochemical methods (centrifugation or chromatography). Their inductive capacity was tested by Niu et all (1953 and 1956). Yamada (1958) extracted inducing substances from liver and bone marrow of adult guinea pig. Teidmann (1961-62) prepared purified extracts of nine-day old chicks. These purified extracts of inductors were macromolecules of proteins or ribonucleoproteins. These have molecular weight between 43,000 and 1,00,000 (Teidmann - 1962).

These extracts were found to be very potent. Even very small quantities like 1 to 2Y (Y = 1/1,000 mg) is enough for successful induction in bringing out neurulation in *Triturus* (Teidmann 1962). However, fractions that contained only deoxyribonu-cleoproteins were found to be totally inactive.

Thus it is clear that the inducing substance is found in the form of both proteins and ribonucleoproteins. It is possible that these ribonucleoproteins may be involved in the transferring of information from inducing cells to the reacting cells. In some experiments the inducing tissues were initially treated with ribonuclease and after incubation it was used for induction and it was found that the tissues and extracts which had very less ribonucleic acid content (less than 1% of the normal quantity) had the same inducing capacity as before. This shows that ribonucleoproteins are not very essential for induction. In another experiment the inductor tissue was treated with proteolytic enzymes like pepsin, trypsin or chymotrypsin. Hyashi (1958) treated liver extract with trypsin many times and found that they lost completely their inductive ability. Tiedmann and his co-workers also obtained similar results. Therefore, the inducing principle is in the form of protein only. Though they may be coupled with ribonucleic acid. The inductive action is due to proteins alone.

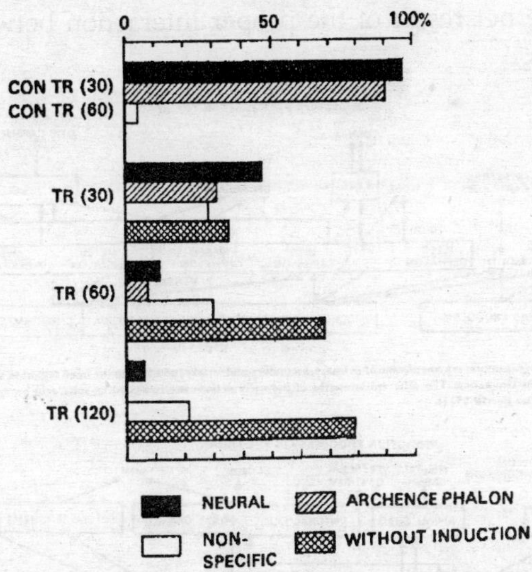

Diagram showing progressive suppression of the inducing power of liver homogenate by repeatedly treatment with the proteolytic enzyme trysin. From above first tier represents control without trypsin.

Mechanism of Neural Induction : The intricate mechanism of neural induction has been explained by five theories by the different embryologists.

Gradient Theory: Toivonen (1955 and 1968) and Yamada (1961), by denatured bone marrow and liver tissue as the inductors concluded that two chemically different factors are the cause for primary induction. These were named neuralizing agent and mesodermalising agent. These agents are found distributed in gradients.

The neuralizing factor has its maximum concentration at the posterior end. In the anterior region only the neuralizing agent is present which induces archencephalon (forebrain). No notochord and no somites are formed in this region. In the middle region both neuralizing and mesodermalising agents act together to produce midbrain, hindbrain and otic vesicles. In the posterior part the mesodermalising agent alone acts to produce the spinocaudal structures. Thus the induction in total is the net result of the proper interaction between both the factors.

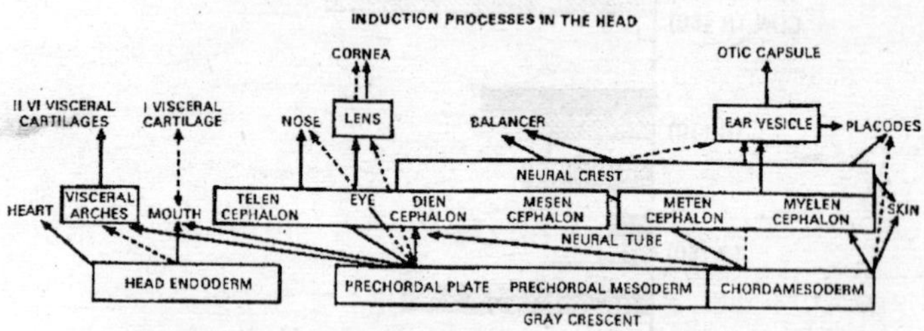

Diagrammatic representation of primary, secondary and teriary inductors in the head region to show their inductive action. The different strengths of inductive actions are indicated by solid and broken arrows (After Berrill 1971).

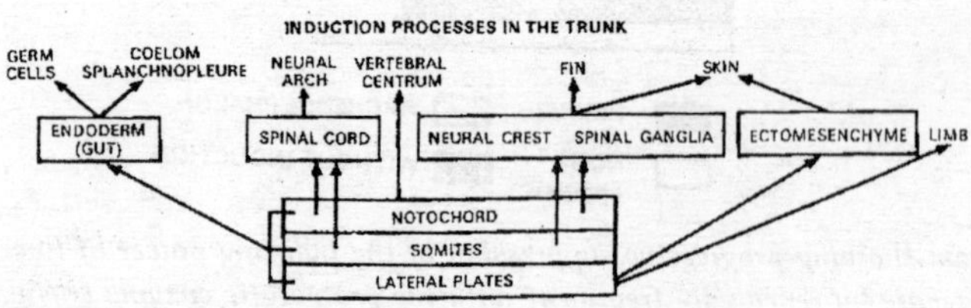

Inductive action of trunk organizers in frog (After BERRILL, 1971)

Protein Denaturation Theory: According to Ranzi (1962-63) the neural induction is due to protein denaturation. In amphibians, the gray crescent which forms the notochord and induces neural tube is also the site of intense metabolic activity. It also corresponds to the site of protein denaturation.

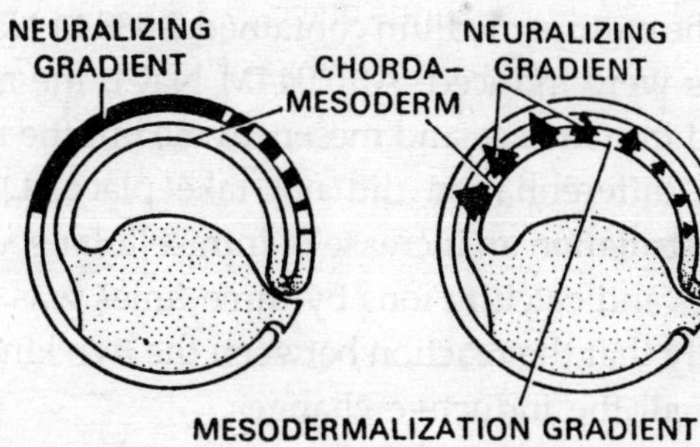

A—Diagram to show the distribution of neuralisation gradient in the ectoderm overlying mesodermalisation gradient in frog gastrula. B—Distribution of mesodermalisation gradient

Saxen and Toivonen (1962) analysed inductions and noted the following : (i) Inductively active tissues can be separated chemically into fractions that possesses different inductive action. (ii) The fractions that form archencephalic inductors are chemically different from those spinocaudal or mesodermal inductors.

Combined inductors like deuterencephalic or spinocaudal inductors, when subjected to chemical or physical treatment loose their ability to induce caudal structures and become pure archencephalic inductors.

One-Factor Hypothesis : Nieuwkoop (1966) used living notochord as an inductor and found that it induces the ectoderm to form neural tissue first and later causes the ectoderm to be transformed into posterior and mesodermal structures. In another experiment he used the live notochord as inductor for different length of time and found that about five minutes' exposure was sufficient to transform ectoderm into brain and eye structures.

Ionic Theory of Barth : L. G. Barth and L. J. Barth (1968) proposed that induction is brought about by release of ions from bound form, which changes the ratio between bound and the free ions inside the cells of gastrula. It was observed in frog gastrula that the induction of nerve and pigment cells of the prospective epidermis depends on the concentration of sodium ions. When the culture medium contained 0.088 M NaCl, nerve pigment cells were induced. At 0.044M NaCl, the mesoderm differentiated into muscle and mesenchyme but the nerve and pigment cell differentiation did not take place. During the process of gastrulation an increase of intracellular sodium ions by forty times and calcium ions by three times was recorded. It is very likely that the reaction between the two kinds of ions brings about all the inductive changes.

From these observations it was concluded that normal embryonic induction depends on endogenous source of ions.

Genes and Inductors

Nieuwkoop (1966) proposed genic theory of neural induction based on the following observations.

1. The component tissues of neural inductor (i.e. chorda mesoderm and endoderm) become differentiated prior to ectodermal cells.
2. During blastula the transcription of mRNA and differential activation of genes in the presumptive chordo-mesodermal and endodermal cells increases many folds.
3. Differentiation process in presumptive ectodermal cells sets in only after mid gastrulation.

Oscar E. Schotte (1940) showed an interesting relationship between genes and inductores. The salamander larvae have temporary structures on the lateral side of the head called balancers. The Axolotl larva of Ambystoma does not have such structures. If a small piece of axolotl ectoderm is transplanted into the head region of salamander gastrula no balancer is formed. However, if the competent salamander ectoderm is transplanted into the head ectoderm of the axolotl larva a balancer is always formed. This shows that the tendency to form balancer is present in the Axolotl ectoderm but it is not competent to respond, the competent ectoderm forms a balancer. These experiments show that any tissue if competent when transplanted responds to a new location on the basis of its genetic constitution alone.

Organizers in Different Chordate Groups : Although primary organizer (chorda-mesoderm) was first discovered in urodele amphibians, it induces differentiation of nervous system in all vertebrates.

In Ascidians : The differentiation of ectoderm into neural tube is induced by the presumptive notochordal tissue and the anterior endoderm. In ascidians the organizing action of notochordal rudiment is restricted, because it can induce differentiation of cells of neuroectoderm. The cells of presumptive epidermis fail to respond.

In Amphioxus : In *Amphioxus,* the tissue from the inner surface of dorsal lip of blastopore of early gastrula has a neuralizing effect and can induce any part of ectodermal rudiment to differentiate into a neural tube.

Tung, Wu and Tung (1962) transplanted pieces of chorda-mesodermal tissue from the inner surface of dorsal lip of blastopore into the blastocoel of another embryo of the same stage. A secondary embryo was developed in the ventral region having a notochord, mesoderm and neural tube.

In Cyclostomes & Amphibians : In these groups also the dorsal lip of blastopore that contains chorda-mesodermal cells acts as primary organizer.

In Fishes : In bony fishes, which have large yolky eggs, the posterior edge of blastodisc which corresponds to the dorsal lip of blastopore or amphibian acts as an inductor. Oppenheimer (1963) has conducted transplantation of posterior edge of blastodisc in the blastocoel of another embryo.

In Birds : In birds, the primary organizer is located in the anterior half of primitive streak, which corresponds to the lips of blastopore of amphibians.

Competence : The concept of competence in embryology was introduced by Waddington (1932). According to him:

Competence *is the physiological state of an embryonic tissue during a particular period when the tissue can respond to the inductive action of a determinate stimuli in a morphogenetically specific way.* For example, the ectodermal tissue is competent with respect to neural induction of chorda-mesoderm for a specific period, after which it becomes competent to other types of inductions like that of lens.

According to molecular biological concept, competence is the sum ability of the enzyme component of the embryonic cell to adapt to a particular ratio of metabolites.

Competence is always a corresponding response to a particular stimulus. Competence with regards to primary induction is called primary competence, e.g. differentiation of neuroectoderm in response to primary inductor (chorda-mesoderm).

In experiments ectoderm was transplanted from various developmental stages starting from blastula to early neurula to other embryos. In all these cases the ectoderm showed gradual loss of competency to become neural tissue with advanced age in response to the inductive action of chorda-mesoderm. When the ectoderm was transplanted at a very late stage, it became only epidermis and nothing else.

In the same way dorsal lip tissues transplanted under

ventral ectoderm at various stages of development, shows that neural competence drops sharply towards the end of gastrulation and is lost by the onset of neurulation.

The decrease in neural competence with ageing of embryonal tissue was tested by another series of experiments. The fragments of gastrula ectoderm were isolated and kept in isolation for different length of time and then they were transplanted to different locations in a neurula, where inductors were active. The result showed that the competence to form brain decreased at the late gastrula stage and ectoderm at the late neurula stage fails to respond to neural induction. Though the ageing tissue losses its competence for one type of induction, it attains competence for newer type of inductions. Thus the ectoderm which loses neural competence responds to the induction to form lens, ear vesicle and nasal pits, etc. These successive states of competence appear to be synchronised with the appearance of primary and secondary inductions.

A study of induction and competence reveals that an interaction of both at the right time is essential for a proper growth and differentiation of the embryo. Once neural induction starts and progresses properly all other inductions follow in the right order.

Competence is not found in the early cleavage stage or blastula stage. It occurs only in the gastrula stage, because transcription of rRNA occurs only at gastrulation, though tRNA transcription starts a little earlier in the late cleavage stage (Brown 1961). The mRNA transcription also starts just before gastrulation. It means competence is closely associated with the starting of the transcription of RNA from the genome. Thus, competence is the passing phase of intense activity in the tissues of a growing embryo in response to the effective inducement provided by the different types of inductors from time to time.

Reciprocal Action

Inductor tissues have power to induce others while the reacting tissue always responds. This gives an active role to the inducer and a passive role to the competent tissue. The initiating or inducing component represents the action system and the reacting tissue forms the responding system. However, in the interacting systems in different animals, a stimulus response sequence is found in both directions. This is called reciprocal action. Morphogenesis of the vertebrate limb provides an example. At about 60 hours of incubation in chick embryo, the ectoderm at the apex of the wing bud thickness forming the apical ectodermal ridge. This ridge is formed as a response to the inductive action of the mesoderm. When mesoderm is grafted on any wound, the ectoderm on the wound forms a similar ridge, although the competency of the ectoderm to form the ridge is lost by about 65 hours of incubation. The mesoderm also loses its ability to induce by the same period of incubation. The newly-formed apical ridge acts as a powerful inductor. In an experiment the ridge was removed from the growing limb bud and further development of the limb stopped. On the other hand if another extra-apical ridge is grafted to a limb bud, two limbs begin to grow from the single primordium. This proves that the apical ectodermal ridge induces mesodermal outgrowth.

The mesodermal bulge now reacts with the ectodermal ridge and supplies a maintenance factor to enale it to continue the inductive action till the terminal parts of the limb are completely formed.

The study of limb morphogenesis gives us an idea about the reciprocal interaction that exists between two sets of tissues. This type of a two-way action is very essential for the proper development of the embryo.

4

The Herdmania

The embryology of simple Ascidian presents an example of retrogressive metamorphosis. The detailed account on the development of Indian genera-*Herdmania* has not been worked out completely. The following is the general account of the embryogenesis of a simple Ascidian.

Gonads (Ovotestes) : *Herdmania* is hermaphrodite and the gonads are known as ovotestes. Herdmania possesses a pair of tabulated ovotestes, one an either right and left side of the body. Each lobe of gonad has testicular tissue on the outer side and ovarian tissue towards inner side. Their genital ducts open into the atrium. The gametes are released in the atrium, from where these are discharged in the sea water. Gonads are protogynous, because the ova mature first.

Gametes

Sperms: Sperms are minute about $4\,\mu$ in length. Each is differentiated into acrosome or beak, head, neck and tail. The sperm are of three different types: — (i) having acrosome and neck of equal size, (ii) acrosome three times of neck, (iii) neck three times longer than the acrosome.

Unfertilised Egg (Ovum) : Egg of *Herdmania* is about 0.3 mm. in diameter. It is microlecithal and isolecithal. The yolk is little and uniformly distributed. The egg is enclosed in three distinct coverings : (i) Vitelline membrane (ii) inner chorion and (iii) outer chorion.

In between the vitelline membrane and inner chorion is the perivitelline space, filled with previtelline fluid. A large number of inner follicle cells with red pigment are found floating in the previtelline fluid. Outside the outer chorion is the outer layer of follicle cells. These are conical and vacuolated.

The cytoplasm or ooplasm is distinctly differentiated into two regions :

Outer Cortical Region or Hyaloplasm : It is the transparent peripheral layer of egg cytoplasm. It is devoid of yolk granules but contains numerous mitochondria. It contains yellow pigment spherules in *Styela* and orange pigment granules in *Boltenia echinata.*

Inner or Central Region : It is slate-gray in colour and contains yolk granules. The nucleus is large and lies eccentrically in the central region of ooplasm. The animal and vegetal poles are not distinct. The presence of nucleus serves to identify animal pole, because it lies towards the animal pole.

Fertilization : Fertilization is external in ascidians. Self fertilization is avoided because of protogynous condition. Sperm enters the ovum at its vegetal pole and initiates the following events:

(1) Fertilization membrane is formed around the egg.

(2) Second maturation division of the egg nucleus is completed.

(3) The egg cytoplasm gets differentiated into specific regions which have rigidly fixed fate. These move from their original position and get rearranged in a definite

pattern. These areas are known as organ-forming areas or presumptive areas and such an egg is called a mosaic egg.

(4) Imparts bilateral symmetry to egg.

Embryogenesis

Differentiation and Rearrangement of Organ-specific Regions of Egg Cytoplasm : The sperm entry into the egg initiates movement of ooplasm. The cortical layer of yellow hyaloplasm moves towards the vegetal pole and collects there to form a cap-like structure. When the sperm nucleus moves towards the centre, it draws the layer of yellow cytoplasm. The yellow hyaloplasm finally assumes a crescentric appearance and lies just below the equator of the egg. This is named as yellow crescent. It represents the presumptive mesoderm.

Simultaneously, the clear cytoplasm provided by the nucleus or germinal vesicle also flows towards the vegetal pole and comes to lie between the yellow cap and gray-coloured cytoplasm. As a result the food-laiden gray cytoplasm occupies the upper two-third of the egg. When yellow cytoplasm moves with the sperm nucleus, the clear cytoplasm also moves along with it. It forms a crescent just above the yellow crescent and is called clear crescent.

When yellow and clear cytoplasm have moved towards the vegetal pole, the gray cytoplasm is shifted towards the animal pole and constitutes anterior two-third of the egg. As the yellow and clear crescents are formed the gray cytoplasm again moves back to the vegetal ple. Finally it forms the gray crescent.

Fate Map of Fertilized Egg

As a result of these migratory activities in the ooplasm, three distinct prospective or presumptive areas are developed. These are:

(i) Presumptive ectoderm present in the form of a clear cytoplasm at the animal pole with little granules. It is formed from the clear crescent.

(ii) Presumptive mesoderm visible as yellow crescent extending posteroventrally near the equator.

(iii) Presumptive endoderm represented by gray crescent at the vegetal pole and placed anterodorsally.

Conklin has named these areas as ectoplasm, mesoplasm and endoplasm respectively. In addition to these three regions, the gray crescent cytoplasm is also differentiated into an upper prospective neural ectoderm (neuroplasm) and a lower presumptive notochord area (chordaplasm).

The prospective organ-specific regions have biochemical differences which control their differentiation into the parts they develop into. It can be demonstrated by centrifuging the fertilized eggs before they undergo cleavage. Centrifugation reshuffles the regions and they occupy abnormal positions. The embryo developing from such an egg has all those its rudiments which develop in the normal embryo but in an entirely different arrangement. This chaotic arrangement corresponds to the position of cytoplasmic precursor occupied in the centrifuged egg.

Cleavage in ascidians is of determinate* type. It begins about half an hour after fertilization. Cleavage is holoblastic and approximately equal.

First Cleavage : It is meridional (vertical). It passes through the polar axis and bisects the mesodermal and chordaneural crescents. The two blastomeres, thus formed, are exactly alike and establish bilateral symmetry.

Second Cleavage: Second furrow is also meridional but at right angles to the first. It cuts off two slightly smaller blastomeres on the posterior side and two larger ones in front.

Third Cleavage : Third cleavage is horizontal and a little above the equator. Of the eight blastomeres thus formed, the upper four are slightly smaller and are known as micromeres.

The lower four blastomeres are larger and are macromeres. At this stage the material of mesodermal crescent lies mainly in the two posterior lower blastomeres and the chordaneural material lies mainly in the anterior macromeres. The future of eight blastomeres can be enumerated as under :

(i) two anterior micromeres produce head epidermis, adhesive papillae and the brain with sense organs,

(ii) the two posterior micromeres produce epidermis only,

(iii) two anterior macromeres form notochord, spinal cord and part of intestine,

(iv) two posterior macromeres (vegetal blastomeres) give rise to intestine, mesenchyme and muscle tissue.

Reverberi concluded that the territories of all other structures of the embryo are fixed at eight-cell stage, the destiny of presumptive neural ectoderm is not fixed. Its differentiation is dependent on the inductive action of chorda cells.

Blastuala : Fourth, fifth and sixth cleavage furrows result in the formation of 64-celled embryo. It encloses a central cavity, the segmentation cavity or blastocoel. The embryo at this stage is known as blastuala or coeloblastuala. Its blastomeres are arranged in a single layer around the blastocoel.

Peculiar Features of Cleavage in Ascidian Egg: Ascidian egg is microlecithal and isolecithal but the cleavage produces unequal blastomeres. This suggests that the position of cleavage furrows in ascidians is not dependent on the amount of yolk. Here cleavage furrows are laid down to separate the egg cytoplasm into areas of distinctive biochemical composition. These areas are enclosed in specific blastomeres. Therefore, these balstomeres have precise developmental potentialities.

Gastrulation

Gastrulation takes place by the process of invagination. It follows the sixth cleavage and is completed by the time of seventh cleavage. The presumptive endoderm cells gradually sink into the blastocoel. The blastocoel becomes progressively reduced and finally disappears and the endoderm comes to lie in contact with the presumptive ectoderm. Thus a single-layered blastula is converted into a two layered, cup-shaped gastrula. Its cavity is known as archenteron and its opening to the exterior is termed blastopore. The blastopore marks the posterior end of the embryo. The gastrula elongates in the anteroposterior axis.

The fully-formed gastrula has an elongated two-layered body with a large archenteron. Its outer layer is formed of presumptive ectoderm cells all over, except a bond of presumptive neural plate on the dorsal side. The inner layer is formed of presumptive endoderm together with cells of presumptive notochord and middorsally and presumptive mesodermal strips dorsolaterally.

Post-gastrular Development

Neurulation (Neural Tube Formation) : The upper surface of the neural plate gets flattened and finally invaginates along the median line. It marks the beginning of neural groove. Its margins grow and complete the formation of neural tube. The embryo at this stage is known as neurula.

The closure of neural tube starts from the posterior end and moves forward. The anterior portion remains opened to the exterior for a short period. This aperture is knows as neuropore. At the posterior end the neural tube communicates with the archenteron. The connection is known as neurenteric canal.

The anterior end of neural tube remains comparatively

wider and develops into the brain vesicle. The remainder of neural tube forms the spinal cord or nerve cord.

Notogenesis : Notochord is formed from the presumptive chorda cells which lie in the roof of archenteron in the median line. These get constricted off from the archenteron and round up to form an elongated rod-shaped notochord. It lies immediately underneath the neural canal.

Mesoderm : Simultaneously, the mesoderm separates from the wall of archenteron dorsolaterally as a pair of solid plates of cells one on either side of notochord.

Formation of Larva

The embryo becomes pear-shaped and its posterior end forms the tail rudiment. This enters the larva stage. The body of larva is differentiated into a large-rounded anterior trunk region and a narrow posterior tail rudiment.

Development of Tail : The tail part of young larva consists of a surface layer of ectoderm, a neural canal and a median row of notochordal cells and a strand of endoderm cells. The mesodermal pouches are formed from the band. These mesodermal pouches form the musculature of the tail. The tail musculature comprises of longitudinal rows of striated muscles on either side of the notochord. The tail elongates rapidly and curves downwards.

Development of Trunk Region : The trunk region also increases in size and assumes oval appearance. The neural canal in the trunk region dilates into a thin-walled cerebral vesicle. It develops a dorsal pigmented eye and a ventral otocyst. The neural canal behind the vesicle thickens into a trunk ganglion. Rudiments of neural gland appear as a ciliated diverticulum from the anterior end of cerebral vesicle.

The archenteron differentiates into the anterior wider part which develops into a large pharynx and the posterior narrow part differentiates into oesophagus, stomach and instestine. The pharynx develops a ventral thickening, the endostyle. Mouth develops anterodorsally near the embryonic neurospora as an ectodermal invagination. An endodermal diverticulum from the archenteron joins it completing the anterior part of alimentary canal.

The atrial cavity appears anteriorly as a pair of dorso-lateral invaginations of the ectoderm which grows inwards into pouches and spreads out laterally around the pharynx. These unite dorsally and open by a single atrial aperture. Ventrally, the two pouches remain distinct. The wall separating the pharynx and atrium gets perforated by a part of slit-like openings, the stigmata. These increase in number both by the formation of new ones and by the division of those already present.

The rudiment of pericardium is nipped off as hollow outgrowth from the archenteron. Heart arises within the pericardium as an invagination from its dorsal wall.

Embryology of Simple Ascidian

The ectoderm cells secrete a cuticular test. Anteriorly it grows out in a dorsal and two lateral adhesive papillae. In the caudal region ectoderm forms two transparent longitudinal flaps, a dorsal and a ventral fin.

Hatching : The larva hatches out of the egg at this stage. It is known as ascidian tadpole. It swims freely with its tail and helps in dispersal.

Ascidian Tadpole

Morphology : Ascidian tadpole exhibits highest degree of chordate organisation. A fully-formed ascidian tadpole measures about 1.5 mm. Its body is differentiated into tail and trunk. It is covered by a thin test.

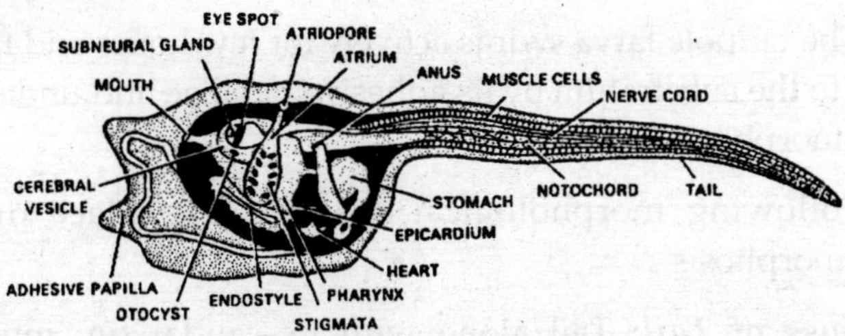

Tadpole larva of Herdmania

Tail: The tail encloses structures which are found in a typical chordate. It encloses a tubular dorsal nerve cord, a centrally-placed notochord and lateral muscle bands. The test covering the tail is prolonged into a tail fin having oblique striations.

Trunk : In the trunk region neural tube of the tail is enlarged to form a sensory vesicle or cerebral vesicle. It contains eye and statocyst. The eye contains a retina, pigmented layer, lens and a cornea. Eye is light sensitive, whereas statocyst is an organ of equilibrium. Alimentary canal lies below the brain. It contains mouth, small buccal cavity, large pharynx, swollen stomach and slender intestine. Rectum opens into the left part of atrium. Pharyngeal wall is perforated by two pairs of gill-slits. The trunk also encloses heart, pericardium and mesenchyme cells.

The anterior end of trunk bears three adhesive papillae. These help the larva for attachment during metamorphosis.

Retrogressive Metamorphosis

'Retrogressive metamorphosis' is a peculiar type of metamorphosis in the life-history of certain individuals, in which certain advanced characters shown by the larva disappear in the adult leading towards the simplification of its organization. Since certain larval organs like notochord, nerve cord, cerebral vesicle, otocyst, etc. degenerate during metamorphosis to assume the adult organization, the life-history of an ascidian affords a very good example of retrogressive metamorphosis.

The tadpole larva swims actively for few hours and finally fixes to the substratum by its adhesive papillae and undergoes metamorphosis.

Following morphological changes take place during metamorphosis :

Loss of Tail: Tail along with its caudal fin, muscles, notochord and nerve cord begins to reduce and finally disappear. It is partly re-absorbed and partly cast off.

Loss of Adhesive Papillae : The adhesive papillae are lost.

Development of Test: The test increases enormously and forms the foot at the posterior end of the body. It is meant for attachment. The test increases in thickness and becomes tough and translucent.

Shifting of Mouth and Atrial Aperture : The body between the point of attachment and mouth grows rapidly. This causes rotation of the body in posterodorsal direction at an angle of nearly 180°. As a result mouth and atrial aperture are carried to the free end and intestine becomes U-shaped.

Formation of Siphons : The part of the body around branchial and atrial apertures gets elongated to form siphons.

Alimentary Canal: The pharynx grows enormously and the number of stigmata increases. It is now known as branchial sac. The stomach and intestine increase in length. Liver is formed.

Completion of Heart: Heart completes its development and acquires connection with the blood sinuses.

Development of Gonads : Gonads and their ducts develop from the mesodermal cells.

Changes in the Nervous System : (i) The cerebral vesicle with ocelli and statocyst is lost. (ii) Anterior part of cerebral vesicle which communicates with the pharynx develops into a neural gland. (iii) Visceral ganglion of the larva is reduced to a small ganglion placed above the neural gland. (iv) Larval trunk ganglion forms the visceral nerve of the adult. (v) Part of the nerve cord lying in the trunk also disappears.

As a result of all these changes *an active, free swimming larva with complex organization and chordate characters (i.e.* possessing notochord, nerve cord and organs of special sense) *metamorphoses into a sedentrary adult ascidian having simple degenerate organization with no traces of chordate characteristics.* Such type of metamorphosis is described as retrogressive or retrograde metamorphosis. As a result of retrogressive metamorphosis photosensitive and geo-negative larva changes into a photo negative and geo-positive adult.

Significance of Embryology of Ascidian : The embryological studies of ascidian is of great significance because :

1. Ascidian egg provides the best example of mosaic eggs. Its ooplasm is well-organized and differentiated into organ-specific areas or prospective areas on account of the presence of naturally occurring pigments.
2. The ascidian development provides an example of determinate type of cleavage.
3. Ascidian development exhibits retrogressive metamorphosis.
4. Highly developed larval organization with distinct chordate characteristics has a taxonomic importance. It helps in establishing the chordate relationship of ascidians.

The Anascidian : The ascidians or sea-squirts are marine primitive animals that are more chordate-like in the larval than in the adult stage. Class Ascidiacea of sub-phylum Urochordata comprises approximately 2,000 species. The common representatives of this class *are Ascidia, Hermania, Ciona, Styela, Botryllus* and *Molgula.* The adults are sendentary, without notochord, nerve-cord and tail. Pharynx is large and perforated by numerous gill-slits. Life-history includes a free-swimming tadpole larva with notochord and dorsal nerve cord in tail. It undergoes retrogressive metamorphosis to become an adult.

A detailed account of the embryogenesis of the Indian ascidian species, Herdmania is not available. Therefore we shall follow a general account of the development *of Styela partita* worked out by Conklin (1905,1911).

The Unfertilised Egg : In ascidians, the egg is relatively small, averaging from 0.1 to 0.2 millimetre in diameter, and is of the microlecithal, isolecithal variety. Their cytoplasm is well differentiated by a natural pattern of pigmentation and distribution of yolk. The fate of every part of the egg becomes fixed or determined without liable to change, before or at the time of fertilization, each giving rise to a definite organ of the embryo. This type of eggs are called determinate or mosaic eggs.

The immature egg *of Styela* exhibits a yolk-free peripheral layer of orange-yellow cytoplasm and a central area, slate gray in colour, through which yolk granules are scattered. The egg's nucleus, termed the *germinal vesicle* at this time, is quite large and rests eccentrically within the central area and closely beneath the yellow peripheral layer. The position occupied by the germinal vesicle serves to identify the animal pole of the egg. The side opposite the germinal vesicle, therefore, is the vegetal pole.

Fertilization : When the egg is released from the ovary, the investing membrane of the germinal vesicle dissolves releasing a clear residual plasm, and the spindle for the first maturation division is formed. But the maturation divisions do not take place until the ovum is penetrated by the spermatozoon. Entrance of the spermatozoon which usually occurs at the vegetative pole, not only incites the maturation divisions but sets off movements within the cytoplasm. The cortical layer of yellow cytoplasm streams rapidly towards the vegetal pole where it collects as a cap . Simultaneously, all but a small portion of the clear plasm provided by the germinal vesicle also flows to the lower pole where it accumulates between the yellow cap and the gray yolk-laden cytoplasm which now occupied the upper two-thirds of the egg.

After the clear and yellow substances have collected at the vegetal pole, the sperm nucleus starts to move toward that side of the egg which future development shows to be posterior. In the meantime, the egg will have completed its maturation divisions and the egg nucleus descends to meet the sperm nucleus just below the equator. As the sperm nucleus moves centroposteriorly, it appears to draw the layers of yellow and clear protoplasm along with it. The yellow substance, which remains largely at the surface, then assumes the form of a crescent with its broad dimension directed posteroventrally and its arms extended a quarter of the way around each side of the egg. The clear substance extends more deeply into the centre of egg, but it also forms a crescent immediately above the yellow crescent.

Formation of Prospective Organ Regions (Fate Map) : As the egg prepares to begin cleavage, a further sorting out of cytoplasmic areas takes place.

The substance comprising the clear crescent gradually diffuses into the animal hemisphere, and the gray yolky plasm becomes confined to the vegetative region. Coincidentally, the gray plasm differentiates into two areas, a dark gray mass at the vegetative pole and a lighter gray crescent immediately opposite the yellow crescent. At this time, therefore, four general regions may be distinguished in the egg :

(i) an upper hemisphere of light protoplasm, (prospective epidermal ectoderm) which originated in the germinal vesicle.

(ii) A yellow crescent (prospective mesoderm) posteroventrally,

(iii) A gray crescent anterodorsally and

(iv) A vegetative area of dark gray yolky substance (prospective endoderm). The gray crescent actually encircles two developmental prospects—an upper neural ectoderm and lower notochord.

The assumption may be made, therefore, that the development of the parts of the embryo enumerated is caused by the kind of cytoplasm that is contained in the cells. This can actually be proved by centrifuging the eggs before they begin cleaving (Conklin, 1931). Such treatment serves to shuffle the regions, so that they come to occupy abnormal positions. An embryo will still develop from a centrifuged egg, but its tissues and rudiments of organs have a chaotic arrangement. It is an orderly chaos, however in the sense that each part develops in the position where its cytoplasmic precursor came to lie to the result of centrifugation.

Cleavage and Formation of Blastula : Cleavage begins about half an hour after fertilization. It is holoblastic and slightly unequal. The first cleavage plane of *Styela* is meridional and it passes through the polar axis and bisects the mesodermal and chordoneural crescents. As it has been determined that the first cleavage plane corresponds to the median axis of the embryo to come, the first two blastomeres represent the material source of the right and left halves of the embryo. These blastomeres are exactly alike and establish the bilateral symmetry, one producing the right half and the other the left half. The second set of divisions is at a right angle to the first, but is again vertical, cutting off two slightly smaller blastomeres at the posterior side and two larger ones in front. This results in the prospective mesoderm coming to lie in the two posterior cells and the chordaneural material in the two anterior cells. The third cleavage is horizontal and passes a little above the equator. It produces an eight-cell stage that consists of an upper (apical) tier of slightly smaller blastomeres and four larger basal cells below. The smaller ones are called micromeres and the larger ones the macromeres or megameres. The third set of cleavages serves to parcel out the prospective organ materials in such a way that the prospective mesoderm lies in the posterobasal pair of blastomeres, the chorda in the anterobasal, blastomeres and the neural ectoderm in both anteroapical and basal cells. The two posteroapical cells and parts of the anteroapical ones provide the epidermal ectoderm; the endoderm lies in the four basal cells.

The eight-celled embryo undergoes three more sets of cleavages. This results in the formation of a flat coeloblastula. It has a fluid-filled cavity, the blastocoel, which is enclosed by a single layer of blastomeres.

Special Features of Ascidian Cleavage: Although cleavage in *Styela* is holoblastic, the resulting blastomeres are only approximately equal in size. Despite small amount of yolk, division is not absolutely equal but reflects the cytoplasmic architecture of the egg. Cleavage serves to parcel into individual blastomeres areas of cytoplasm of distinctive biochemical composition. That this parcelling is real indeed has been demonstrated by experiments in which certain blastomeres are injured so as to prohibit them from further developmental participation. If, for instance, the four right hand blastomeres of an 8-cell stage are injured, the left-hand blastomeres produce only a left half-embryo; or if the four rear blastomeres are immobilized, the four in front produce only those parts they are normally destined to produce, namely epidermis, neural tube, notochord, and endoderm. As for the origin of these "organ-forming stuffs", modern studies in developmental genetics suggest that the genome of the original oocyte prescribes the biochemical substances deposited in the egg. These substances then selectively specify or regulate gene activity in the individual blastomeres so as to promote continuing differentiation.

Gastrulation and Formation of Neurula : The coeloblastula gastrulates by embolic invagination. Gastrulation begins after the sixth cleavage and is completed by the time of the seventh cleavage *i.e.* between the 64-cell and 128-cell stage. Blastopore, present on the ventral side of the gastrula, closes and the embryo begins to lengthen along the embryonic axis indicated by the plane of the first cleavage. The *neural plate* of the elongating gastrula then invaginates along the midline to form a groove which subsequently takes the form of a tube, the *neural tube.* The stage during which this process occurs is called the neurula.

Formation of the Larva : With further development the neurula transforms into a minute tadpole-shaped larva. It is equipped with a typically chordate tail having central notochord, dorsal neural tube, lateral muscle bands and a trunk containing a sensory vesicle with sense organs and a neural gland. The changes that occur during this transformation are as follows :

1. *Tail:* The future dorsal and lateral parts of the embryo wall near the blastopore proliferate posteriorly to form the tail rudiment.
2. *Notochord:* The notochordal cells invaginated during gastrulation and lying in the roof of the archenteron come to form a single longitudinal row in the tail and they constitute the future notochord.
3. *Tail Musculature and Body Mesenchyme:* Concurrently with the formation of the tail rudiment and the notochord, a solid band of mesoderm cells is budded off from each side of the archentron. These bands develop into *body mesenchyme.* They also extend into the tail, where they give rise to the tail *musculature.* The

latter consists of three longitudinal rows of muscle cells on either side of the notochord.

4. *Nerve Cord and Brain Vesicle:* A neural tube arises by the infolding of the presumptive neural plate occupying the middorsal line of late gastrula. The anterior part of the neural tube enlarges into a *cerebral vesicle* which later develops two *ocelli* and an *otolith*. The neural tube extends into the tail dorsal to the notochord as the future nerve-cord.

5. *Neuropore:* At the forward end of the cerebral vesicle a neuropore comes to open in the developing pharynx. This pore represents the forerunner of the pharyngeal opening of the adult neural gland.

6. *Atrium:* Just behind the cerebral vesicle, the dorsolateral ectoderm on each side of the larva invaginates, initiating the formation of atrium. It starts enveloping the developing pharynx.

7. *Alimentary Tract:* The archenteron differentiates into the various parts of the alimentary tract. Pharynx develops an *endostyle* in the ventral wall and three pairs of gill slits in the lateral walls. The gill-slits establish communication between the pharyngeal cavity and the atrial chamber.

8. *Gill-slits:* Number of gill-slits increases later, by subdivision of the first three pairs of gill-slits.

9. *Heart:* Rudiments of *heart* and *pericardium* appear as a hollow outgrowth from the ventral wall of the pharynx.

10. *Adhesive Papillae:* Anteriorly, the tadpole develops three adhesive papillae.

11. *Test:* Leaving the adhesive papillae, everywhere else the surface of the larva gets covered by the rudiments of the test or tunic. It also covers the mouth and makes it non-functional.

Hatching : About eight hours after fertilization larva gets fully formed. It bursts the egg membranes and swims away. The free-swimming tailed larva is called the ascidian tadpole or appendicularia. The tadpole swims about for only a short period—from minutes to a few hours at the most. It serves primarily as a dispersal and site-selection device.

Structure of the Tadpole Larva

The fully developed larva of Herdmania is about 1.5 mm long. Its exterior is covered by a thin test. The body of tadpole is differentiated into two distinct regions :

(1) a short anterior trunk and

(2) a long posterior tail.

Trunk: It is much short in comparison to the tail. In its mid-dorsal region, the anterior part of the nerve cord is expanded to form the brain which shows three regions :

(i) Anterior narrow solid *cerebral cone.*

(ii) Middle swollen, oval hollow *sensory vesicle* and

(iii) Posterior narrow solid *visceral* or *trunk ganglion.* The sensory vesicle encloses three sense organs : a *postero-dorsal ocellus,* an *antero-ventral ocellus* and a *statocyst.* The latter contains a central *otolith* and is an organ of equilibrium. The ocelli are sensitive to light.

The mouth is located on the anterior part of the dorsal surface of the trunk. It is covered by test and is, therefore, non-functional. The larva gets its nutrition from the yolk reserves of endodermal cells of the embryonic gut. The alimentary canal is well differentiated into a short *buccal cavity,* a large *pharynx,* a short narrow *oesophagus,* a swollen *stomach,* a curved slender *intestine* and a small *rectum* opening into the left part of the atrium. The pharynx has pairs of gill slits or *stigmata* and a ventral *endostyle.*

The atrium is an ectodermal pouch lying on the sides of and dorsal to the pharynx. It opens to the exterior by a dorsally situated *atrial aperture.* The heart, enclosed in a pericardium lies below the pharynx. A group of undifferentiated mesenchyme cells is found in the hind region of the trunk. Towards the end of the free-swimming life, the ectoderm protrudes out at the anterior end of the trunk to form three stalked adhesive papillae, two being dorso-lateral and one ventro-lateral in position.

Tail: The tail of the ascidian tadpole is laterally compressed and about 1.0 mm long. The test covering the tail is produced into a wide median vertical tail-fin that shows oblique striations looking like fin-rays. The tail contains an axial skeletal rod, the notochord, a part of which projects into the trunk. Above the notochord is a hollow nerve cord that extends into the trunk anteriorly. Below the notochord is present a strand of endodermal cells. On both sides of the nerve cord, notochord and endodermal strand are present *three* muscle bands in the anterior and *two* in the posterior part of the tail.

The tail serves as a locomotory organ of the larva. .The ascidian tadpole larva swims about actively in the surface waters by vibrating its long tail for about three hours after hatching. It then, sinks to the bottom and fixes to some substratum by the help of its adhesive papillae. The fixed larva stands upside down on the substratum, slowly brandishing its tail in water. After attachment, the larva undergoes a peculiar kind of metamorphosis.

Retrogressive Metamorphosis

The retrogressive metamorphosis of ascidian tadpole comprises following morphogenetic changes:

Loss of Tail: Metamorphosis involves degeneration of the tail, including notochord, nerve cord and tail muscles. These tissues are autolised and resorbed by the metamorphosing larva. As a result the tail begins to shorten and ultimately disappears altogether.

Changes in the Brain: The sensory vesicle with its sense organs breaks down. The anterior part of the sensory vesicle gives rise to the neural gland, whereas its posterior part, in conjuction with the trunk ganglion, forms the nerve ganglion of the animals the trunk ganglion transforms into the visceral nerves.

Perfection of Alimentary Tract: The pharynx enlarges, the stigmata increase in number and are vascularised by blood-channels. Stomach grows bigger, intestine becomes U-shaped and liver is formed.

Formation of Ectodermal Ampullae: Ectoderm and test extend from the four corners of the trunk of attached, metamorphosing larva over the substratum in the form of outgrowths called ectodermal ampullae. They serve a double role of respiration and anchorage.

Shifting of Mouth and Atrial Aperture: The portion of the larval body between the point of attachment and mouth proliferates rapidly. This causes the body to rotate dorso-posteriorly through an angle of nearly 180°. Due to this, mouth and atrial aperture are carried to the opposite free end.

Loss of Adhesive Papillae: The adhesive papillae not of any functional significance in the adult disappear.

Development of Test: The test grows to enclose the entire animal. It becomes thick, tough and translucent.

Elaboration of Blood-vascular System: The heart completes its development and gets connected with the blood-sinuses at both the ends.

Formation of Gonads: Gonads and their ducts develop in the mesoderm.

Opening of Mouth: The test is resorbed in the region over the mouth so that an adult ascidian feeding by ciliary currents, becomes established.

Thus an active free-swimming larva with many typical chordate features like an axial notochord, dorsal hollow nerve cord and ventral gut changes into an inert, sessile adult with little characterization of chordate nature. When metamorphosis includes such morphogenetic changes that convert an advanced larva into a primitive adult animal, then such metamorphosis is called degenerative or retrogressive metamorphosis.

A free swimming larva with obvious chordate characters formed in the life-history of ascidians is of a great phylogenetic significance. It proves the chordate nature of the adult tunicates despite the fact that they do not exhibit common features encountered in the chordate animals.

5

The Nutrition

Nutritional Requirements of Embryo

Embryonic development includes cell-multiplication, cell-growth and cell-differentiation. Energy, new protoplasm and enzymes are required for the accomplishment of these processes. Therefore, a continuous supply of oxygen and nutrients like carbohydrates, amino acids and certain minerals is essential. The reproductive cells and the embryo lack the means of obtaining nutrients from the environment. 'The embryonic nutrition is the supply of required nutrient material for the synthesis of more protoplasm and other compounds for cell differentiation and for the production of energy.'

Modes of Embryonic Nutrition

There are basically three ways of embryonic nutrition —

1. Animals with indirect development have eggs with very little food reserve. So their embryonic development is very brief and in few hours to a few days the larva or juvenile hatches out of the egg. This utilizes food

from the environment to sustain growth. The larva then grows and metamorphoses to become adult. It is seen in majority of aquatic animals, majority of invertebrates and all amphibians.

2. Many animals produce yolky eggs. The developing embryo utilizes this reserve food stuff either directly or indirectly from the reserved yolk. This is found in fishes, reptiles, birds and primitive mammals.
3. In higher mammals (eutherians) and in certain fishes (sharks) the embryo receives nourishment from mother through a structure called placenta and is retained in the womb (uterus) of mother.

Oviparity, Ovoviviparity and Viviparity

Oviparous : Animals that lay or spawn eggs are known as oviparious. Majority of invertebrates, and all the chordates except eutherian mammals are oviparous.

Viviparous : In mammals (Eutherians), sharks and some invertebrates the eggs are retained within mother's body during the embryonic development. Therefore, they give birth to young ones. These are called viviparous.

Ova-viviparous: In ova-viviparous forms, the embryo develops within the uterus of female and gets protection, but does not receive any nourishment. e.g. Echidna.

Food Reserve and Embryonic Nutrition

Nature of Reserve Food in Egg : The reserve nutrient material in the egg cytoplasm is called yolk. As a matter of fact yolk is not a definite chemical substance, rather a mixture of proteins, neutral fats, phospholipids, glycogen and certain other carbohydrates. When yolk contains proportionately more protein, it is called 'protein yolk' and yolk mainly with phospholipids and fats is called 'fatty yolk'. Both types of yolks are present side by side in the eggs but their ratio varies.

Protein yolk is more abundant in eggs of many invertebrates and lower chordates, while fatty yolk is more abundant in polylecithal eggs of bony fishes, reptiles and birds.

The yolk is stored in the eggs either as granules or as platelets. The yolk-platelets are formed of phosvitin and lipovitellin.

Formation of Yolk

The yolk may be synthesized in the eggs or elsewhere in the body and then transported by blood to the egg or to the surrounding follicle cells.

(1) In the first case (e.g. Spirorbis eggs) the metabolites required for the synthesis for yolks are taken up by the oocyte by pinocytosis. These enter the rough E.R. and then Golgi complex and are converted into yolk.

(2) In insects the partially phosphorylated phosvitin (yolk-protein) is synthesized in the intestine and in mammals inside the liver. It is then transported by blood to follicle cells which transfer it to the developing oocyte.

The partially phosphorylated yolk protein- phosvitin is soluble in water but in fully phosphorylated form, it is insoluble. Inside the mitochondria of oocyte the partially phosphorylated phosvitin is phosphorylated by receiving phosphate molecule from ATP in presence of enzyme protein-kinase.

Utilization of Yolk

1. In mesolecithal, holoblastic eggs (frog's eggs) in which the yolk is comparatively less and somewhat uniformly distributed the yolk is utilized in a very simple way. During cleavage, the yolk gets distributed mechanically into the daughter cells or blastomeres of vegetal pole. Enzymes present inside the blastomeres break up the complex molecules of yolk into simpler substances which are then utilized in the formation of proteins

(enzymes) and new protoplasm by micromeres and macromeres.

2. In macrolecithal eggs with meroblastic cleavage (eggs of reptiles, birds, prototherians and fishes), the cleavage furrows are restricted to the blastodisc (embryonic area) only which lies over the yolk. Thus the embryonic cells remain in direct contact with the yolk. Therefore, in early stages of development, the dividing blastomeres spread over the yolk and absorb underlying yolk by diffusion.

In later stages of development, when the extraembryonic membranes (amnion, chorion and allantois) develop around the embryo, the splanchnopleure (endoderms-planchnic mesoderm) of the midgut spreads over the yolk mass, encloses it completely and forms the yolk-sac.

Though, the yolk sac is connected to the digestive tract by a yolk stalk. The yolk as such is not transported to the embryo by this route. This endodermal surface of the yolk-sac is thrown into folds that penetrate the yolk mass. Its endoderm cells produce digestive enzymes that change the insoluble yolk into soluble form. This solubilized yolk is absorbed by the endodermal lining of the yolk-sac and is transported to the embryo through a pair of vitelline veins. The yolk-sac has a network of capillaries from vitelline arteries and vitelline veins.

Embryonic Nutrition from Mother : In viviparous animals, the egg is with hardly any food reserve. The developing embryo has to depend on mother for nourishment to a lesser or greater degree. So the embryo develops inside the uterus (womb) of mother gets attached to the uterine wall and obtains nourishment from her until birth through placenta.

Placenta is a structure or organ that establishes an organic connection between foetus and mother. It is formed of maternal and foetal tissue jointly and serves for the transport of nutrient substances and oxygen from maternal blood stream and eliminates nitrogenous wastes into it.

Occurrence : Placenta is not found exclusively in mammals but also occurs in animals belonging to different groups which are basically oviparous, for example placenta is formed in *Peripatus* (Onychophora), *Salpa* (Tunicata), *Mustelus laevis* (Elasmobranchia) and certain lizards and snakes (Reptilia). The nature of foetal tissue that forms placenta with maternal uterine wall is different in all these cases.

Composition of Placenta

Structurally, placenta consists of two different parts lying in close approximation-

1. *Maternal Part of Placenta:* This part of placenta is furnished by the uterine endometrium.
2. *Foetal Part of Placenta:* It is derived from the extra embryonic membranes of the embryo. The foetal membrane-chorion establishes contact with the endometrium of uterus. Its vascular supply comes either from the vitelline circulation of yolk sac or from the allantoic circulation provided by the allantois. Based on this, the placenta can be following two types:

Chorio-vitelline or Yolk-sac Placenta : In this type of placenta, the connection is established between the uterine wall and that part of chorion which is lined with the yolk-sac and has a network of vitelline blood vessels of the yolk sac. The allantois remains relatively small. In some metatherian mammals (Marsupialia-*Didelphis* and *Macropus),* though the eggs are small and without yolk, these develop a large and highly vascular yolk-sac. It fuses with the chorion and makes it vasular. Such a foetal association is known as yolk-sac placenta. The uterine wall secretes a viscous fluid, the uterine milk. It is absorbed by the villi of yolk-sac placenta and through vitelline circulation is carried to the embryo.

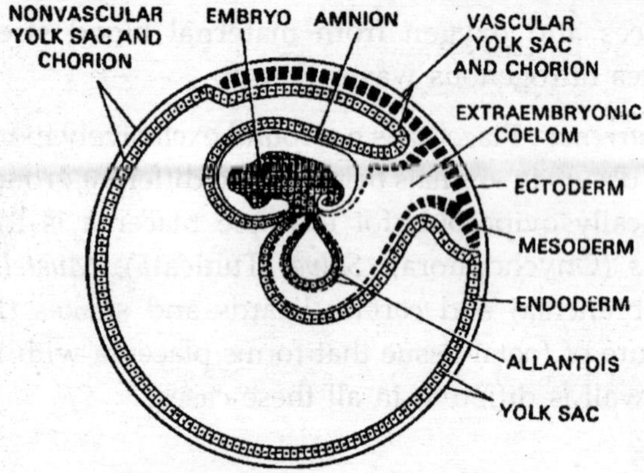

Yolk-sac placenta in Didelphis.

Chorio-allantoic Placenta (True Placenta) : In chorio-allantoic or allanto-chorionic placenta, the connection is established between the uterine wall and the chorion lined with allantois and has a network of allantoic blood vessels. The yolk-sac remains rudimentary and non-functional. It is found in some marsupials *(Dasyurus* and *Parameles)* and all eutherian mammals.

Implantation : The egg is fertilized in fallopian tube and immediately starts dividing. Simultaneously, it descends down the oviduct to reach the uterus. On reaching the uterus the zona pelucida surrounding it gets dissolved and the embryo now enters the blasocyst stage. It gets attached to the uterine wall. This attachment of blastocyst to the uterine wall is known as implantation. The time taken for implantation varies in different groups of mammals, being 6 days in rats and 8-10 days in man. Before implantation, the blastocyst is nourished by a secretion of the tubular uterine glands called the 'uterine milk'. It contains organic substances used as nutrients.

Formation of Placenta (Placentation) : After implantation, at first the embryo obtains its nourishment by enzymatically breaking down the cells of the uterine lining immediately around it. Later on, a placenta is developed through which embryo extracts nutritional elements from maternal blood stream.

The blastocyst penetrates deep into the uterine wall. At this time the extraembryonic membrane-chorion that surrounds the trophoblast is produced into finger-like projections, called villi that penetrate into depressions in the uterine wall. Later on, these villi are penetrated from allantois which forms connective tissue and blood vessels of the foetal placenta. These allanto-chorionic villi become highly vascular and grow into the uterine wall, which in the area of contact form crypts and receives the trophoblastic villi. This interdigitate structure of embryonic (allanto-chorionic villi) and maternal part (uterus wall) is called a placenta and the process of formation of placenta is known as placentation. The association may become more intimate by dissolution or erosion of some of the layers of uterine wall or trophoblastic villi or both.

Thus, in implantation, the attachment of the embryo and uterine wall is superficial whereas in placentation the association is more intimate with trophoblastic villi eroding deep into the uterine wall, eventually breaking through the maternal blood vessels.

Structure of Placenta

The most primitive type of true placenta as found in cow, goat, etc. is formed of following layers of embryonal and maternal tissues-

	1. Foetal blood capillaries	— Derived from allantois
Embryonal	2. Foetal connective tissue	
Layers	3. Foetal chorionic epithelium	— Derived from chorion
	1. Uterine epithelium (mucous epithelium of uterus)	
Maternal	2. Uterine connective	
Layers	3. Maternal blood capillaries	

Classification of Placenta

A. Based on Mode of Implantation

In placental mammals, the 'elation of chorionic sac to the uterine wall varies greatly and can be distinguished into following three types.

Superficial Implantation : The chorionic sac lies in contact with the lining of main uterine cavity but it is not burried in it. This type of implantation is also called central implantation. It is found in ungulates, carnivores and monkeys.

Eccentric Implantation : The chorionic sac lies in a fold or pocket which losses off from the main uterine cavity. It is found in beaver, rat and squirrel.

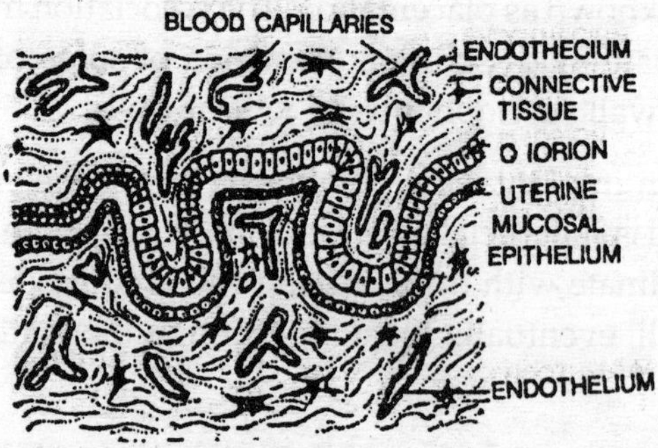

T.S. of placenta showing its maternal and foetal components.

Interestitial Implantation : The chorionic sac penetrates into the substance of uterine lining and establish deep contacts, *e.g.* hedgehog, guinea pig, apes and man.

B. Classification Based on the Degree of Association

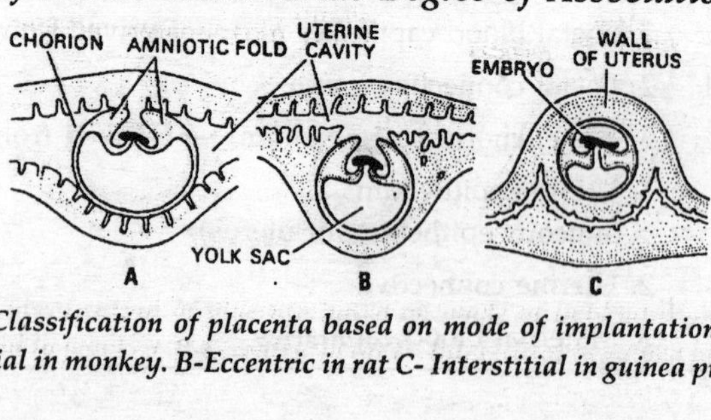

Classification of placenta based on mode of implantation.
A-Superficial in monkey. B-Eccentric in rat C- Interstitial in guinea pig and man.

The degree of closeness between foetal and maternal tissues varies within the eutherian mammals. Based on the degree of their intimacy three types of placentae are recognized.

Non-deciduate Placenta : In non-deciduate placenta the implantation of embryo in the uterus is superficial. The foetal chorionic epithelium lies in contact with the uterine epithelium. At the time of birth the foetal villi are drawn out completely without tearing or causing any injury to the uterine wall and no bleeding occurs. This type of placenta is called non-deciduate or non-deciduous placenta. It is found in pigs, cattle, horse and other ruminants.

Deciduate or Deciduous Placenta : In deciduous placenta, the degree of contact between foetal and maternal tissue is more intimate. The wall of the uterus becomes eroded to various degrees, so that the foetal chorionic epithelium may come to lie either in the connective tissue or into the maternal blood. At the time of parturition, when foetal part of placenta separates from the uterine part of placenta, there is more or less extensive haemorrhage and tearing of tissues from the uterine wall. The placentae of this type are known as deciduous and the uterine wall as decidua. It can be differentiated into three regions :

Decidua Basalis : the part of decidua between chorionic vesicle and the muscles of the wall of uterus.

Decidua Capsularis : the part of decidua which surrounds the chorionic sac and separates it from the cavity of the uterus.

Decidua Parietalis : the part which forms the inner lining of the rest of the uterus. The deciduous placenta is found in man, rabbit, dog, cat, etc.

Contra-deciduate Placenta : In *Parameles* and *Talpa* (mole) the association between foetal and maternal tissue is intimate as in deciduous placenta. But at the time of parturition both maternal as well as foetal tissue are lost and absorbed in situ by maternal leucocytes. This modified deciduate placenta is called contra-deciduate placenta.

C. Classification Based on Distribution of Villi on Chorion

Diffused type with villi scattered all over the surface of chorio.

Examples : in ungulates—horse, mare, lemur, pig, etc.

Cotyledonary Type : with villi distributed in isolated patches as in goat and ruminants like deer, sheep, cattle.

Zonary Type : with villi arranged in a definite band or girdle encircling the middle of blastocyst or chorionic sac.

Example : Zonary placenta is found in carnivores—cats, dogs, etc.

Discoidal Type : with villi located in one or two discoidal areas. It is called mono-discoidal placenta when the villi form one patch and bidiscoidal if the villi are present in two disc-shaped areas. Examples — Discoidal placenta is found in mouse, rats, rabbit, money, anthropoid apes, and man.

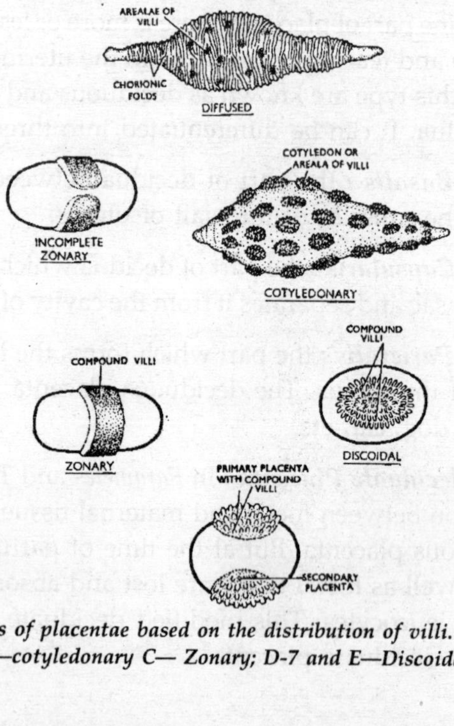

Different types of placentae based on the distribution of villi. A—Diffused ; B—cotyledonary C— Zonary; D-7 and E—Discoidal.

D. Histological Classification of Placenta

Based upon the histological relationship of embryonic villi with the uterine wall and the degree of erosion the mammalian placentae are classified into five types:

Epitheliochorial Placenta : In this type of placenta the embryonic trophoblast and the uterine epithelium remain in close contact but both of them retain their original layers. The chorio-allantoic villi lie in the pocket-like depressions of the uterine wall.

(i) Endothelium of foetal blood vessels. Foetal layers

(ii) Chorionic connective tissue

(iii) Ectoderm of chorion (chorionic epithelium).

(iv) Uterine epithelium maternal layer

(v) Endometrial connective tissue

(vi) Endothelium of maternal blood vessels.

The chorio-allantoic villi lie in the pocket-like depressions of the uterine wall. Since epithelium of uterine wall lies in contact with the chorionic-epithelium. This type of placenta is called epithelio-chorial placenta. It is found in marsupials, ungulates (pig and horse, etc.) and lemurs. It is the most primitive type of placenta.

Syndesmo-chorial Placenta : In this type of placenta the chorionic villi erode the uterine wall, so that the uterine epithelium is ruptured and the chorionic epithelium lies in contact with the connective tissue of the uterine wall, e.g., sheep and cow. (i.e. ruminant ungulates).

Endotheliochorial Placenta : Not only the uterine epithelium but the uterine connective tissue is also eroded to the extent that the chorionic epithelium of villi comes in contact with the endothelium of maternal blood vessels, e.g. dog, cat and other carnivores.

Haemo-chorial : Here uterine epithelium, connective tissue and the endothelial wall of the maternal blood capillaries are eroded with the result that the chorionic epithelium comes in direct contact with the maternal blood which circulates in the lacunae formed in thickened trophoblast of the villi, e.g. man.

Haemo-endothelial : In this type the uterine epithelium, uterine connective tissue, endothelium of maternal blood capillaries and the trophoblastic epithelium are eroded with the result that the foetal capillaries lie freely in maternal blood, e.g. rabbit.

Physiology of Placenta

The mammalian eggs are with almost no yolk. Therefore, for nutrition, the mammalian embryo depends entirely on the supplies from the maternal body through the placenta. Hence, a close contact is established between the maternal and foetal tissue and the maternal and foetal vascular supply are in communication but never in direct contact. The maternal blood does not enter the blood circulation of the embryo or vice-versa. The two circulations are separated by a placental barrier. Morphologically, the placental barrier is composed of the maternal and foetal tissues of the placenta lying between the maternal and foetal blood spaces.

The composition of placental barrier varies in different types of placenta. It may be formed of all the three layers of foetal and maternal tissues i.e. trophoblastic epithelium, connective tissue, endothelium of foetal capillaries, uterine epithelium, connective tissue, endothelium of connective tissue and endothelium of maternal blood capillaries or in the last stages only the endothelial layer of foetal and maternal blood capillaries. Physiologically, the placental barrier acts as semi permeable membrane, allowing some substances to pass through but keeping out others.

Therefore, in mammals, the embryo depends completely on mother for its nourishment and oxygen supply throughout the developing period. Mother also removes nitrogenous wastes, and carbon dioxide from the embryo. The pregnant mother, therefore, acts as stomach, intestine, liver, lungs and kidneys for the foetus. It is, therefore, obvious that good health and proper nourishment of mother is essential.

Functions : The primary function of placenta is the interchange of materials present in the blood streams of mother and embryo. All the substances have to pass through the placenta either by simple diffusion, pinocytosis, or by active transport, etc.

The mode of transmission is associated with the size of molecules. Small molecules of oxygen, carbon-dioxide, water, soluble inorganic materials such as chlorides and phosphates of sodium, potassium and magnesium and soluble organic substances like glucose, etc. monosaccharides, hormones, vitamins and nitrogenous wastes, etc. pass through placenta by diffusion. Macromolecules of polysaccharides, lipids and proteins are absorbed by the cells of trophoblastic villi which are obtained by pinocytosis. Thus, the placenta carries out following functions :

1. *Nutrition*: Placenta brings about the transportation of nutrients (monosaccharides, disaccharides, amino acids and small lipid molecules) from maternal blood stream into the foetus.

2. *Respiration*: Placenta helps in the exchange of oxygen and carbon-dioxide between foetus and mother and thus helps in respiration. Oxygen from maternal blood diffuses into the foetus blood, where oxygen concentration is comparatively less than in maternal blood. Similarly diffusion of CO_2 from foetus blood into the maternal blood stream is also facilitated.

3. *Excretion :* The nitrogenous waste products produced as a result of metabolic activities of the embryo diffuse through placenta into maternal blood steam.
4. *Immunity*: The antibodies developed in the blood of mother against certain diseases like diptheria, measles, smallpox, scarlet fever, etc. are passed from mother into the foetus. These introduce passive immunity and insusceptibility to these diseases.
5. *Transport of Pathogens:* Certain pathogenic organism like viruses diffuse through plancenta. If mother during pregnancy is infected with some virus, its organisms manage to enter the foetus and cause infection. Viruses causing syphilis, measles, smallpox, chickenpox, rubella, etc. infect the foetus if mother gets infected during pregnancy. Some of them may even cause congenital deformities, if these enter the foetus during early pregnancy.
6. *Transport of Drugs:* Some drugs taken by mother during pregnancy cross the placental barrier and may even cause developmental deformities. The sleeping drug, thalidomide, which was used by ladies as a sedative and to avoid nausia and morning sickness during early pregnancy (25 to 44 days) was found to cause deformities in limb development of the foetus, perforation of anus and development of defective heart. The children born to such mothers had flipper-like limbs, a condition known as phocomelia. The children are called thalidomide babies. Drugs like quinine and aspirin are also teratogenic.
7. *Storage of Substances*: Placenta stores materials such as fat, glycogen and iron and participates in the metabolism of proteins.
8. *Secretion of Hormones*: Like endocrine glands placenta secretes many hormones such as progesterone,

estrogen, gonadotropin, placental lactogens, etc. Progesterone helps in the maintenance of pregnancy and prevents premature parturition. Relaxin helps in birth by relaxation of pelvic ligament and contraction of muscles of uterus and urethra.

9. Protection of foetus against bacterial infection of mother- Placenta during first half of pregnancy is impermeable to bacteria and macromolecules. It, therefore, reduces chances of appearance of many influences of maternal ill health on the foetus. However, in the later half of pregnancy, the placenta becomes more permeable and there are chances of passing the germs from mother to foetus.

6

The Regeneration

During the life-time of an animal organism some of the parts of its body may become damaged or lost either accidentally in natural conditions or wilfully imposed by the experimenter. The damage may be a wound which partially destroys the tissues of the animal's body, or it may involve the loss of an organ or larger part of the body. Most animals have to some degree, the ability to replace defective or missing parts. This process of repair and renewal of the lost parts of the body is known as regeneration.

Among animals, the power of regeneration was first discovered in Hydra by Abraham Trembley in 1744. Since then, it has been found to occur in all animals, though in varying degrees. Regeneration is more pronounced in the lower than in higher animals.

Types of Regeneration

Animals exhibit 4 types of regeneration. They are as follows:

Epimorphosis or Epimorphic Regeneration (Morgon, 1901): This type of regeneration is exemplified by the renewal of limbs in salamanders and the replacement of the broken tail of a lizard. In salamanders, if a limb is amputated, it can be regenerated within a few weeks. The regenerated organ is thus an addition to the other parts of the animal's body. It is the common type of regeneration found in higher animals.

Morphallaxis or Morphallactic Regeneration: In this type of regeneration the new individual is produced not by addition of parts to the residue of the animal's body but by remodelling the entire available mass of cells into a new whole. For example, a small section of the body of *Hydra,* comprising as little as 1/200 part of the original individual, can regenerate a complete whole animal. This type of repair involving a reorganization of the remaining part oi the body of an animal is known as morphallaxis or morphallactic regeneration. It is exhibited by lower animals.

Heteromorphosis or Heteromorphic Regeneration: When a different organ develops from the one that has been removed, the phenomenon is called heteromorphosis or heteromorphic regeneration. For example, in the shrimp *Palinurus,* the eye may regenerate after being removed if the cut be made through the eye stalk, just proximal to the eye and distal to the nerve ganglion. It may be remembered that the ganglion lies at the base of the eye inside the stalk. However, if the cut is made at the base of the stalk, the ganglion is removed together with the eye, and the eye will not regenerate. A regeneration bud is definitely formed, but instead of the lost eye, it gives rise to an antenna like organ. In this case the ganglion and the eye constitute together a regeneration territory (Guyenot and Ponse, 1930) or regeneration field (Weiss, 1926). If a part of the territory (the nerve ganglion in the aforementioned example) remains intact, the complete system may be replenished. If the whole "field" is lost, it cannot be regenerated at the expense of other parts of the body.

Super-regeneration: The development of a superfluous

number of organs or parts of the body, (heads, tails, limbs) as a result of regeneration, is known as super-regeneration. In planaria, a lateral incision may cause the development from the wound surface of either a new head or a new tail, or both. If both a head and a tail are regenerated, the head develops that portion of the wound surface which faces anteriorly. The tail, on the other hand, develops from the wound surface facing posteriorly. Similarly lateral incisions near the head end of the earthworm give rise to additional heads ; incisions in the middle parts of the animal cause the development of both heads and tails ; while incisions in the posterior part of the body result in the formation of tails only. In these cases the regenerated parts are additional and, therefore, superfluous to the animal.

Mechanism of Regeneration, the Renewal of a Limb in a Salamander **:** The limbs of newts and salamanders, in the adult as well as in larval stages, are capable of extensive regeneration. Limbs of larvae are sometimes bitten off by other members of the same species or the limbs of adult animals may be cut off at different levels for various experiments on the subject.

Regeneration involves a complicated sequence of histological transformations in the region of injury or amputation ;

The Closing of the Wound: The immediate effect of injury is the exposure of tissues and cells lying normally in the interior of the body on to the surface. Some of these cells are crushed, torn or become destroyed by being subjected to an unfavourable environment. Thus the surface of the wound is covered with the scattered bits of dead cells. In animals provided with blood vessel system, the blood from the severed vessels flows into the wound and clots there. This prevents further loss of blood.

The first repair process is the covering of the wound surface with skin epithelium. The epidermis from the edges of the wound spreads over the wound surface and penetrates under the clot between the latter and the intact living connective tissue. The epithelium spread and covers the open wound surface due to amoeboid movement of the cells. No growth, whatsoever, is involved in this process at the edges of the wound.

The time required for the epithelium to close the wound surface depends on the size of the wound and the size of the regenerating animal. In the salamander larva, after the amputation of a leg the wound is closed in the course of one or two days.

Dedifferentiation: After the closure of the wound, the tissues adjoining the cut surface undergo dedifferentiation, i.e., they loose their distinctive histological character. The intercellular matrix of bone and cartilage gets dissolved so that the cells come to lie freely under the epidermal cap of the wound. The connective tissue fibres disintegrate, and the connective tissue cells undergo apparent dedifferentiation. The myofibrils in the muscles disappear and the nucleo-cytoplasmic ratio greatly increases. The cells of all tissues attain an undifferentiated state like the embryonic cells.

Formation of the Blastema or Regeneration Bud: Undifferentiated cells accumulate under the epithelial layer covering the wound. The combined cap of epithelial and subjacent cell mass is known as the blastema. Two main theories have been proposed regarding the origin of the cells of the blastema :

(a) According to one school of thought, the cells of the blastema are all of local origin, i.e., they are derived from the tissues immediately adjoining the wound surface. With the exception of the epithelial covering of the wound, all other cells in the blastema are set free from the dedifferentiating skeleton, connective tissue, muscles etc.

(b) According to a second theory, the blastema is derived not from the dedifferentiated cells at the wound level, but from special reserve" cells migrating to the regeneration site from distant parts of the body. These cells are supposed to be brought here either by amoeboid movement or with the blood stream.

It is now established that neither of these two theories have a general application but that both sources of cells of the blastema may occur in different animals.

Dedifferentiation: While the processes of dedifferentiation of tissues underneath the epidermal cap are still going on, cells in the region adjoining the wound start proliferating and dividing by mitosis. This is followed by distinct period of growth. With the passage of time, the cells of the regenerating limb become organized and redifferentiated into the cartilage, bone, nerve and the connective tissue which make up the functional leg. On the outside, rudiments of digits appear, separated by slight indentations.

Regenerative Ability in Animals

The ability of animals to regenerate missing parts differs greatly in the various groups of animals. In some of them, almost any part of the body lost or damaged can be regenerated, while in others this power is limited.

Invertebrates

Coelenterates: In the coelenterates, the regenerative ability is very high. Hydra, being a lower animal, shows regeneration to an amazing degree. If cut into two or more parts, each part grows into a new and complete individual of diminished size. Hydra show spolarity or antero-posterior differentiation in regeneration. Polarity is the fact that the anterior side of any section of the animal grows a head while the posterior side of the section grows a tail. Thus the posterior end of a cut hydra regenerates the mouth and tentacles ; the anterior part of the body regenerates the posterior end with the foot or basal disc. Even a fragment as small as .004 mm in diameter can grow into entire animal provided it contains a portion of both epidermis and endodermis. If only the head is split into two, a peculiar "two-headed" or Y-shaped, hydra is formed.

Hydra is normally in a continuous state of "physiological regeneration". According to Brien (1953), just below the tentacles and the hypostome there is found a growth zone, where *interstitial cells* give rise to all other cells of the body, *e.g., onidoblasts, sex cells,* epithelio-muscular cells etc. Most of the mitoses in the body of the Hydra occur in this zone. With the formation of new cells, old cells are pushed toward the hypostome and tentacles and, to the peduncle and foot where they are discarded and shed to the outside. In about 40 days, the older cells are replaced by new cells. This process of cell replacement is a continuous process and due to this Hydra is potentially immortal.

Platyhelminths: Planarians among Platyhelminths possess unique powers of regeneration. Planarians may be cut across or lengthwise, and each part of the body will regenerate the missing half. A planarian can regenerate the entire organism from a middle section with the pharynx. If the anterior end of planaria is cut along the length into 2 or more parts, each part develops into a new head resulting in a many-headed monster.

In planarians, power of regeneration is maximum near the head and minimum near the posterior end. This is correlated with the metabolic rate which is highest is the head and becomes progressively lower towards the tail. This variation in metabolic rate and associated regenerative power is called the metabolic or axial gradient. The concept was first conceived by CM. Child in 1941.

When the cut is made, undifferentiated cells derived from

the parenchyma migrate to the cut surface, form a regeneration blastema and give rise to the lost portion.

Complete planarian can develop from small sections of the worm. The regeneration in planaria is thus carried out in a way that combines epimorphosis and morphallaxis.

Nemerteans: These animals possess a high regenerative ability. Very small fragments of heir body can give rise to a complete worm by regeneration.

Annelids: In Annelida, polychaetes and oligochaetes have the ability to regenerate anterior and posterior ends after an amputation. If an earthworm is cut in two halves, the posterior hall regenerates the anterior end with the mouth, and the anterior end regenerates a new posterior end. In most of the annelids regeneration is, however, somewhat restricted. At the anterior cut surface only a limited number of segments are formed. This number is typical for every species. For example, in the earthworm *Allolobophora foetida*, only four or five segments will be regenerated at the anterior end after amputation.

The process of regeneration is an epimorphosis. A regeneration bud is formed by a special type of cells called neoblasts found normally in the perithoneum of the posterior surface of the intersegmental septa.

Hirudinea do not regenerate at all.

Arthropods: In Arthropoda, regeneration is restricted to the renewal of lost appendages. Some crustaceans like *lobsters* can regenerate lost limbs at any stage of development, including the adult, whereas insects could replace them only in larval stages. Crabs and some spiders exhibit autotomy.

Autotomy or self multilation is a special adaptation which helps the animal to escape being overpowered by a predator. They shed their leg when seized by the enemy at a perforated breaking point, across the second leg joint. The leg is broken off by the violent contraction of the extensor muscle. It is regenerated at leisure.

After the loss or amputation of an appendage in an arthropod, the wound is covered by a chitinious cap. A regeneration blastema is formed underneath this cap. The blastema later reproduces the limbs by way of epimorphic regeneration.

Mollusca: The regeneration is relatively poor in molluscs. In gastropods, eyestalks with eyes, and parts of the head or of the foot may be regenerated. Cephalopods may regenerate their arms only.

Echinoderms: The starfishes, brittle stars, and sea lillies can regenerate arms and parts of the disc. A star-fish can regenerate an entire organism from just one arm and the central disc. An isolated arm, however cannot develop the central disc and other arms in *Asterias*. Star-fish also exhibits autotomy if an arm is injured or held up. The Holothuroidea are capable of regenerating the respiratory tract and the alimentary canal, which are often ejected through the anus.

Vertebrates

Fishes: In fishes, regeneration is restricted to the fins only.

Amphibia: *(a) Anurans:* Regeneration takes place during the larval stage only. When, legs first appear on a frog tadpole, they can be regenerated easily if lost. After metamorphosis, however, a frog is normally unable to regenerate a missing leg.

(b) Urodeles: In vertebrates urodele amphibians possess unique powers of regeneration. In newts and salamanders and especially in their larvae, limbs as well as tails and external gills can regenerate. Furthermore, the upper and lower jaws, and parts of the eye *e.g.*, lens and the retina also regenerate.

Reptiles: Among reptiles, the lizard *Gecko (Hemidactylis flavivirdis)* is known to regenerate its tail following autotomy.

The tail is broken off at a preformed level near the base. To release the mechanism of autotomy, the distal part of the tail must be injured or seized with such force as to cause distress to the animal. As a result the lizard parts with its tail. After the tail is shed, a regeneration blastema is formed on the wound surface, and this gives rise to a new tail. The regenerated tail, however, differs from the original tail; the normal segmentation of the vertebral column is not restored and the scales covering the regenerated tail differ from the normal ones.

Birds: In birds regenerative ability is rather poor ; only parts of the beak can be regenerated.

Mammals: Mammals cannot regenerate entire organs. They can, however, regenerate tissues, i.e., the restoration of defect and lesions in various tissues. A few examples are as follows:

1. Wound healing is equivalent to tissue regeneration.
   (a) Skin wounds may be covered by newly formed epidermis and connective tissue.
   (b) In the case of large skin wounds, the newly regenerated connective tissue differs from the normal dermis and can be distinguished as *scar tissue.*
2. The skeletal tissue possesses extensive powers of regeneration. Large defects in the bones especially those of the limbs, can be corrected after fractures etc.
3. If parts of individual muscles are removed, the defects can be repaired by a proliferation which takes place at the cost of the remaining part of the muscle.
4. Lesions in the tendons can be replaced by connective tissue in the first step. Later on, the connective tissue acquires the structure and mechanical properties of the tendon.

5. The digestive glands, especially the liver is capable of extensive regeneration after damage.
6. The replacement of blood after blood loss is another example of tissue regeneration in mammals.

Reconstitution from Isolated Cells : Reconstitution is the reaggregation of isolated cells into a new whole animal. This phenomenon was discovered *in sponges* by H.V. Wilson (1907). When a sponge is rubbed through bolting silk, the entire organization of the animal is broken up, and the tissues of the sponge are reduced to a residue consisting of isolated cells and cells debris. The isolated cells can be distinguished into archeocytes, choanocytes and pinacocytes of the adult sponge. After some time the isolated cells aggregate into larger masses which eventually become organized into new sponges. When the cells reaggregate, each type of cells take up a definitive position in the new aggregate. For example, the pinacocytes cover the whole aggregate from without ; the choanocytes join together and rebuild the radial canals ; the archeocytes take up their normal position. Galtsoff (1925) estimated that about 2000 cells are necessary to produce a new sponge.

Reconstitution of a new whole from isolated cells may be compared to regeneration by morphallaxis, as the individual cells into which the sponge is broken up retain their specific histologic character. The entire process rests mainly on a rearrangement of the cells in space rather than on a progressive differentiation.

Physiological Process involved in Regeneration : Physiologically, regenerating animals have two periods with a different type of metabolism : (1) destructive metabolism and (2) constructive metabolism.

Destructive Metabolism: The period of destructive metabolism is of greater significance in animals having a considerable dedifferentiation at the beginning of regeneration, as in amphibians. The physiological changes occurring during this phase can be summarised as follows :

(1) There is an abrupt increase in the activity of proteolytic enzymes. Protein in the regenerating tissue becomes decomposed by the action of these enzymes. Among the proteolytic enzymes, the increase of *kathepsin* is remarkable. The activity of the *dipeptidases* also increases sharply during the first few days after amputation.

At first, the cells damaged by amputation are destroyed through the activity of proteolytic enzymes, but the main function of these enzymes is to cause dedifferentiation of a part of healthy tissue adjacent to the wound surface. Destruction of intercellular substances and the highly differentiated parts of cells, e.g., muscle fibrils, is an important aspect of this process.

(2) As a result of protein catabolism, the amount of free amino acids increases to about double the amount in normal tissues— from 16.8% to 35.1% of the total nitrogen.

(3) A qualitative change in the structure of the proteins and their products also takes place. This is exhibited by an increase in the amount of reduced sulphydryl compounds.

(4) The respiratory quotient, R. Q. (CO_2/O_2) falls abruptly, reaching the level of 0.57 immediately following respiration. This may be due to incomplete oxidation in the tissues.

(5) Anaerobic glycolysis replaces oxidation, therefore, lactic acid increases in regenerating tissue as compared with normal tissue.

(6) The enzymes which in normal tissues carry on the oxidation, *e.g., cytochrome oxidase,* show a low level of activity in regenerating tissues.

(7) The absolute amount of oxygen consumed may fall in the early stages of regeneration.

(8) The catabolic changes occurring in the earlier phases of regeneration—accumulation of free amino acids, of lactic acid, of free-SH groups, all lead to lowering of pH in the tissues of the cut limb and the regeneration blastema.

Constructive Metabolism: The metabolism of the constructive phase of regeneration is characterized by following features :

(1) There is an increase in oxidation.

(2) pH returns to normal.

(3) Respiratory quotient (R. Q.) becomes higher.

(4) Free-SH groups and lactic acid decrease in amount.

(5) The cells of the regeneration blastema become very rich in cytoplasmic ribonucleic acid mainly due to newly synthesized RNA. When the stage of differentiation of the regenerating part is reached, the amount of RNA in the cells diminishes again.

(6) The size of the nucleoli increases in cells participating in regeneration.

Factors Influencing Regeneration : The regeneration is influenced by a number of external as well as internal factors :

Temperature: The rate of regeneration is dependent on temperature. Increase of temperature, upto a certain point, enhances regeneration.

Food: Regeneration is not much affected by food. Even a starving animal will regenerate its lost parts at the expense of internal resources. The energy for regeneration is provided by the metabolism of stored food materials. As a result the regenerating animal, though completely rebuilt, is very small in size, *e.g., Planaria lugubris* (Morgon, 1901).

Nervous System: It has a special influence on regeneration. The nervous system influences mainly the earlier stages of regeneration. In the *amphibians,* the early states of regeneration proceed normally only if the region of the wound receives an adequate nerve supply. If the nerves are cut before amputating the leg or arm of a newt, processes of dedifferentiation set in but the redifferentiation does not start at all. In *planarians* the regeneration blastema is formed in conjunction with cut nerve cords. It is believed that the regeneration is caused by some chemical substance released by the nerves. The nature of this chemical substance, however, is not known. Moreover, nervous system may be used cause regeneration of otherwise non-regenerating parts. When the sciatic nerve of a young metamorphosed frog was dissected and deviated into a freshly amputated forelimb, a blastema was formed which developed into an incomplete limb with rudiments of hand or fingers (Singer, 1950).

In a newly born *Opossum* (marsupial), regeneration of a hindlimb may be stimulated by in planting a piece of brain tissue into the limb before amputation. As a result of this operation, distal parts of the limb undergo regeneration, but a perfect normal limb is not formed.

Age: The power of regeneration usually diminishes with increasing age. Among the vertebrates, there appears to be a progressive loss of regeneration power with increasing age. It is a well-known fact that bone fractures and skin wounds heal in a child much more rapidly than in an elderly person. This phenomenon may be explained by a hypothesis that aging tissue simply losses the ability to respond to the regeneration promoting chemical substance released by the cut nerves.

X-rays: X-rays are found to retard or stop the process of regeneration because they are known to inhibit or suppress the mitotic activity of cells. However, the inhibiting effect of X-rays depends upon the amount of irradiation administered. Although there may be some individual variation, yet a dose of 5000 to 7000 rontgen suppresses regeneration in every case. An irradiated regeneration blastema does not grow. Instead of developing the skeleton and muscle of the limb, it becomes filled with connective tissue.

Physiological and Reparative Regeneration : Physiological regeneration includes regular replacement of cells that are lost due to day-to-day activities, as for example, replacement of R.B.Cs., cells in the epidermis of skin or in the lining of gastro-intestinal tract. In our body approximately 25x10 red blood corpuscles are present in active circulation. About one per cent of them die and are replaced daily.

Reparative regeneration is the process of replacement of lost parts or repairing of damaged body parts, as for example, the regeneration of limb in *Salamander*, or regeneration of lost tail in lizard or replacement of the damaged cells and healing of the wound.

Epimorphosis and Morphallaxis

Epimorphosis or epimorphic regeneration is the replacement of lost part of the body by growth and differentiation of cells from the remainder piece of the part. e.g. renewal of amputed limb in salamander or starfish.

Morphallaxis or morphallactic regeneration is the regeneration of new individuals by remodelling the available undifferentiated cell mass from the pieces of an animal body. It involves reorganization of various parts of an organism from few cells to form a new organism. For example, regeneration of whole sponge body from few archaeocytes, or of a new *Hydra* from a small piece of bodywall, comprising just 1/200th part of original individual. Morphallaxis is seen only in lower animal groups.

Heteromorphosis and Super Regeneration : In heteromorphosis or heteromorphic regeneration, the regenerated organ is different from the one that has been removed. For example, in shrimp, *Palinurus,* the eye regenerates only if the eye-stalk is cut proximal to the eye and distal to nerve ganglion. If the cut is at the base of eye-stalk and the ganglion is removed along with the eye, the eye fails to regenerate. The regeneration bud formed at the cut and grows into an antenna-like organ. The ganglion and the eye together constitute the regeneration field (Weiss, 1926) or regeneration territory (Guyenot and Ponsil 1930). If the field as a whole is lost, it cannot regenerate into that part, but even if a part of this field is intact, it is capable of regenerating the complete system.

Super-regeneration is the development of a superfluous number of organs or parts of the body as a result of regeneration. For example, in *Hydra* or *Planaria,* a lateral incision at the anterior end causes the development of one head on each wounded surface. Same way in earthworm the lateral incision near the head end produces additional head. Incisions in the middle parts *of Hydra* or *Planaria* cause the development of both heads and tails, while incisions in the posterior part of the body result in the formation of tails only.

Regeneration of Salamander Limb as an Example

Morphological Events During Regeneration : Limbs in salamander and newt exhibit high power of regeneration both in the adult and in larval stage. The process of regeneration involves following events :

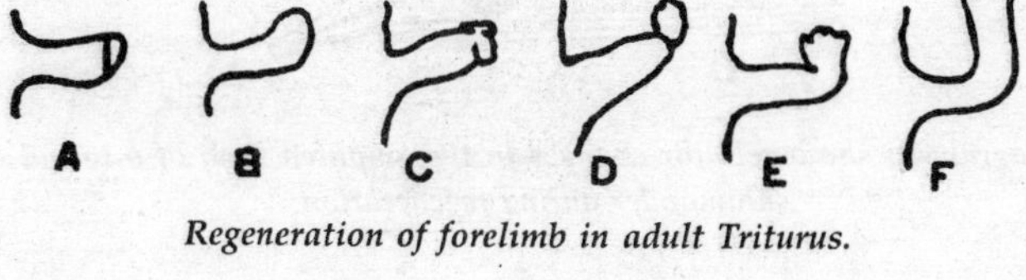

Regeneration of forelimb in adult Triturus.

Wound Healing (Closing of Wound) : As a result of amputation, the tissues that normally occur in the interior of limb, are exposed on the surface. Some of them are squeezed and damaged. The blood flows out from the cut vessels and spreads over the wounded surface. The blood coagulates over the wound. The epidermal cells from the edges of the cut migrate and spread over the exposed surface underneath the blood clot. This process is wound healing. This process is very quick and takes 1-2 days. The time required for epithelium to close the wound depends on the size of wound.

Formation of Blastema (The regeneration bud) : A few days after the healing of the cut or wound, the epidermis covering the wound bulges out forming a stumpy outgrowth. This is known as blastema or regeneration bud. A blastema is formed by the accumulation of undifferentiated mesenchyme cells below the epidermis. It continues to grow in size for some time before differentiation sets.

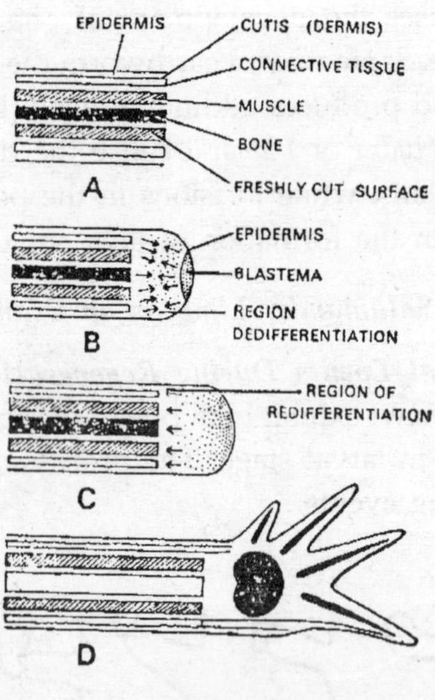

Diagram to show cellular changes in the amputed limb of a larval salamander during regeneration.

The blastema has the properties of a limb bud formed in the embryo, because it has the potentiality to grow and differentiate into a limb.

Morphogenesis (Formation of limb) : The limb lastema passes through several distinct stages during the course of differentiation. (i) In an adult newt at 20°C, 15 days after amputation, the blastema is filled with undifferentiated cells. (ii) by 20 days blastema becomes cone-shaped. (iii) by 25 days, the palette stage is reached when the blastema appears a flattened cone. (iv) Within 30-35 days, the first sign of digits appears. This is notch stage. (18.1D) (v) From these digit-rudiments new digits are formed. (vi) Within 75 days the complete limb is regenerated, which is essentially similar to the normal limb.

Histological Events During Regeneration

Dedifferentiation : After the wound is covered with epithelium, the differentiated tissue of the stump adjoining the cut surface (cartilage, nerve, connective tissue and muscles in case of limb) undergo extreme degeneration and become undifferentiated mesenchyme cells, this is called dedifferentiation.

The intercellular matrix of the skeleton dissolves and the cells are released. These enlarge and assume the appearance of embryonic mesenchyme cells. These migrate and accumulate beneath the ectodermal cap. Similarly, mesenchyme cells are released by the dissolution of connective tissue fibres and the fragmentation of multinucleate muscle cells. The cells from all these sources are histologically indistinguishable and are said to be dedifferentiated. Continuous dedifferentiation causes more mesenchyme cells to accumulate beneath the apical cap, converting the early blastema into a conical structure (cone-stage).

Proliferation : When blastema reaches certain size, the process of dedifferentiation stops. The cells of blastema in the region adjoining the wound start proliferating and dividing by mitosis. As a result blastema grows in size. The growth is maximum immediately after blastema formation and gradually declines.

Redifferentiation : The differentiated tissues of the limb stump induce the undifferentiated cells of blastema to redifferentiate the lost parts of the limb in conformity with their own organization. The process of redifferentiation starts in the cone-stage. Initiation for redifferentiation comes from the pre-existing limb tissues is supported from the following experiment. The young blastema fails to differentiate when transplanted to some foreign site, whereas an older blastema differentiates into limb parts even when it is transplanted to some new site.

Physiological Processes during Regeneration : Physiological processes involved during regeneration are separated into two different periods with a different type of metabolism :

(A) Destructive or Catabolic Phase

The early phase of regeneration or the phase of dedifferentiation is the period of destructive metabolic activities. The physiological activities of this phase are :

Increase in the Activity of Proteolytic Enzymes : Immediately after amputation, there is increase in the activity of proteolytic enzymes, specifically kathapsin and dipeptidases. The proteolytic enzymes perform following functions : —

(i) These destroy cells damaged due to amputation.

(ii) These cause dedifferentiation of healthy tissue adjacent to the wound surface.

(iii) These destroy inter-cellular substances and the highly differentiated parts of cells.

Increase in Free Amino Acids : As a result of protein catabolism the amount of free amino acids is almost doubled (16.8% to 35.1%).

Respiratory Quotient (R. Q.) : The respiratory quotient in the degenerating tissue falls abruptly reaching a level of 0.57. This is due to incomplete oxidation.

Anaerobic Glycolysis : Due to incomplete oxidation, lactic acid, the end product of anaerobic glycolysis accumulates in the degenerating tissue.

Respiratory enzymes like cytochrome oxidase, shows a lower level of activity during early stage of regeneration.

The absolute amount of oxygen consumption also falls in early stages of regeneration.

Lowering of pH : The catabolic changes occurring in the early stages cause lowering of *pH*.

(B) Constructive or Anabolic Phase

During constructive phase, the dedifferentiated cells again differentiate into corresponding tissues. This phase shows following characteristics

(i) Increase in oxidation

(ii) Return to normal *pH*

(iii) Increase in respiratory quotient (R.Q.)

(iv) Decrease in the amount of lactic acid

(v) Increase in ribonucleic acid (specially RNA)

(vi) Size of nucleoli increases in cells participating in regeneration.

Injury affects metabolism of carbohydrates and proteins. The electrolytic balance is altered. The tissue releases large quantities of K^+ ions and retains Na^+ and Cl^- ions. All the physiological changes are under hormonal control.

Origin of Cells of Blastema

Two different theories have been proposed regarding the origin of cells of blastema: —

Local Origin of Blastema Cells : According to some embryologists, the cells of blastema are derived from the highly organized tissues immediately adjoining the cut surface. The fully differentiated muscle, nerve, cartilage and connective tissue cells undergo dedifferentiation. Their matrix is dissolved and the more specialized parts of the cells disintegrate changing them into undifferentiated mesenchyme cells.

The theory is based on the following experiment :

(i) If entire animal is exposed to X-rays and then the limb is amputed, the amputed limb fails to regenerate.

(ii) If limb alone is irradiated and amputed, it does not regenerate.

(iii) If the limb is protected from X-rays by a lead shield and rest of the body is irradiated, the limb regenerates normally.

(iv) If only a portion of limb is irradiated the limb fails to regenerate in case the cut is in the irradiated part and regenerates normally in case the cut is made below or above the irradiated zone. This shows blastema cells originate locally.

Distant Origin of Blastema Cells : According to another view, the undifferentiated mesenchyme cells migrate to the regeneration site from distant parts of the body. Either they move by amoeboid movement or are brought by the blood stream. Experiments on *Planaria* support this view. If a Planarian is irradiated with X-rays and then wounded, no regeneration occurs because exposure to X-rays makes the cells incapable of regeneration. (i) If a small part of the body is protected against radiation and rest of the body is exposed to X-rays; any amputation will be regenerated, irrespective of the location of wound. This shows that the unexposed cells are capable of migrating long distances to form blastema.

Regeneration Ability in Animals

The ability to regenerate lost parts is present throughout the animal kingdom but to various extent. It may involve replacement of damaged cells, healing of wound, or a complete replacement of the organ lost or formation of a complete animal from small fragments.

Regeneration power is especially more in sponges, coelenterates, flatworms, annelids and tunicates. In some cases fragmentation and regeneration are the usual methods of asexual reproduction. In starfish and holothurians regeneration is a means of protection. Among vertebrates the power of regeneration is limited to the regeneration of limbs, jaws, gills and tail, while in higher vertebrates it is limited to healing of damaged tissue only.

A. Regeneration in Protozoa

Protozoans can regenerate even from very small segments if these contain a part of nucleus, ectoplasm and endoplasm. In them it is morphallectic regeneration. In many ciliates, like *Stentor*, *Blepharisma* and *Spirostomum*, the cell cortex (ectoplasm) plays the most significant role in regeneration. If cortex is stripped off in *Stentor*, it rounds off and survives only for a while. In ciliates macronucleus is necessary for regeneration.

B. Regeneration in Porifera

Regeneration from Small Segments : Small body fragments containing both the layers can regenerate into a new sponge.

Reconstitution from Isolated Cells : In sponges the whole organism can be reconstituted from a few undifferentiated cells (archeocytes) of sponge body. When a sponge is rubbed through bolting silk, its cells get isolated. These isolated cells include pinacocytes, choanocytes, archeocytes. These aggregate into masses and organise into the whole organism.

C. Regeneration in Coelenterata

In Coelenterata, the regeneration ability is exceedingly high. Trembley in 1744 showed that if *Hydra* is cut into two or more parts, each part develops into a complete *Hydra*. The anterior part of *Hydra* regenerates the basal disc and posterior segment regenerates the hypostome and tentacles. The middle segments regenerate both hypostome and basal disc. Sections as small as 1/200th part of the body with both ectoderm and endoderm can regenerate into a complete *Hydra*. The interstitial cells are the embryonic reserve cells having totipotency. These proliferate and migrate to the damaged end and form blastema. Regeneration in *Hydra* exhibits polarity or antero-posterior differentiation.

In other coelenterates, the regenerative power is highest in polypoid forms but is much reduced in medusoid forms.

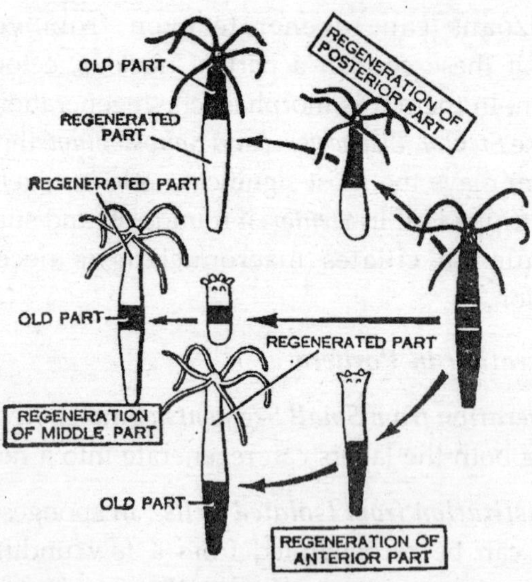

Regeneration in Hydra.

D. Regeneration in Flatworms

Planarians among flatworms have remarkably high regeneration power. Like *Hydra,* each cut part of body regenerates into a complete organism. The regenerated organisms are comparatively smaller than the original one. A multiheaded planarian can also arise if head is incised lengthwise. The presence of undifferentiated totipotent neoblast cells is responsible for the remarkable regeneration power. These cells are derived from the parenchyma that fills the body cavity.

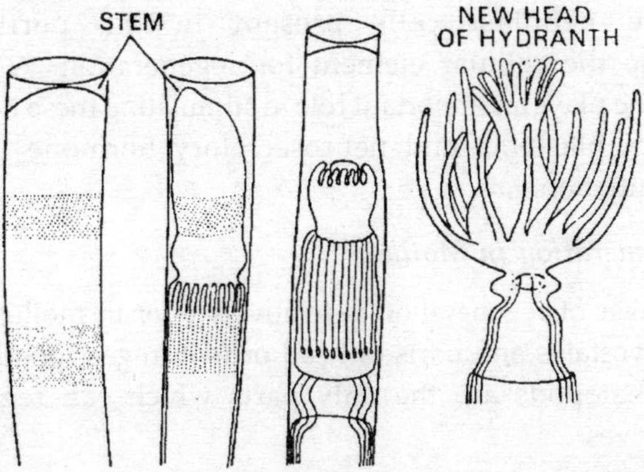

Regeneration of a new head of a hydranth from the distal part of the Tubularia stem.

Other platyhelminthes do not regenerate.

Regeneration in Nemertines : Nemertines also possess remarkable regenerative ability. Even a very small fragment can regenerate into a complete worm.

E. Regeneration in Annelida

Both polychaetes and oligochaetes can regenerate their amputed anterior and posterior ends. But at the anterior end only limited number of new segments could be added. This number is characteristic of each species. In earthworm-

Allolobophora foetida, only first four or five segments can regenerate. The caudal regeneration is more common in them. *Chaetopterus* can regenerate a complete individual from only one of its first fourteen segments. Leeches lack regenerative capability.

The neoblast cells present in the peritoneum provide the cellular element for regeneration. A wound hormone plays an important role in stimulating these neoblasts to form blastema and neurosecretory hormone initiates differentiation.

F. Regeneration in Molluscs

Power of regeneration is relatively poor in molluscs. The eyes, eyestalks and parts of head or foot in gastropods, arms of cephalopods are the only parts which can regenerate themselves.

G. Regeneration in Arthropods

In arthropods regeneration power is limited to the renewal of lost appendages. Crustanceans can regenerate lost limbs at any stage of development but insects can replace them only during larval stages. Crabs and spiders exhibit autotomy. On being caught by the enemy, they shed their limb at a prefixed breaking point across the second joint by the violent contraction of the extensor muscle.

H. Regeneration in Echinoderms

Starfishes, brittle stars and sea lilies can regenerate their lost arms and even parts of the disc. Starfishes with more than five arms are quite frequent. Holothurians can eject their viscera, specially the respiratory tree and alimentary canal through anus and regenerate them afterwards.

I. Regeneration in Vertebrates

Fishes : In fishes, regeneration is restricted to the fins only.

Amphibia: (a) In anurans regeneration takes place during the larval stage only. When legs first appear in a frog tadpole, they can be regenerated easily if lost. After metamorphosis, however, a frog is normally unable to regenerate a missing leg.

(b) *Urodeles:* In newts and salamanders and especially in their larvae, limbs as well as tails and external gill can regenerate. The upper and lower jaws, and parts of the eye e.g., lens and the retina also regenerate.

Reptiles : Among reptiles, the lizard Gecko (*Hemidactylus flaviv*irdis) is known to regenerate its tail following autotomy (self mutilation). The tail is broken off at a preformed level near the base. To release the mechanism of autotomy, the distal part of the tail must be injured or seized with such force as to cause distress to the animal.

As a result the lizard parts with its tail. After the tail is shed, a regeneration blastema is formed on the wound surface, and this gives rise to a new tail. The regenerated tail, however, differs from the original tail; the normal segmentation of the vertebral column is not restored and the scales covering the regenerated tail differ from the normal ones.

Birds : In birds regenerative ability is rather poor; only parts of the beak can be regenerated.

Mammals : Mammals cannot regenerate entire organs. They can, however, regenerate tissues, i.e. the restoration of defects and lesions in various tissues. A few examples are as follows :

1. Wound healing is Equivalent to Tissue Regeneration :
   (a) Skin wounds may be covered by newly-formed epidermis and connective tissue.
   (b) In the case of large skin wounds, the newly-regenerated connective tissue differs from the

normal dermis and can be distinguished as scar tissue.

2. The skeletal tissue possesses extensive power of regeneration. Large defects in the bones, especially those of the limbs, can be corrected after fractures etc.
3. If parts of individual muscles are removed, the defects can be repaired by a proliferation which takes place at the cost of the remaining part of the muscle.
4. Lesions in the tendons can be replaced by connective tissue in the first step. Later on, the connective tissue acquires the structure and mechanical properties of the tendon.
5. The digestive glands, especially the liver is capable of extensive regeneration after damage.
6. The replacement of blood after blood loss is another example of tissue regeneration in mammals.

Factors Affecting Regeneration

The regeneration ability of an organism, in general, is determined by:

(i) its constitution,

(ii) by the degree of its tissue differentiation, and

(iii) the stages of ontogenetic development.

However, the ability may be altered by certain environmental factors such as temperature, food, etc. or by special treatments.

Temperature : Similar to other biological activities, the rate of regeneration is altered by change in the temperature. The increase in temperature up to a certain limit accelerates regeneration, while at low temperature it either slows down or diminishes completely. For example, in *Planaria,* total regeneration either does not occur at 3°C or it is faulty, but it is most rapid at 29.7°C. A temperature of 32°C is lethal for the animal.

Food : Food does not affect regeneration. Even the fasting animals will regenerate the lost parts by metabolizing constituents of their own body. This was shown by Morgan (1901) in *Planaria lugubris.* It was cut lengthwise and the left half was fed and right half was kept entirely without food, both the halves regenerated. However, the animal regenerated from right half was smaller.

Oxygen Concentration : In hydroid colonies, the length of hydranth blastema increases with increased concentration of oxygen.

Radiation : If a regeneration blastema is exposed to X-rays it fails to regenerate. A dose of 5000 to 7000 r (r = roentgen) is found to have a suppressive effect. X-rays inhibit or suppress mitotic activity of blastema cells, so that the irradiated cells fail to divide and blastema gradually diminishes in size. Localized irradiation with UV light at elbow region of larval *Ambystoma* causes a regression of development of upper arm and forearm but initiates the development of a supernumerary limb at irradiate site.

The treatment of regenerating cells with mustard gas also inhibits regeneration because of arrest of mitotic cell division.

Electric Current : Small direct currents and electric fields stimulate tissue regeneration and healing of fractures. According to Backer (1974) both electric conduction and regenerative processes are fundamental properties of organisms independent of and antedating the presence of sophisticated nervous system.

Sea Water **:** According to Zwilling (1939) if the outer perisarc of a hydroid hydrorhiza is cut, exposing an area of inner coenosarch to water, regeneration of a secondary hydranth takes place.

Stimulation of Regeneration

According to definition, the regeneration is the replacement of lost part. From this, it could be concluded that loss of a part acts as a stimulus for its regeneration. But experiment conducted by Bodemer (1958-60), Ruben (1960), Polez-hayev (1933) have shown that a number of factors may be responsible to stimulate regenerative activities.

1. *Traumatization* : Polez-hayev (1933) suggested that traumaization of muscle is essential for the regeneration of limb in *Salamander*. A deep incision on the side of a salamander limb leads to the formation of a regeneration blastema on the cut surface which grows out into an additional limb as in ordinary regeneration of lost limb.

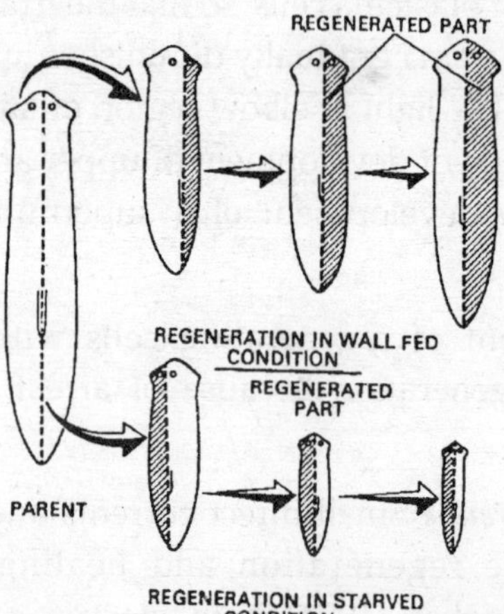

Regeneration in Planaria to show effect of starvation. This shows that regeneration is given top priority in the utilization of body reserve.

In a planarian, a lateral incision at the anterior end induces the development of an additional head from the cut surface. An incision at the posterior end causes the development of an additional tail. Similarly, an additional head or tail or both may develop in earthworm by a cut near the anterior end, posterior end or in the middle part of the body. Traumaization by pricking with a needle stimulates regeneration in *Hydra*.

In all above cases, the original parts of the animal (limb, head or tail) had not been removed. It is, therefore, evident that the stimulus for regeneration is provided by the presence of wound rather than the absence of an organ. The development of additional organs or parts of the body, as a result of regeneration is called 'super-regeneration'.

***Tissue Destruction Byligature*.:** Nassonov (1930) has shown that the presence of an open wound is also not essential for regeneration. The damaged and disintegrating tissues are said to liberate some substance or substances that induce regeneration. The damage to the tissues may be caused by tight ligature.

***Nervous System* :** Nervous system plays an influential role on regeneration. For example,

(A) In Newt

(i) If the nerves supplying the leg or the arm of a newt are destroyed at the time of amputation of limb or during early stages of regeneration, the process of regeneration stops and the blastema formed may be reabsorbed. If nerves are cut before amputating the limb, processes of dedifferentiation set in and continue unchecked leading to the destruction of limb.

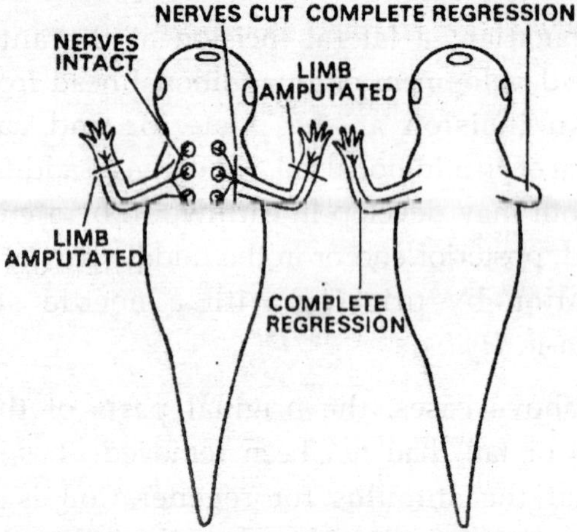

Diagram to show the arrest of regeneration of Newt's limb when Its nervous supply was cut off (After Schotte, 1926).

However, in newt the nervous system influences only during early stages of regeneration. If redifferentiation has already commenced the damage to the nerve will have no effect on the regenerating limb.

(ii) Bodemer (1959) has suggested that the deviated nerve promotes dedifferentiation in the musculature of shoulder and leads to the formation of blastema. In successful cases this grow out into a complete supernumerary limb. If a limb nerve is transplanted to a place away from shoulder or pelvic level, it causes the formation of a limb at a spot where no limb development could have been expected.

In Planariuns : Santos (1931) has shown that when cerebral ganglion of a planarian is excised along with a piece of surrounding tissue and is transplanted to some different part of the body, it causes the formation of a new head at the site of transplantation, this shows that in planarians, the regeneration blastemas are formed in conjunction with the cut nerve cords.

In Annelids : In annelids neoblast cells migrate along the ventral nerve cord to reach the wound, to form regeneration blastema. If the nerve cord is excised some distance from the cut in earthworm, no regeneration occurs at the cut level. However, a new head develops from cut end of the nerve cord.

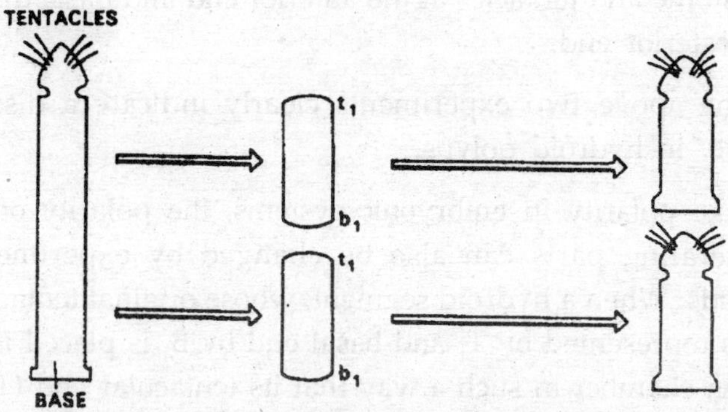

Regeneration and polarity in coelenterate polyp.

Polarity in Regeneration

Similar to animal-vegetal polarity of the egg, the body of organisms and their parts also exhibit distinct polarity. The same axial organization is maintained in the regenerating parts. For example, the body of *Hydra* or of *Tubularia* polyp has a distinct hypostomal region with tentacles (designated by t) at the anterior end, a basal disc (designated by b) at the posterior end and a long body or stem. If the stem is cut into two equal parts, the posterior or basal end of the first piece regenerates the basal disc for attachment and the anterior or hypostomal end of the second piece regenerates hypostome and tentacles.

A—By exposing the original tentacular and basal ends of polyp segment to low and high concentration of oxygen respectively. B—By ligaturing the polyp stem in the middle.

Similarly, if the stem of hydroid or polyp is cut into three segments, the first segment (anterior) regenerates basal disc at the lower end, the third segment (posterior segment) regenerates the hypostomal end at the upper end and the middle segment regenerates both, hypostome and tentacles at the anterior end and the middle segment regenerates both hypostome and tentacles at the anterior end and basal disc at the posterior end.

The above two experiments clearly indicate a distinct polarity in hydroid polyps.

Like polarity in embryonic systems, the polarity of the regenerating parts can also be changed by experimental methods. When a hydroid segment, whose original tentacular end is represented by T_1 and basal end by B_1 is placed in an oxygen chamber in such a way that its tentacular end (T_1) is exposed to low oxygen concentration and basal end (B_1) to high oxygen concentration (Fig.A). It was observed that the end exposed to high oxygen concentration developed a set of tentacles and the end kept in low oxygen concentration developed into basal disc. This shows that the polarity of two ends was reversed.

When a piece of polyp is ligated in the middle, both T_1 and B_1 ends develop tentacles and the ligatured ends develop into basal discs. Thus two individuals are obtained from one segment. The results can be compared to obtaining two embryos by dividing the egg by a ligature.

Inductive Interactions in Regeneration : The damaging and disintegrating tissues of a wounded body part release some chemical substances which act as stimulus for regeneration. Some different kinds of inductive interactions also occur in various animals.

Inductive Interaction in Regeneration of Hydroid Coelenterates : In hydroids, there exists an axial gradient of the level of metabolic and mitotic activities. It is highest in the hypostome or head region and the lowest being in the basal region. A transplanted head region suppresses the formation of another head region in its immediate vicinity by producing growth-inhibiting substance. This substance diffuses downward though the body column and become gradually ineffective as it moves to the basal end.

Burnett and others (1966) have shown the presence of a single inhibitor that diffuses from the hypostome and inhibits the differentiation of hypostome in the nearby region. However, it does not inhibit regeneration of other organs. In *Hydra,* the inhibiting substance is found to be a polypeptide. It remains associated with the neurosecretory granules.

In addition to inhibiting factor, growth-stimulating principle is present in the hypostomal region. This inducer stimulates division of interstitial cells forming a growth centre. The growth centre produces inhibitory principle only when the metabolism and mitotic activity of an area is high. It is effective in the area where it is produced. It diffuses downwards into the peduncular area, where it is no longer active and a basal disc is formed.

Inductive Interaction in Regeneration of Planaria : In freshwater *Planarians,* the regeneration blastema and cut surface of the wound interact during regeneration in the morphogenesis. During morphogenesis there are successive inductions and inhibitions which interact and prevent repetitive regeneration of an organ.

It has already been mentioned that the morphogenetic steps in regeneration of anterior part in Planarian transected just posterior to the genital aperture. The tissues at the cut surface form blastema. Brain is the first tissue that differentiate in the blastema. The brain then induces the differentiation of eyes and other head structures. The pharyngeal region (II) is induced by the head and it, in turn, induces the formation of pharynx. The inhibition mechanism acts parallel to the inductive processes and prevents repetitive regeneration of an organ.

Induction in Regeneration in Annelida : The neurosecretory hormones produced by the brain greatly influence the regeneration. The nerve cord exerts a local trophic effect of regeneration. If it is deflected, it leads to abnormal regeneration. By this method regeneration can be induced along the whole body length in *Myxicola aesthetica* and *Nereis diversicolor*.

Inductive Interaction in Limb Regeneration in Vertebrates: In vertebrates the neural-trophic factor liberated by the nerves at the cut end, is responsible for regeneration. Therefore, nerve supply to the amputed limb is essential. The nerve endings form synapse-like contact with the epidermal cells of the blastema cap. If a limb is first denervated and then amputed or the nerves are blocked to enter the epidermis by any means, the regeneration fails to occur. If dedifferentiation and blastema formation has started before, the nerve supply is cut, the regeneration continues normally, because the neural-trophic factor has already penetrated the regeneration blastema. This type of regeneration is nerve dependent.

7

The Egg

The fully developed female sexual cell is termed the ovum (L. *ovum*, egg). When fecundated by union with the male element, the egg or female germ cell gives rise to a new individual. The eggs of different animals vary widely in size, in the size and arrangement of yolk and in their coverings. They are relatively large in size and inert as compared with the male reproductive cell. An animal egg-cell has three basic functions : (i) it supplies a haploid set of chromosomes to the future embryo ; (ii) it provides most of the cytoplasm to the embryo; and (iii) it supplies food reserves that will enable the embryo to attain a status where it can launch off to feed upon exogenous food materials.

Size : Marine invertebrates usually produce small eggs in enormous numbers. Their size ranges from about 50 μ *(e.g., polychaete annelids)* to about 150 μ in diameter *(e.g., tunicates)*. In vertebrates, they vary in size from 0.07 mm. in the *mouse* to about 3.5 inches diameter in the *Ostrich*. The size of the egg chiefly depends upon the amount of yolk reserves in it. Sharks and rays among fishes, reptiles and birds generally lay eggs of larger dimensions. On the contrary, the eggs of mammals are minute, with very little yolk, and measure about 100 u in diameter.

Shape : Typically, the mature eggs are spherical in shape, but in a few animals, as in insects, the eggs are elongated. Among vertebrates, the eggs of hagfish *Myxine* and the *ganoid fishes* are oval in shape. Although the eggs of birds are also oval in shape externally, but their egg cells (yellow portion) are actually spherical in shape.

Organisation of a Mature Graafian (Ovarian) Follicle (Mammal) : The outermost layer of a mature graafian follicle is called the theca externa which consists of concentrically arranged fibres and fusiform cells. Inside the theca externa the cells appear large and avoid or spindle-shaped and are known as the theca interna. This layer is thought to secrete *estrogens* and its cells show the typical features associated with cells secreting steroids. There is also a rich capillary plexus in the theca interna.

Follicles about 0.2 mm in diameter begin to collect pools of fluid. This follicular fluid called liquor folliculi is rich in mucoproteins and is secreted by·the follicle cells. It comes to occupy a single cavity, the antrum. The fluid pushes the ovum and its neighbouring follicle cells, to one side. A peripheral shell consisting of many layers of cuboidal follicle cells surrounds the antrum. It is known as stratum granulosum. Smaller isolated intercellular accumulations of follicular fluid may occur in the membrana granulosa. These may form rounded vacuoles which stain deeply. The basal row of granulosa cells is separated from the theca interna by a basement or glassy membrane.

The mass of granulosa cells enclosing the mature ovum projects into the antrum, forming a hillock, the cumulus oophorous or discus proligerous. The ovum is surrounded by the prominent zona pellucida. The corona radiata is a well-defined, radially arranged layer, of columnar cells immediately surrounding the zona pellucida. The cells of the carona radiated are peeled off from the zona pellucida when the oocyte passes down the oviduct following ovulation.

The Egg Membranes

The egg cell like all other cells, is covered by a plasma membrane, or plasmalemma. In addition to the plasma membrane, eggs of most animals are surrounded by one or more accessory envelopes called *egg membranes.* These are classified into three different groups with reference to their origin.

Primary Egg Membranes:. The primary egg membranes are those membranes which are formed by the ovum itself. These develop around the plasma membrane of the egg in the space occupied by the interdigitating microvilli of the oocyte and follicle cells. In the initial stages of its formation the primary membrane consists of mucopolysaccharide but in later stages it may incorporate fibrous proteins. The primary egg membrane bears different names in different animals :

(a) *Vitelline Membrane:* The primary egg membrane of insects, molluscs, amphibians and birds is called vitelline membrane. It is usually thin and transparent and is closely applied to the surface of the underlying plasma membrane.

(b) *Zona Rediata:* It is so called because of its striated appearance and represents the zone of interdigitating microvilli around the oocyte. Zona radiata has a wide distribution among vertebrate eggs, notably those of the shark, certain bony fishes, amphibians and reptiles. In birds a zona radiata is not evident, but in mammals it is usually conspicuous around an early oocyte.

(c) *Zona Pellucida:* It is unstriated and takes the place of the zona radiata of young mammalian oocyte. Towards the time when the oocyte reaches its full size a denser material of fibriller structure (mucoprotein) appears in between the interdigitating processes of the oocyte and the follicle cells. The material becomes consolidated, eventually fills most of the space between the follicle cells and the oocyte, and becomes the *zona pellucida.*

(d) *Jelly Envelope:* The eggs of sea-urchin and many other marine invertebrates are surrounded by a thick, structureless jelly coat which belongs to the category of primary egg membranes.

The primary egg membranes are generally closely applied to the surface of the oocyte, but at a later stage a space filled with fluid may appear between the cytoplasm and the membrane. This space is known as the perivitelline space.

Secondary Egg Membranes : The secondary egg membranes are produced by the follicle cells immediately surrounding the developing oocyte. These membranes are usually hard and impermeable. The secondary envelopes are of the following types :

(a) *Chitinous Shells:* These surrounds the eggs of insects, ascidians and cyclostomes (e.g., *Petromyzon).*

(b) *Chorion:* In insects and ascidians the follicle cells secrete a second thicker membrane around the vitelline membrane. This second membrane is called the chorion. As the chorion is tough and impermeably it is provided with a single opening called *microphyl* at the anterior end.

There are no secondary membranes around the eggs of urodele amphibians, reptiles and birds.

(c) *Ovarian Follicles in Mammals:* Although true secondary egg membranes are lacking, around the zona pellucida (primary membrane) in the mammalian oocyte but the cells comprising the ovarian follicle, within which the egg lies, are ovarian in nature. Thus, theca (externa and interna), membrane granulosa, and corona radiata are designated as secondary egg membranes in mammals.

The mammalian egg, when released from the ovary, is commonly surrounded by a layer of follicle cells, termed the corona radiata. The cells of the corona radiata are peeled off later at fertilization.

Tertiary Egg Membranes : Tertiary membranes are secreted by the oviducts or other accessory pails of the female genital system while the egg is passing from the ovary to the exterior. They are not immediately connected with either ovum or ovary. Tertiary membranes are of various kinds :

(a) *Albumen Coats*: The eggs of amphibians are surrounded by albuminous (mucin-jelly) coverings. There are, in all, three distinct layers of jelly which are secreted as the eggs are propelled through the oviducts. When the amphibian egg is deposited in water, the jelly absorbs water and swells. It protects the egg and sometimes serves to make the eggs adhere to one another and to submerged objects in the water.

(b) *The Mermaids Purse: Mermaid is* a mythological figure having the head and trunk of a woman and the tail of a fish. In the oviparous sharks and rays the egg is surrounded by a protective egg-case called the mermaid's purse. It is a hard shell secreted by the shell glands present in the oviduct. The shell is drawn out into four long twisted horns which serve to entangle the eggs among submerged plants.

(c) *Albumen, Shell membranes and Calcareous shells* of reptilian and avian eggs.

(i) *Albumen* or *white of the egg.* 85% of the egg-white is water; remaining 15% is a mixture of several proteins, mostly albumins. It forms two dense strands known as the chalazae, which help to keep the egg cell in the centre of the egg white.

(ii) *Shell Membranes.* There are present two layers of shell membranes next to the egg white. The two membranes adhere closely over most of the surface of the egg but are separated by an air space at the blunt end of the egg. The inner membrane adheres to the egg white whereas the outer membrane adheres to the shell. The shell membranes consist of fibres of keratin.

(iii) *Calcareous Shell.* It is the outermost egg membrane consisting chiefly of calcium carbonate ($CaCo_3$). The shell is pierced by about 7000 fine pores.

Tertiary membranes are lacking in mammals, with the exception of the Prototheria.

(d) *Egg Capsules* of molluscs and selachians belong to the group of tertiary membranes.

Types of Eggs

The animal eggs are classified according to four criteria. They are (I) the amount of yolk, (II) the distribution of yolk, (III) the presence or absence of shell, and (IV) the type of development.

According to the Amount of Yolk

Microlecithal Eggs: The eggs containing small amount of yolk are called microlecithal eggs (Torrey, 1970). Some embryologists described them as alecithal eggs (Kent, 1969) or oligolecithal eggs (Romer, 1962 and Balinsky, 1970).

Examples : Amphioxus, tunicates, and eutherian mammals.

Mesolecithab Eggs: Some eggs acquire a moderate amount of yolk and are described as mesolecithal.

Examples : Amphibia, Dipnoi and Petromyzontia.

Macrolecithal Megalecithal or Polylecithal Eggs: The eggs which contain enormous food reserves (yolk) are called macrolecithal eggs. *Examples.* Myxinoidea, Chondriohytyes, Osteichthyes, Reptiles, Birds and Prototherian mammals.

According to the Distribution of Yolk

Isolecithal or Homolecithal Eggs: In isolecithal eggs, the amount of yolk laid down is small and it is scattered fairly evenly throughout the cytoplasm. *Examples :* Sponges, Amphioxns, tunicates and eutherian mammals.

Telolecithal Eggs: The distribution of yolk is unequal. It is collected eccentrically in the lower part of the egg (vegetal pole). Many annelids and molluscs and most amphibia have eggs of this type.

Centrolecithal Eggs: The amount of yolk is large and it is concentrated in the centre of the egg cell. Cytoplasm is distributed as a clear, layer around the outside of the yolk. A tiny mass of cytoplasm containing the egg nucleus is also present in the centre of the egg. Eggs of this type are characteristic of some coelenterates and most arthropods.

Discoidal Eggs: In these eggs, the amount of yolk is so enormous that it occupies the largest portion of egg except a small disc-shaped area of the cytoplasm called *blastodisc.* The latter is found at the top of the yolk mass. Such eggs are characteristic of squids and octopuses, fishes, reptiles, birds and prototherian mammals.

According to the Presence or Absence of Shell

Cleidoic Eggs: Cleidoic means boxlike. The eggs of reptiles and birds which are laid on dry land become self-contained, fully laden with yolk and surrounded by albumen and a water proof shell. Such eggs, which have become self-sufficient (with the exception of O_2 intake and CO_2 outflow) are called *cleidoic* eggs. Some terrestrial arthropods have also evolved cleidoic animals.

Non-cleidoic Eggs: The non-cleidoic eggs are not protected by shells. This type of eggs are characteristic of animals wherein the development is internal.

According to the Type of Development

Determinate or Mosaic Eggs: In the development of certain animals the fate of every part of the egg becomes fixed without liable to change, before or at the time of fertilization. The head-tail, left-right axes and dorsal-ventral of the future embryo are pre-determined in the zygote. If a particular portion of the egg is removed experimentally, the developing embryo will be deficient in a particular organ.

This type of egg, therefore, is called a determinate or mosaic egg because once it has become determined, the egg behaves like a mosaic, in which the fate of the egg parts cannot be changed after fertilization. This types of eggs are encountered in acoelomates *(Protozoa, Porifera, Platyhelminthes)*, pseudocoelomates *(Aschelminthes)*, schizocoelomates *(Annelida, Arthropoda* and *Mollusca)*, and tunicates.

Indeterminate or Regulative Eggs: In this type there is no predetermination and the fate of various egg portions is usually not fixed until three cleavages have produced eight cells. If blastomeres are separated before this stage, each develops as a whole embryo, and not as a partial one. The egg of coelenterates and most enterocoelomates *(Echinoderms* and *Chordates)* are of the regulative variety.

Polarity of Egg

Definition: Polarity or bipolar differentiation *refers to an unequal distribution of various substances (e.g., yolk RNA molecules, pigment granules) and cellular constituents in the advanced oocyte and later, in the egg in respect to the two opposite poles and the main axis of the egg.*

The line connecting the two poles of the egg is considered to be the main axis of the egg. The nucleus of the egg lies close to one pole. It is termed the animal pole. The opposite pole is called the vegetal pole as it accumulates yolk which provides nutrition to the developing embryo. When the oocyte undergoes meiosis, the three polar bodies are always formed at the animal pole. This features helps in identifying the animal pole in oligolecithal and telolecithal eggs wherein the concentration of the yolk at the vegetal pole is often not very distinct.

Instances of Polarity

Polarity in Amphibian Egg: The polarity is clearly marked in the amphibian eggs. At the animal pole of the oocyte, the yolk platelets are small and are not packed very densely. At the vegetal pole, the yolk platelets acquire a larger size and they come to lie very close to each other. As a result very little cytoplasm is left between them and the vegetal half of the egg is filled by a densely packed mass of yolk. Besides, there is much more pigment in the animal hemisphere of the amphibian oocyte than in the vegetal hemisphere. The animal hemisphere is dark brown or black while the vegetal hemisphere appears clear white.

Polarity in the Egg of Dentalium: In the elephant tusk mollusc *Dentalium,* two areas at the opposite sides of the egg are devoid of pigment and are, therefore, colourless. One of the two colourless areas lies on the side with which the egg is attached to the wall of the ovary. This side, represents the vegetal pole of the egg. It is seen to be made up of clear protoplasm which does not contain yolk granules. This yolk-free and unpigmented cytoplasm at the vegetal pole is called the vegetal polar plasm. The pigment-free cytoplasm at the animal pole is termed animal polar plasm. It is only partly free from yolk.

The fully grown oocyte contains a pigment which varies from olive green to brick red. As mentioned above the pigment is absent at the two poles.

Polarity in Mammalian Oocyte: A polar organization exists in the early mammalian oocyte because its nucleus lies close to one pole of the egg which is designated as the animal pole. The position of the animal pole is further affirmed at the time of the meiotic divisions because polar bodies are discharged here. Besides, the mammalian oocyte also possesses a bilateral organization. The side of the egg which is rich in RNA corresponds to the dorsal side of the embryo whereas the side with vacuolated cytoplasm will become the future ventral side.

Origin of Polarity

The polarity of the egg is determined by the position of such parts in the egg cell as the nucleus, yolk and other cytoplasmic substances. Two main hypotheses have been proposed to explain the factors that are responsible for the unequal distribution of the egg cell parts :

1. Many embryologists believe that the polarity is determined by the position of attachment of the growing oocyte to the ovary. In *molluscs* and *echinoderms* the vegetal pole of the egg develops from that end of the oocyte by which it remains attached to the wall of the ovary. Obviously, the greater amounts of yolk are deposited in the part of the egg cell which is nearest to the proximal surface of the ovary. Therefore, this part becomes the vegetal pole and the opposite side develops into the animal pole. This explanation is plausible for the eggs which are attached to the ovary by a single point. In the case of amphibians and mammals, the oocytes are surrounded by follicle cells from all sides. In these eggs polarity is not discernible on this basis.

2. Child (1941) gave a different explanation of the origin of polarity. According to him the animals pole is a more active place of metabolism and hence requires a better oxygen supply. It should, therefore, develop on that part of the oocyte which is nearest, to a blood vessel and, to the place of attachment with the ovary. Conversely, the opposite end develops into the vegetal pole. According to Balinsky (1970) the polarity is not always determined by the direction of blood flow because some of the cells, in addition to eggs, also exhibits a distinct polarity. For example, in nerve cells the polarity is manifested by the opposite differentiations of axon and dendrites. Likewise, there is a distinct difference between the proximal and distal ends of epithelial cells. Further, in the interior of any cell, the position of the centrosome in respect to the nucleus establishes a general form of polarity. Here, the line drawn through the centrosome and the nucleus represents the *main axis*. This polarity affects the distribution of cytoplasmic inclusions. For example, the Golgi bodies are often found grouped around the centrosome. Moreover, it may also influence the nuclear structures. When the oocytes are in the meiotic prophase, the chromosomes converge to that side of the nucleus which is nearest to the centrosome.

8

Fate Maps

The animal egg is a relatively large and dense, more or less spherical mass of protoplasm. In some primitive animals such as ascidians *(Ciona, Cynthia)*, some annelids, *Amphioxus*, some molluscs and frog the egg cytoplasm is differentiated into distinctive regions having natural colour differences. For example, the egg cytoplasm of *Stylea* is distinguished into four general regions: (i) the upper hemisphere of light protoplasm, (ii) a crescentric posteroventral region of yellow colour, (iii) a crescentric antero-dorsal region of grey colour, and (iv) vegetative area of dark grey colour.

Because of this natural differential pigmentation, it is possible to follow the fate of these regions and the complete cell lineages. The upper clear light-coloured protoplasm develops into epidermal ectoderm, the yellow crescent into the mesoderm, grey crescent gives rise to neural ectoderm and the dark grey vegetative region develops into the endoderm.

These areas are described as prospective organ regions, such as prospective epidermal ectoderm, prospective mesoderm, prospective neural ectoderm, notochord and prospective endoderm. The representation, showing the fate of each part of an early embryo, is called a fate map.

Construction of Fate Maps by Artificial Markings : The natural differential pigmentation of the egg cytoplasm either does not occur or it presents such an ambiguity that the determination of fate of all the blastomeres is not possible. In such cases some artificial markers are used which introduce artificial demarcation and help in the construction of fate maps. Following two methods are used to introduce differentiation by artificial means:

Vital Staining Method : Vogt (1925) devised vital staining procedure. The method includes staining the cytoplasm with some vital dyes like nile blue sulphate, neutral red, Bismarck brown. These dyes can stain the cytoplasm without injuring it.

A piece of agar is soaked in a vital dye and is applied to the surface of the embryo at a specific position. The dye diffuses from the agar and in no time the parts or cells of the embryo adjacent to agar are stained. Several areas can be marked simultaneously by using different pieces of agar dipped in different vital stains.

The vitelline membrane is permeable to the vital stains. Therefore, the embryo can be stained even without removing it. The presence of stain does not change the normal development of the embryo. The position of stained cells in the differentiated embryo clearly shows the future of the stained area and their migration to their prospective positions.

The dyes used for vital staining do not spread. These remain localized to the cells or cytoplasmic area to which agar piece is applied VOGT was able to construct the fate map showing the position of future ectoderm, mesoderm and endoderm, and the position of presumptive neural tube and notochord, etc.

on the surface of blastula of frog. Now the fate map of teleost fishes, reptiles and birds, etc. have been prepared.

Carbon Particle Marking : Spratt (1946) devised another method for marking cells of a developing embryo. The tiny particles of carbon are applied to the surface of the embryo. The carbon particles stick to the surface of cells and are used as markers for tracing the movement and lineage of cells and for drawing the fate map.

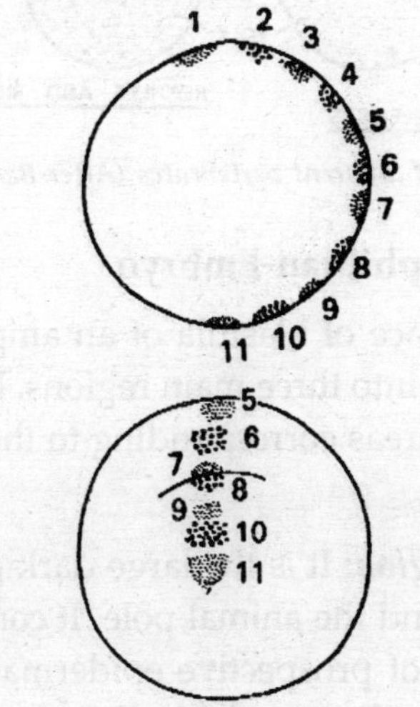

The future displacement of nine areas marked by vital stain during gastrulation.

Radioactive Labelling : Recently, the radioactive labelling of blastomeres has been employed to as certain their prospective destiny. Tritiated thymidine marker is used for constructing the fate map in eggs with excessive amount of yolk.

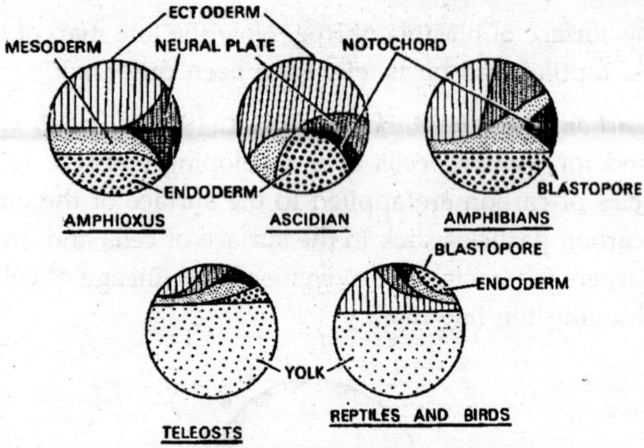

Fate maps of different vertebrates (After Berrill, 1971).

Fate Maps of Amphibian Embryo

The whole surface of blastula of an amphibian (frog) can be roughly divided into three main regions. Inside each region can be recognised areas corresponding to the future organs of the animal.

The Animal Region: It is the large dark grey or black part of the blastula around the animal pole. It consists of two main regions: (i) Region of prospective epidermal ectoderm which develops into the epidermis of the skin of embryo. (ii) Region of prospective central nervous system which contains material for brain, spinal cord and the sub-areas for the sense organs like eyes, ears and nose.

The Intermediate or Marginal Zone : It is the grey-crescent area that extends all around the equator of the blastula and contains following sub-regions : (i) Notochordal region or the region of prospective notochord present on the dorsal side of blastula. (ii) Prechordal plate which lies next to notochordal region towards the vegetal pole and develops into the prechordal connective tissue of the embryo. (iii) The area for anterior part of alimentary canal lies below the prechordal plate and gives rise to the endodermal lining of the mouth, gill region and pharynx. (iv) Region of segmental muscles that lies on both the sides of the notochordal area and develops into trunk muscles or somites. (v) Ventro-lateral-mesoderm consists of the lateral and ventral parts of marginal zone and gives rise to the mesodermal lining of the body cavity, the kidneys and reproductive organs.

Vegetal Region : It occupies the vegetal half of the embryo and is formed of unpigmented large macromeres. The region develops into the midgut and hindgut.

Fate Map of Chick Embryo

In chick blastula the blastoderm is bilaminar, consisting of epiblast and hypoblast. Both of them participate in organ formation. Therefore, the fate map of chick blastula, are made for each of the two layers, by vital staining (Wetzel 1929; Pasteels, 1940) and by using carbon particles (SPRATT, 1946).

The epiblast of the blastula of chick embryo may be differentiated into following areas:

Anterior half or Animal half of epiblast of the area pellucida contains the sub-regions of: (i) Presumptive epidermal ectoderm that develops into the skin epithelium. (ii) Presumptive neural plate that lies in the anterior half slightly anterior to the middle. It occurs as a crescentric transverse band that will give rise to central nervous system and sense organs.

Presumptive Notochordal Region : It lies in the middle line just below the equator. It develops into the notochord.

Presumptive Somite Region: It lies in the middle line just behind the notochordal area and develops into the musculature of the body.

Ventro-lateral Mesodermal Area: It occupies most of the posterior half of the area pellucida. It gives rise to the mesodermal lining of body cavity.

Presumptive Extra-embryonic Mesoderm : Produces the extraembryonic mesoderm and helps in the formation of extraembryonic membranes.

The hypoblast layer forms the presumptive endoderm and a part of it contributes to the formation of notochord. The presumptive endoderm forms the wall of gut and also the lining of the yolk sac.

Utility of Fate Maps

The fate maps are very significant in clearly understanding the mechanism and significance of gastrulation. The cellular components of blastula are all arranged on its surface. During gastrulation these components or areas migrate from their existing positions to the prospective positions.

Cell-Lineage

Various methods have been devised to study cell-lineage in animal eggs. The most important of them are:

1. Study of cell-lineage by tracking down the peculiarities found in each cell.
2. Alphabetical nomenclature of cells
3. Use of stains
4. Extirpation method
5. Isolation experiments.

1. *Following the Cell Peculiarities* : All blastomeres do not have the same shape, colour and appearance. They have many differences. A careful observer can note down these peculiarities and follow them during the course of development to know which organs they give rise to. This can be easily done with the eggs of certain animals like the frog, the ascidian *Cynthia* and the mollusc *Dentalium*.

2. *Alphabetical Nomenclature*: The blastomeres can be labelled in the alphabetical order and followed. This method can be applied to eggs having spiral mode of cleavage as in polyclads, nemertines, annelids and molluscs (other than Cephalopods). The blastomeres are usually named in the clockwise direction.
3. *Use of Stains* : Various stains have been used to follow the course of the development of cells. Best results were obtained when vital dyes were used. W. Vogt (1925) first used vital dyes like Nile blue sulphate and Neutral red in embryological studies. The method involves the pressing of small pieces of agar impregnated with vital dyes against the surface of the blastula and then closely following the changes in the shape and migration of the blastomeres.
4. *Extirpation Method* : CHABRY (1887) drew the fertilized eggs of the ascidian-*Ascidiella* into a capillary tube of smaller diameter and pricked off one or other blastomere with the help of a glass needle under a good dissection microscope. The embryo can then be followed to find out the tissues and organs that are found missing.
5. *Isolation Technique* : Certain blastomeres are isolated and their development is followed to find out their potentiality. Vital stains like, Janus green, Nile blue or neutral red are applied at the blastula stage and then the isolated cells can be conveniently studied.

Cell-lineage in Planocera

The polyclad *Planocera* exhibits spiral cleavage. The first cleavage plane is meridional and the second is also meridional but at right angles to the first. The four blastomeres thus formed are not equal in size. One is much larger and is slightly posterior in position. The other three blastomeres also possess some peculiarties which make them easily identifiable. The blastomeres are named clockwise as A, B, C & D. These four blastomeres are called a quadrant. The third cleavage is horizontal and is slightly above the equator resulting in the formation of four small micromeres above and four larger macromeres below. The micromeres are named as la, 1b, 1c and 1d while the macromeres are named as 1A, 1B, 1C and 1D. The blastomeres la, 1b, 1c and 1d form the first quartet of micromeres.

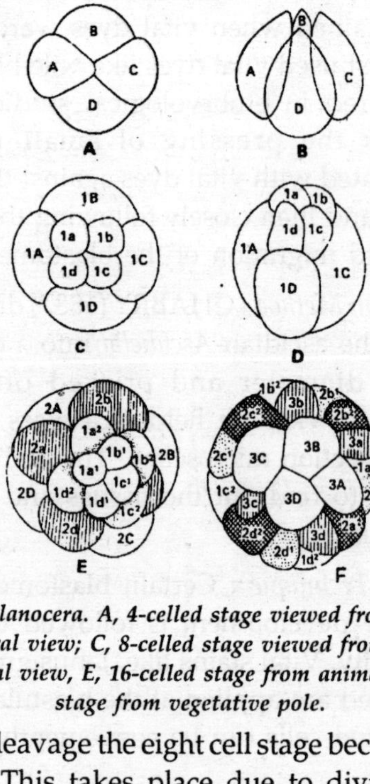

Spiral cleavage in Planocera. A, 4-celled stage viewed from animal pole. B, 4-celled stage in lateral view; C, 8-celled stage viewed from animal pole, D, 8-celled stage, lateral view, E, 16-celled stage from animal pole, F, 32-celled stage from vegetative pole.

On further cleavage the eight cell stage becomes the sixteen-celled embryo. This takes place due to division of the first quartet of micromeres and macromeres. Each micromere gives rise to two cells, 1a becoming la and la^2, 1b as 1b^2 and 1b^2, 1c as lc^1 and 1c^2 and 1d as 1d^1 and 1d^2. The four macromerea 1A, 1B, 1C and 1D form four micromeres 2a, 2b, 2c and 2d that form the second quartet and four macromeres 2A, 2B, 2C and 2D.

The sixteen-celled embryo reaches the 32-celled stage by a further division of cells. The micromeres of the first two quartets divide into two. At the same time the macromeres 2A; 2B, 2C and 2D divide to form the third quartet of micromeres-3a, 3b, 3c, and 3d and the four macromeres 3A, 3B, 3C and 3D. The ectomeres which later give rise to the ectoderm is formed of the first three quartets of micromeres and their derivatives. Slowly the ectomeres spread over the surface of the embryo and form a single layer—thick envelope except a small gap, which forms the blastopore. Now the embryo is in the gastrula stage.

The fourth quartet is formed by a further division of macromeres and consists of the micromeres 4a, 4b, 4c and 4d and the macromeres 4A, 4B, 4C and 4D. Of the eight cells seven cells viz. 4a, 4b, 4c, 4A, 4B, 4C and 4D divide and form small cells of yolk to become the food for other cells. The cell 4d which is much larger than other cells and even bigger to 4D forms the mesentoblast. It gives rise to the endoderm and mesoderm.

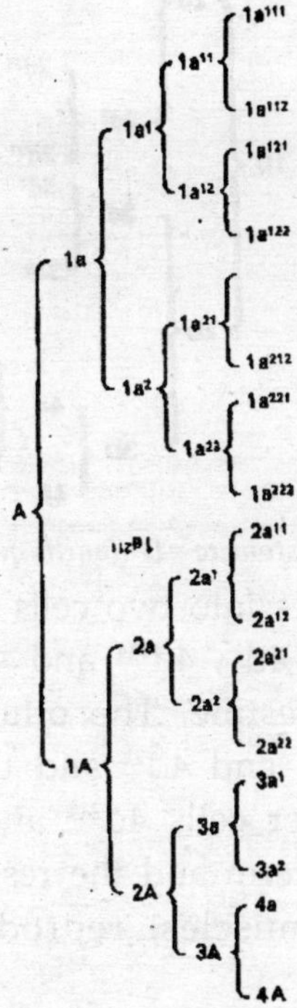

Cell products of blastomere—A (First quartet) in Planocera.

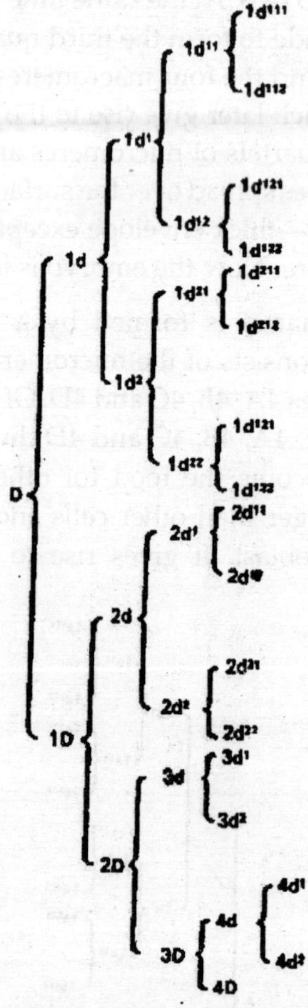

Cell products of blastomere—D (fourth quartet) in Planocera.

The cell 4d divides into two cells $4d^1$ and $4d^2$.$4d^1$ gives rise to the cells 4d , 4d , $4d^{111}$ and $4d^{121}$, which form the endoderm of the intestine. The other cell 4d divides to form larger cells $4d^{21}$ and $4d^{22}$ and the smaller cells $4d^{211}$ and $4d^{221}$. The smaller cells $4d^{211}$ and $4d^{221}$ contribute to the pharyngeal endoderm and the rest form the mesoderm that gives rise to muscles, reproductive tissues, and mesenchyme, etc.

Cell-lineage studies were mostly done with invertebrates, such as *Celepsin, Nereis, Trochus* and *Ascaris.* The first attempt on chordates was made by E. G. Conklin (1905) on the ascidian *Stylea (Cynthia) partita,* later followed by VOGT (1925 ; 29).

Positional or Presumptive Determination : Studies of cell-lineage explain the process of determination. According to Nelson (1953) determination is "the unknown and invisible changes that occur within a cell or cells which effect a limitation or restriction of potency". The way in which the determination of individual organs or parts of organs is brought about is called individuation.

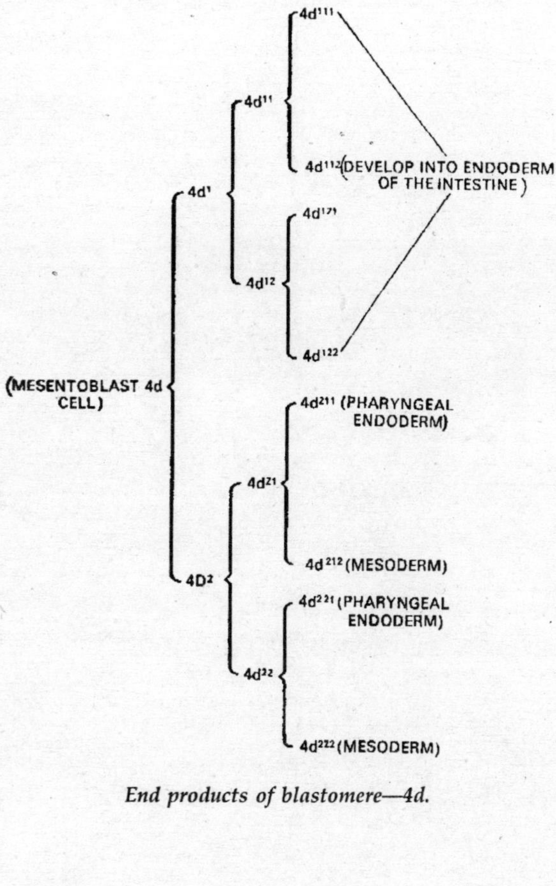

End products of blastomere—4d.

The limitation of potency to be reduced to that of a general organ system like nervous system, etc. with the ability to determine organs of that system is termed rigid or irrevocable determination. However, in many cells determination is dependent upon their location in an organism and not their inherent ability to differentiate is referred to as positional or presumptive determination.

The ectodermal cells of amphibian blastula divide into epidermal and neural area during gastrulation due to the activities of the Chorda mesodermal area. Another interesting aspect of determination is potency expression which means the release of potency to facilitate development.

9

Growth and Differentiation

The development of either a multicellular or a unicellular organism involves two interrelated processes ; differentiation and growth. Cellular differentiation involves the change of a cell from an embryonic to a specialized type. Growth refers to an increase in protoplasmic mass.

***Differentiation*:** The term differentiation refers to the events by which cells and other parts of an organism become different from one another and also different from their previous condition. It is a broad expression that encloses a host of operations responsible for increasing diversification of form and function.

Types of Differentiation

Differentiation may broadly be classified into three types: 1. Morphological differentiation. 2. Physiological or histological differentiation and 3. Chemical differentiation.

Morphological Differentiation: During the course of multiplication individual cells and groups of cells become structurally different from other cells and groups of cells. For example, from a common starting point in generalized ectoderm, nerve cells and epidermal cells acquire distinguishing features of size, shape and internal architecture. Morphological differentiation occurs in various ways viz, (i) *cell migration* (ii) *cell aggregation* (iii) *localized growth* (iv) *enlargement* (v) *constriction* (vi) *fusion* (vii) *splitting* (viii) *folding* (ix) *evagination* (x) *invagination* etc. For example, the notochord is formed by *cell migration* and *aggregation,* optic cup by *invagination* and metanephric duct is formed as *an outgrowth* from the hind end of the mesonephric duct.

Physiological or Histological Differentiation: Histologic differentiation is the process as the result of which the parts of the organism acquire the ability to perform their *special functions.* In the case of multicellular animals, the parts in questions are the eel and groups of cells.

The special functions of cells in this definition are distinguished from the basic functions of life which are common to all living cell. Every cell is capable of performing the processes of metabolism (e.g. respiration, synthesis, etc.), possesses to a certain degree the ability for ameboid movement, shows irritability and is able to react external stimuli. These functions are found in undifferentiated as well as in differentiated cells. Differentiated cells, however, are able to perform special functions, or to perform them in such a way, the other cells cannot. Thus the nerve cells are capable of conducting) *nervous impulses* to great distances and at a high speed. The live cells secrete *bile* (besides their other functions). The melanophoric produce granules of *pigment* in their cytoplasm. These are the special functions of nerve cells, hepatic cells and melanophores.

The ability to perform special functions is dependent on the existence to specific mechanisms in the differentiated cells. These mechanisms are sometimes visible in the form of organoids of the cells, such as the *myofibrils* of muscle cells, *cilia* of epithelial cells the trachea, long *processes* of nerve cells. These obvious morphologic: properties of the cells are also called differentiations. They are actually the visible expression of the process of differentiations. In other tissues, the differentiation becomes visible not so much as change in the structure of cells itself but as the result of the production by the cells of intercellular structures, such as fibers in the connective tissues, *matrix* of cartilage and bone, *cuticle* on the outer surface of the skin in invertebrate animals. These extracellular parts are called differentiations in the same sense as the organoids of the cells. The special function of a cell may be the secretion of some substance that does not remain in the tissue as a permanent part but is removed or dissolved in the surrounding medium. In this case, granules of secretion may sometimes be seen in the histological preparations as a morphological expression of the function of the cell.

The functional mechanisms of histologically differentiate cells are cytoplasmic. The building up of these mechanism therefore causes a shift in the relative volume of the nucleus and the cytoplasm. The nuclei of the cells are their conservative part; they do not change essentially with the onset of development. It is believed that even in the case of fully differentiated cells, the nuclei in all the various tissues of the animal's body have the same chromosomes and genes. In differentiated cells, the mass of cytoplasm increases while the nuclei do not increase, or do not increase in the same proportion. The ratio-mass of cytoplasm to mass of nucleus— increases with differentiation. This ratio gives a rough quantitative estimate of the degree of differentiation. The estimate maybe made even more exact if chemical substances and not morphological parts are taken into consideration. The basic substances of the nucleus are the chromosomes, with DNA as their essential component. The cytoplasmic structures are built up of proteins. Furthermore, the enzymes, which are the essential part of the functional mechanism of a cell, are of a protein nature. It is thus possible to substitute the amount of DNA for the basic structure of the cell and the amount of protein for its changing functional mechanisms. Direct measurements show that the relation protein/DNA changes with differentiation in agreement with expectation (Davidson and Leslie, 1950).

Chemical Differentiation: A vertebrate egg, whatever its class, has a complex chemical composition from the very beginning. The same is often reflected in a measure of pattern and spatial arrangement. As the egg cleaves and progressively becomes converted to blastula, gastrula, and definitive embryo individual cells and areas of cells become biochemically different from one another. This is known as chemical differentiation or chemo-differentiation.

The elaboration and assortment of chemical differences lie at the root of the morphologically and physiological differences that ultimately emerge. The acquisition of special biochemical properties by the cells takes place before the appearance of a recognizable neural tube, heart, or whatever else. In other words, there comes a time when a given region of an egg or embryo takes on those chemical qualities that dictate the course of development to be followed by that region. The process by which this fixity of developmental prospect is acquired is called *determination*. Differentiation, therefore, might be redefined as follows : *the series of events by which materials become chemically determined and then assume distinctive form and function.*

Whatever the nature of differentiation of a cell, it is based on the chemical constitution of that cell. In every case where the function of the cells consists in the elaboration of some substances, whether in the form of structural elements or in the form of secretions, there must be a specific enzyme or specific combination of enzymes responsible for the reaction. As the substances produced by cells are very diverse, a correspondingly varied assortment of enzymes may be postulated as being present in different tissue cells. It may therefore be said that *differentiation is the production of unique enzymatic patterns.* (Spiegelman, 1948 ; Boell, 1948, 1955).

All enzymes are known to be proteins, so that the last sentence may be paraphrased to read "differentiation is the production of unique protein patterns." This wording is a more general one, as it includes not only proteins having enzymic properties but also the proteins which are not enzymes. An important group of the latter kind are the structural proteins, which are particularly prominent in some differentiations of cells and tissues. Some of the structural proteins are permanently intracellular, such as the *keratin* produced in the epidermis cells of terrestrial vertebrates. Other structural proteins, although produced by the cells, are eventually extruded from the cells and accumulate in the intercellular spaces. *Collagen* is the best known of such proteins.

Other organic substances such as lipids and carbohydrates, alone or in conjunction with proteins, play a very important role in the life of cells, but between these substances and the proteins there is a very important difference. The synthesis of carbohydrates, lipids and also smaller molecules, such as organic acids (including amino acids), occurs under the control of enzymes and enzyme systems, which are of a protein nature. Given a certain pattern of proteins in a cell, the other components are then determined by the enzymic activities of the proteins.

The proteins of the cell, on the other hand, are not produced by the action of other proteins, but are synthesized under the direct control of nucleic acids. Ultimately, the structure of every protein in the cell is determined by the sequence of nitrogeneous base pairs in the chromosomal DNA.

It is generally accepted that new proteins are synthesized via a complex mechanism that has its start in the genetic material of the cell. Much of the evidence for this mechanism derives from studies on microorganisms, but the conclusions are presumably applicable to all types of animal cells. Nuclear deoxyribonucleic acid (DNA) is the essential material of heredity and it will be recalled that a molecule of DNA consists of a double ribbon of nucleotide units arranged in a linear order. Each nucleotide is composed of a molecule of the sugar deoxyribose, a phosphate groups, and one of four nitrogeneous bases, adenine (A), guanine (G), cytosine (C), and thymine (T). In forming a DNA molecule, the nucleotides are paired so that adenine is linked with thymine and guanine with cytosine. Since the symmetry of the molecule dictates that the A—T combination is different from T—A, and G—C different from C—G, the specificity of any part of the DNA molecule depends upon the order of these four possible combination of bases in the double ribbon.

Now the great diversity of proteins upon which cell differentiation rests is based on 20 *amino acids* : the uniqueness of any given protein molecule depends upon the number and kinds of amino acid units of which it is composed and on the order in which they are strung together. In the final analysis, the sequence of amino acids that characterizes a particular protein is dictated by the order of the nucleotide pairs in a molecule chromosomal DNA. But the translation of the DNA message is an indirect one involving intermediate steps.

The two strands of the DNA molecule separate, but instead of replicating themselves as in the course of cell division, each strand serves as a mould or template upon which, through the mediation of a special enzyme, a slightly different type of nucleic acid is assembled. This is *ribonucleic acid* (RNA) which differs from DNA in that it incorporates the sugar *ribose* rather than deoxyribose and contains *uracil* in place of thymine. The RNA molecule then splits away and passes from the nucleus of the cell into the cytoplasm. Passing as it does into the cytoplasm and being a complementary copy of and thus containing the same genetic information as that in other words, the exact sequence of nitrogenous bases along a DNA strand is transcribed in the molecule of messenger-RNA. As already noted, every protein features a unique sequence of amino acids. It is now known that every amino acid is specified by a sequence of three bases in the messenger-RNA; therefore the total sequence of "triplets" in the messenger-RNA will specify the sequence of amino acids and thus the protein to be formed. But elements other than messenger-RNA enter into this process.

After passing out of the nucleus, messenger-RNA associates itself with small granules in the cytoplasm known as *ribosomes* which are themselves composed of RNA plus protein in about a 60-40 per cent ratio. The genetic information coded in the sequence of bases in the messenger-RNA is translated into an amino acid sequence within the messenger-RNA-ribosome apparatus. This is done in a series of steps. First, free amino acids present in the cytoplasm are activated by special enzymes, one for each amino acid. This complex of amino acid and activating enzyme is then coupled to still another type of RNA known as *transfer-* RNA. The activating enzyme is discarded, and the new complex of amino acid and transfer-RNA is coupled to the messenger-RNA on the ribosome(s).

Coupling presumably involves "recognition triplets" of bases in the transfer-RNA that bond to their complementary coding triplets in the messenger-RNA. The amino acids then detach from the transfer-RNA and, in accordance with the sequence specified by the messenger-RNA and matched by the transfer-RNAs are linked in a chain to form a specific protein.

Growth

Definition: The energy that a cell derives from metabolic processes is largely used in the synthesis of cellular material. As cellular material is synthesized, the protoplasmic mass of the cell increases. *This increase in cellular mass is called growth:*

It results from synthesis of new protoplasm, both the cytoplasmic and nucleic, and protoplasmic products are called apoplasmatic substances such as the fibres of connective tissue and the matrix of bone and cartilage. Because the physiological economy of the individual is based on the cell and because there are minimum requirements of cells surface volume ratio, increase in mass is usually accompanied by cell division. Cell multiplication, then is a distinguishing characteristic of growth.

Growth is the result of the excess of the anabolic (synthetic) over the catabolic (destructive) processes in the organism. If synthesis and decomposition go on at the same rate, there is no increase in the bulk of the organism i.e., no growth will take place. In certain conditions, decomposition dominates over synthesis, as for instance in prolonged senselessness, when synthetic processes are impossible because of lack of food supply, while catabolic processes (oxidations, etc.) continue to satisfy the current requirements for energy. After the internal food reserves e.g., fat in the adipose tissue, have been exhausted, the energy is produced at the expense of the proteins of the protoplasm. This results in a decrease in the mass of living matter which may be called degrowth (Needham, 1942).

Measurement of Growth and its Graphic Representation: By weighing a growing animal at regular intervals and plotting the weight against time on a diagram, a growth curve is obtained which shows the increase of the mass of the animal with time. The shape of the growth curve very often resembles the latter S : there is an initial part, where the curve rises very gradually, then a middle part, where the curve rises steeply, and the last part, where the rise of the curve is again slowed down and it asymptotically approaches a horizontal line signifying the limit of growth in each particular case. A curve of this shape is known as the sigmoid curve.

If the increments of growth for equal time intervals are measured, the increase in different periods of life of the same individual may be estimated. The increase, taken as a difference between the final and initial size (weight) of an animal for any period of time, irrespective of other factors, is called the absolute increase. The sigmoid curve is actually a graphic representation of the absolute increase, and it shows that the absolute increase per unit of time is, in this case, greatest in the middle part of the growth cycle.

The rate of growth is measured as the relative increase—the increase related to the initial mass of growing substance. The exact definition of the rate of growth is then

$$v = \frac{aW}{dt} \quad \frac{1}{W}$$

where v is the rate of growth and W is the size (weight) of the animal at any given time .

Growth thus defined is, in its essence, an increase in geometrical progression, the increase being proportional to the initial quantity of growing substance. Increase in geometrical progression is called exponential; growth is thus an exponential process.

Differentiation

"Differentiation is the full sequence of changes involved in the progressive diversification of cell structure and function that is the hallmark of development," Ebert and Sussex 1965.

The process of development involves the division of the fertilized egg into many cells which assume different size, shape, structure and function. The various cells form tissues and organs that together give the correct and complete form of the animal. This whole process is called differentiation. The process of differentiation is irreversible because the differentiated or specialized cells cannot revert back to undifferentiated stem cells.

Zygote

↓

Different types of cells

↓

Different organs of the animals

In a general sense, differentiation is divided into intracellular differentiation and intercellular differentiation. Intracellular differentiation is met with in Protozoa, in spermatogenesis and in orogenesis. Intercellular differentiation occurs in multicellular animals and plants. Some authors refer to intracellular differentiation as non-cellular differentiation or cytodifferentiation and intercellular differentiation as supracellular differentiation. In a broader sense it refers to the differentiation of the different cells, tissues and organs from a single cell, while in a narrow sense it refers to the differentiation of parts of an organism to attain the ability to perform their special functions like the conduction of inpulse in nerve cells or the secretion of bile by hepatic cells. It virtually includes complete process of embryogenesis; because each cell of the developing embryo becomes different from one another and from their original form.

Types of Differentiation

Differentiating cells show unique characters in the form of shape, structure, chemical nature and behaviour. On the basis of origin of these differences the process of differentiation can be divided into four kinds:

Morphological Differentiation: The differences in shape and size of the cells that are acquired during the course of development is termed morphological differentiation.

Physiological Differentiation : This involves the difference in the functional activities of the cells.

Behavioural Differentiation : This differentiation involves a change in the behavioural pattern of certain cells like the nerve cells to be able to transmit impulses and the muscle cells to contract.

Chemodifferentiation or Biochemical Differentiation : This is the most important kind of differentiation. "Chemodifferentiation represents the initial step in the entire differentiating process" — Nelson. During the whole process of cleavage and gastrulation, the different areas of the original egg become biochemically different from each other. This biochemical difference leads to the formation of different cells, tissues, etc.

Origin of Differentiation

All kinds of differentiation are caused by change in the chemical constitution of the cell. All chemical changes are brought about by enzymatic actions. Any change in the enzymatic pattern will naturally lead to differentiation. Spiegelman (1948), therefore, suggested that "differentiation is the production of unique enzymatic patterns'. All enzymes are proteins and, therefore, any change in protein pattern will also bring about chemo differentiation. Balinsky (1970) has described differentiation as the production of unique protein patterns.

There are two types of proteins found in cells viz. Structural proteins and proteins forming enzymes. Most of structural proteins like keratins are intracellular while others are expelled from the cells and get accumulated in the intercellular spaces. Synthesis and metabolism of all components of the cell including carbohydrates, lipids, etc. take place under the influence of enzymes. The synthesis of proteins or the enzymes is controlled by the nucleic acids. Thus the basic structure of all cells is determined by the DNA of the chromosomes.

Totipotency of Nucleus : The countless cells making up the embryo or adult body contain the same type of nucleus with the same chromosome compliment and with same genetic informations as possessed by the original zygote. This has been proved by a number of experiments :

1. Hans Spemann (1928) constricted the fertilized egg of newt, *Triturus* with a loop of fine hair. The constriction was not carried out completely, so that the two halves were still connected with a narrow bridge of cytoplasm. The nucleated half of the zygote began cleavage, the non-nucleated half did not. After 16 cell-stage, a nucleus happened to pass through the cytoplasmic bridge into the non-nucleated half. Henceforth, this half also began to cleave. Spemann tightened the noose, cutting the two halves of the egg. Each half now developed into a normal embryo, except that the half with delayed nucleus was delayed in its development. Spemann concluded that the nuclei remained totipotent.
2. Robert Briggs and Thomas King (1952) activated frog's egg with a fine glass needle. Then they removed its nucleus and replaced it with a nucleus from the cell of more advanced embryo (late blastula or gastrula). The transplanted nucleus underwent nuclear divisions to form blastomeres and subsequently a normal adult. Briggs and King concluded that the nucleiremain totipotent and do not get irreversibly changed in the course of development.
3. In another experiment Fiscberg and Gurdon (1968) transplanted a nucleus from differentiated intestinal cell (endoderm cell) of an amphibian tadpole into the enucleated amphibian egg. A normal adult developed from the transplanted egg.

Role of Egg Cytoplasm during Differentiation : If the nucleus remains totipotent and all the embryonic cells have identical genetic composition, how these become different during the process of differentiation? Presumably, all genes are not equally active in all the cells. There is differential gene expression in different types of cells.

The only possible clue must be found in cytoplasm. The different areas of the cytoplasm of the egg have different influence on the nuclei and make them produce different types of cells. This can be proved by the following experiments:

(i) Danielli (1955) grafted the nucleus of *Amoeba proteus* to an enucleated *Amoeba discoides*. The proteus nucleus assumed the characteristics of discoides nucleus.

(ii) Moore (1941) conducted a series of experiments with *Rana pipens* and *Rana palustris*. The enucleated egg of *Rana palustris* was fertilized by the sperm of *Rana pipens*. The rate of cleavage and blastomere arrangement were that of *R. palustris*. The same effect was seen when the reverse fertilization was done. This clearly showed that it is the cytoplasm that always determined the type of development.

(iii) Brache (1922) noticed that the unripe sea urchin eggs if fertilized, the sperm nucleus that has entered the egg took up the appearance of egg nucleus.

(iv) Hartmann (1924), Prescott (1956) found out that the nucleus of *Amoeba* can be prevented from undergoing nuclear division for a considerable time by removing the cytoplasm from the cell at regular intervals.

(v) Nuclear transference from the blastula stage to the unfertilised egg results in some interesting reactions. The blastular nucleus which synthesized DNA and almost no RNA when shifted into an unfertilised egg produces RNA and no DNA. However,' if the same

The two cells that do possess the full complement of chromatin material later turn out to be the germ cells. Thus different cells of the blastula have different chromatin content and really possess quantitative differentiation. The differential DNA quantum has differential nucleo-cytoplasmic interaction. A similar phenomenon has been noticed in some Diptera.

Gene Amplification : In the formation of amphibian oocytes at certain stage in which the rRNA synthesis is very active. The gene for rRNA exists in a large number of copies. In some cases where the genome of the oocyte was tetraploid it contained not just four nucleoli but nearly 1000. Each one of these nuclei actively synthesizes rRNA. This leads to the conclusion that the oocyte contains many copies of the genes for rRNA. The diploid genome of *Xenopus laevis* contains nearly 1600 copies of the genes for rRNA and all of them are clustered in the nucleolar organizer region.

Another interesting case of gene amplification is noticed in the lampbrush chromosome of Amphibian oocytes. Here again extra copies of tRNA and mRNA molecules are met with that have a regulatory influence over the process of development.

Genetic Lesions: In 1958 researchers at Oxford University found a mutant variety of *Xenopus laevis* that possessed only one nucleolus instead of the usual two. These animals are called 1.nu.individual. This deficiency of nucleolar material does not, however, prevent normal development. When the mutants were mated (1.nu x l.nu) the offsprings were of the followings types: Normal form (2.nu), heterozygous (l.nu) and homozygous mutant (0.nu) in the typical Mendelian ratio of 1:2:1. The (0.nu) individual without any nucleolus does not develop beyond the early stages. The (0.nu) mutant is formed due to the deletion of 28S and 18S rRNA genes from one of the chromosomes.

(B) Chemical Changes of DNA

There are two methods by which DNA may be modified chemically. They are :

(a) Alkylation.

(b) Methylation.

The enzymes necessary for bringing about these reactions are already found within the cell itself. The reactions affect particular nucleotide bases of the DNA which in turn alter other results. Of these methylation takes place only after DNA replication and so this reaction has to take place every time after the DNA replication is completed.

Control of Differentiation during Transcription : At the level of transcription during the process of protein synthesis, the various genes present in the chromosomes of a developing embryo may be controlled by the following methods:

Gene Regulation by Histones : The chromosomes contain nucleoproteins. The nucleic acid part of this is made up of a DNA while the protein part is predominantly made up of a kind of proteins called histones. These histones contain mostly basic amino acids like arginine, lysine and histidine. The DNA molecule has free acidic groups of phosphoric acid on the outer surface, which are able to have firm bonds with the NH_2 groups of the basic amino acids present in the histones. Thus this association becomes intimate.

This association of DNA with histones prevents the DNA from interacting with other substances present in the cytoplasm. This view has been expressed by Stedman (1950) and Bloch (1962). The DNA is thus deprived of the opportunity of serving as templates for the production of mRNA. Experimental proof in support of the above view is available. Cell-free preparations containing DNA from calf thymus and RNA polymerase taken from *Bacillus megagaterium* synthesize RNA in presence of RNA precursors. When histones were added to this mixture RNA synthesis was inhibited. It was also noticed that different fractions of histones affect RNA synthesis differently.

In another experiment isolated calf thymus nuclei were treated with trypsin to remove histones. The RNA synthesis increased three fold when about 70% of the histones were removed (Allfery, Littau & Mirsky, 1963). In a similar experiment on plant material a complete removal of histones from the chromosomal DNA showed a five-fold increase of RNA synthesis (Huang and Bqnner, 1962).

On the basis of all these studies, it is assumed that histones are involved in the regulation of gene activity. Berrill (1971) suggested that histones inhibit DNA-primed RNA synthesis in unrelated forms like bacteria, pea and mammal and generally diminish the activity of DNA polymerase.

It is possible that the DNA-histone relationship may be altered by differences in distribution of histones that may exist in chromosomes. The histones which act as repressors are modified by phosphorylation, acetylation and methylation. These modifications change the DNA-histone interactions and bring about differential transcription (Goodenough & Levine 1974).

Gene Regulation by Heterochromatisation : The heterochromatic region of the chromosome remains inactive during the process of protein synthesis. The active genes are rarely marked in the heterochromatic region. In mammalian females the heterochromatic 'X' chromosome is totally inactive. Another interesting feature is that the paternal chromosome complement in male mealy bugs is genetically inactive. Various studies have proved beyond doubt that transcription of RNA does not take place in heterochromatin.

Therefore, Heterochromatisation is associated with the stoppage of RNA transcription. This is possible because Heterochromatisation controls the degree of condensation or coiling of the chromosomes to render the DNA strands not available for RNA transcription.

Heterochromatisation is clearly evident in some specialized cells. The normal human leucocytes contain large sections of condensed heterochromatin and, therefore, the synthesis of proteins is very less. On the other hand the leucocytes of persons suffering from leukemia lack heterochromatin and, therefore, show protein synthesis at a prolific rate. However, the mechanism of the genes getting "locked up" by Heterochromatisation and also "released" from the condensed state is not properly understood. The studies of J. Freaster have shown that acidic proteins play an important role in this drama (Goodenough and Levine 1974).

Gene regulation by Acidic Proteins : The acidic proteins are non-histone proteins and the most important and abundant acidic proteins are phosphoproteins. The main constituents of the phosphoproteins are tryptophan and tyrosine. The role of acidic proteins in the control of transcription is known only through circumstantial evidence.

The acidic proteins are intimately associated with the DNA helix and their distribution varies from one tissue to another even within the same organism. This makes one to believe that they may play a good role in gene regulation. It is possible that the acidic proteins interact with the basic histones so that the histones are temporarily shut off in their activity as repressors. If a histone preparation with a known inhibitory effect on DNA dependent RNA synthesis is pre-incubated with phosphoproteins its inhibitory effect is reduced (Markert & Ursprung, 1974). In this way they can indirectly promoted transcription.

Control at Translation Level

The message carried by the mRNA has to be decoded and the required amino acids are to be picked up to form the various proteins. This involves several steps and so there is always a possibility of various controls existing at each level. The important regulatory mechanisms that exist at the translation level are the following: —

A. Movement of mRNA from the Nucleus to Cytoplasm

It is possible that all the mRNA that leaves the nucleus may not reach the cytoplasm. There may be loss of bits of mRNA which means that the translation may not be correct. If some of the mRNA is prevented from reaching the cytoplasm then also the translation may be different.

B. Retention or Breakdown of mRNA within the Nucleus

The mRNA may be passed to the cytoplasm or may be degraded or broken down due to various factors. Degradation may occur in some portions of the mRNA strands bringing about differential translation.

C. Masking of mRNA

Once the *m*RNA is masked, translation is not possible. Masking requires the work of another agent to act. Masking may not be entire but partial thereby bringing about differences in translation.

D. Effect of Specific Regulatory Molecules on mRNA

Certain regulatory molecules present in the cytoplasm may associate with the mRNA and thereby prevent the mRNA from playing their role in translation. The association may be partial or complete.

E . Destruction of mRNA

Sometimes the mRNA may reach the ribosomes intact but may be destroyed there due to certain forces that may exist. This prevents or alters the translation work thereby bringing about differentiation.

F. Ribosomal Inactivation

The ribosomes which normally play an important role in protein synthesis may be inactivated so that particular protein may not be formed. After some time the ribosome may also be activated. This phenomenon brings about temporary breaks in translation.

G. Changes in the Folding of Nascent Polypetide Chains

During the process of protein synthesis the polypetide chains form the precursor of proteins. This happens by folding. Any alternation in the folding pattern may alter the structure and bring about differentiation.

H. Change Brought about in the Factors that Influence Protein Synthesis

Many factors like hormones, enzymes, etc. bring about differentiation by influencing the path of protein synthesis. Hormones are found to be very effective in this direction, and they bring about these changes through different pathways.

They may act as gene depressors. When an injection of hydrocortisone was given to rats the rate of RNA synthesis increased in the liver. Similarly, if oestrogens are injected, the uterine endometrium shows great activity. It is noticed that cortisone stimulates the secretions of the four enzymes — *Tryptophan pyrrolase, Tyrosine transaminase, glutamic alanine transaminase* and *Arginase.*

Hormones may also influence enzyme activity at the level of transplantation. Some of the recent experiments tend to support the view that hormones may control translation by producing secondary effects. Hormones affect chromosomal gene activity by getting localized in the nucleus. The hormones are more organ specific than gene-specific.

According to Britten & Davidson (1969), the following are the effects of oestrogen on cells of the uterine wall: —

(i) Increase in total cell protein.

(ii) Increase in transport of amino acids into cell.

(iii) Increase in protein synthesis activity per unit amount of polyribosomes.

(iv) Increased synthesis of new ribosomes.

(v) Alteration of amounts of nuclear protein to nucleus.

(vi) Increased amount of polyribosomes per cell.

(vii) Increase in activity of two RNA polymerases.

(viii) Increase in nucleolar mass and number.

(ix) Increase in synthesis of contractile proteins.

(x) Imbibition of water.

(xi) Increase in synthesis of many phospholipids.

(xii) Increased *de novo* synthesis of purines (dependent on new enzyme synthesis).

(xiii) Alteration in membrane excitability.

(xiv) Alteration in glucose metabolism.

(xv) Increase in synthesis of various mucopolysaccharides.

Levels of Differentiation

According to Berrill (1971) the differentiating system involving different proteins and enzymes falls into three categories. These are : —

1. Fundamental structures and metabolic pathways that exist in all cells.
2. Secondary metabolic pathways found in the cells of a number of tissues.
3. Characteristic function that occurs in single specific cells type.

The concentration level of the proteins in all three categories varies during differentiation. It is clear from this picture that the whole process is the net result of the activation or modulation of the activity of different genes.

Rutter, Wesself and others (1967) who worked on the developing mouse and rat pancreas with reference to both exocrine and endocrine cells recognise four levels of differentiation. They are:

(a) the undifferentiated state

(b) the protodifferentiated state

(c) differentiated state

(d) modulation

Though the levels of differentiation are four in number the changes involved are three. This can be well illustrated with reference to the differentiation of pancreatic cells:

(i) The first change involved is the conversion of the entirely undifferentiated cell to a cell with pancreatic character. Certain specific pancreatic proteins are found in easily detectable levels giving us the clue that the genes required for pancreatic differentiation are going to be switched on. This process involves certain important changes at the genetic level with repercussions in the developmental activities. This leads to the protodifferentiated level.

(ii) The second change involves the conversion of the protodifferentiated level to the differentiated state. This is an active period when cells undergo proliferation. After some time proliferation stops in cells that have begun to undergo differentiation. This secondary regulatory event is marked by the synthesis of ribosomal RNA, the grouping of functioning ribosomes and the development of the endoplasmic reticulum. According to Rutter (1967) there must be a common cause that brings about the formation of endoplasmic reticulum, stoppage of cell proliferation and increased protein synthesis.

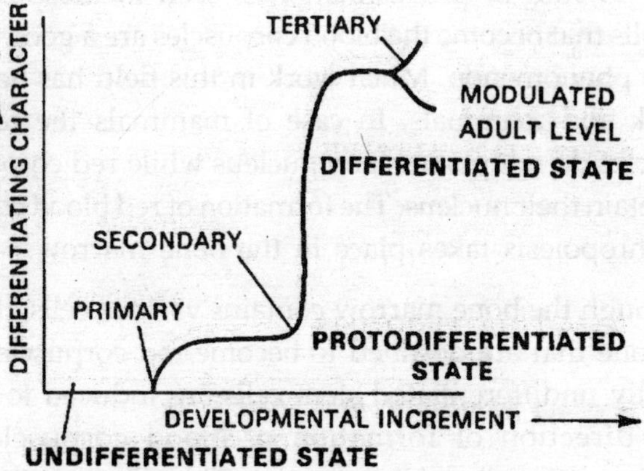

Possible regulatory stages in cytodifferentiation (After Berrill, 1971)

(iii) The third and final change involves certain modifications that make the cell definitely distinct from earlier stages. These are changes that occur at a very late stage in development and can be called modulation. This final differentiated state occurs in response to extracellular factors like metabolites or hormones. According to Wessells (1967), mitosis is not only important for growth but also for differentiation. He suggested two examples to explain his concept.

(i) Cells that can produce antibodies when come across antigens, always divide first before the process of antibody formation takes place.

(ii) The mammary cells when induced by hormones first undergo cell division before the secretion of casein in response to hormone stimulation.

Stem Cell : The "undifferentiated cells" that act as source material for various specialised tissues are found in all parts of the body and are called "stem cells". All structures of the plant arise from the stem cells and as these cells also give rise to various other differentiated cells they are aptly called stem cells. Though stem cells are supposed to take up any role, a certain amount of predestination is seen in these cells. The stem cells that become the blood corpuscles are a good example for this phenomenon. Much work in this field has been done in chick and mammals. In case of mammals the red blood corpuscles do not possess any nucleus while red corpuscles of chick retain their nucleus. The formation of red blood corpuscles or erythropoiesis takes place in the bone marrow.

Though the bone marrow contains various cells, it is some cells alone that are destined to become red corpuscles. These originally undifferentiated stem cells are induced to proceed in the direction of formation of blood corpuscles. This phenomenon is called determination. The substance that brings about this induction is called determiner. In this case the determiner is a hormone called erythropoietin. The stem cells now become proerythroblasts and undergo a series of changes called maturation. During the period of maturation certain interesting chemical changes occur. These include formation of new proteins, carbohydrates, enzymes, lipoproteins, nucleoproteins and the ability to synthesize haemoglobin.

Bessis (1967) suggests that erythropoietin which is found in plasma acts on stem cells by initiating transcription of earlier repressed genetic loci. In this way it acts as a depressor. The hormone causes the accumulation of glucosamine, haemoglobin synthesis and mRNA synthesis. The accumulation of iron is explained by the fact that (i) erythropoietin stimulates the marrow cells to accumulate that is needed for haeme synthesis. (ii) globin removes the haeme and directs its iron towards haemoglobin formation.

A very interesting aspect of the RBC formation is that the RNA synthesis is completely stopped in mature cells. Even in chick RBC, where a nucleus is present RNA synthesis is completely lacking.

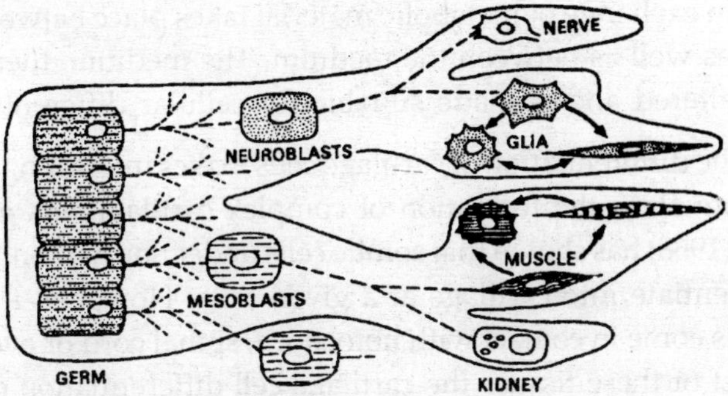

Differentiation of unspecialised embryonic cells (stem cells) into neuron, glea, muscle and kidney cells.

Effect of Microenvironment on Differentiation : Has the microenvironment anything to do with differentiation? Do cells differentiate when they are isolated? These are interesting questions that are well answered by some experiments.

The epidermal cells of the basal layer which proliferate remain unspecialised. Once these cells loose their attachment with the basal membrane they become crowded and are forced into more superficial layers of the epidermis. The cells of more superficial layers synthesize keratin. It is very clear that the cells differentiate and synthesize keratin only where they become separated from the basement membrane or only when they enter a new microenvironment. It shows that environment has a greater impact on the determination of fate and differentiation of undifferentiated cells.

Wilde (1961) did experiments with isolated undifferentiated, pigment cells. He observed that isolated cell kept in a hanging drop in culture medium never differentiates.

On the other hand, if two cells are kept in hanging drop, one of them undergoes differentiation. It is possible that this is due to the influence of the neighbouring cell and also due to the change the micro-environment brought about by the presence of the other cell. If more cells are kept together then the number of cells that differentiate also increases. It is possible that an exchange of metabolic material takes place between the cells as well as between the medium. The medium, therefore, gets altered and is made suitable for cellular differentiation.

The differentiation of cartilage cells makes interesting study as it involves the formation of complex cartilaginous matrix. Lash (1968) has shown that somite cells under normal conditions differentiate into cartilage at a given time. However, if these tissues come in contact with notochord, spinal cord or even the extract of these tissues the cartilage cell differentiation occurs faster. Lash explains this by stating that when somites are exposed to various inducers like notochord, spinal cord or the extract of these tissue the activity of the existing metabolic patterns is increased.

On the whole the problem of cellular differentiation is an interesting phenomenon. According to Khruschev (1981) cellular differentiation is a central problem of developmental biology.

10

Organogenesis

Development of Central Nervous System : The central nervous system in vertebrates develops from the neural tube. Originally, the anterior end of neural tube is expanded and walls are thicker than in its posterior part. The anterior expanded part of neural tube develops into the brain and the remaining part as spinal cord.

Development of Brain

The anterior part of neural tube swells into three brain vesicles:

(i) the prosencephalon or forebrain.

(ii) the mesencephalon or midbrain.

(iii) the rhombencephalon or hindbrain.

Prosencephalon : The pronsencephalon is the anterior-most vesicle. It gets divided into two swellings, the telencephalon and diencephalon. The telencephalon grows bigger and by a middorsal depression lengthwise, it forms two cerebral hemispheres of the adult brain. The cerebral hemispheres grow forward into the olfactory lobes. The diencephalon remains diencephalon. Its roof remains thin and becomes highly vascular. This vascular region is called anterior choroid plexus. From the roof of diencephalon also develops a pineal gland or epiphysis borne on a short thin pineal stalk. The floor of diencephalon grows ventrally into a finger-like projection, the infundibulum. It gets attached to the outgrowth from the roof of buccal cavity. This is known as Rathke's pocket. It grows into the pituitary body.

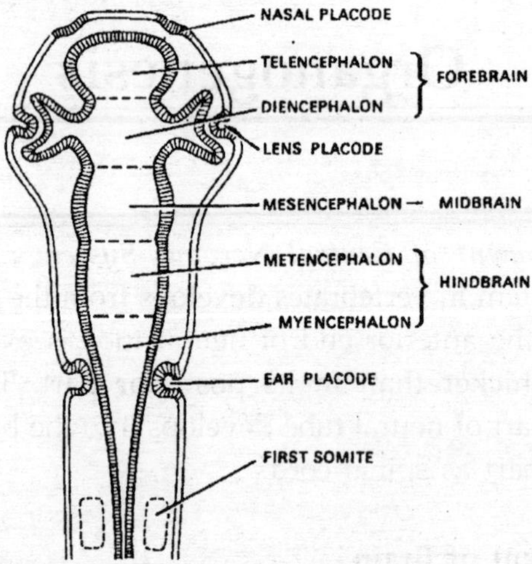

Diagram showing primary brain vesicles

The telencephalon and diencephalon in higher vertebrates (reptiles, birds and mammals) bend downwards. This bend is called cephalic flexure.

Mesencephalon : The mesencephalon does not change very much. It develops into the midbrain. Its side walls become thick. In non-mammalian vertebrates the dorso-lateral walls of mesencephalon swell to form the optic lobes. In mammals the optic lobes are four in number. The optic lobes are formed as two pairs of bulgings arising from the roof of mesencephalon. These are called corpora quadrigemina.

Rhombencephalon : The third brain vesicle gives rise to anterior metencephalon and posterior myelencephalon. The metencephalon is narrow, ring-shaped and develops into cerebellum. In lower vertebrates it is not well-developed. In higher vertebrates, the floor of metencephalon grows down into two swellings which develop into Pons varolii. Two bulgings arising from its dorsal wall fuse to form cerebellum of the adult. The myelencephalon gives rise to medulla oblongata. Its roof is thin and highly vascular. The capillary net in this area forms the posterior choroid plexus.

The Spinal Cord

The remaining part of neural canal modifies into spinal cord. It elongates dorsoventrally and becomes laterally compressed. It swells in girth at the level of arms and legs forming the brachial and sciatic plexus. The neural canal changes into a narrow central canal.

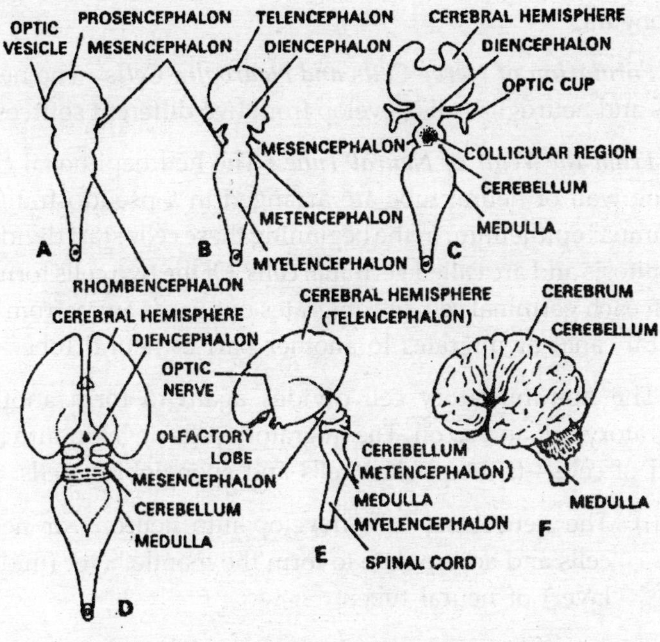

Different stages in the development of brain in man

Cavities of the Brain and Spinal Cord : The neural canal enlarges at various places inside the brain to form the brain cavities or ventricles. In the cerebal hemispheres the neural canal grows as two out-pushings and forms the two lateral ventricles. These are connected with the rest of the neural canal by two short passages.

These are called foramina of Monro. The neural canal inside the diencephalon gets vertically elongated and forms diocoele or third ventricle. Inside the mesencephalon, the neural canal remains a small cylindrical cavity, the iter or aqueduct of Sylvius. The neural canal inside the metencephalon and myelencephalon forms fourth ventricle of medulla oblongata. In all vertebrates except mammals the cavity inside the optic lobes is called optocoel which remains connected with the iter of mesencephalon. In mammals optic lobes are solid.

The neural canal in the spinal cord changes into a narrow central canal. It is connected with the fourth ventricle of medulla oblongata.

Formation of Nerve Cells and Neuroglia Cells : The nerve cells and neuroglia cells develop from two different sources —

From the Wall of Neural Tube : The neuroepithelial cells in the wall of neural tube are arranged in a pseudostratified columnar epithelium. In the beginning these cells start dividing by mitosis and are called germinal cells. Of the two cells formed from each germinal cell, one migrates outwards away from the neural canal or migrates to another part of neural tube.

The non-migratory cell divides again to form another migratory cell and so on. The migratory cells develop into two kind of cells—(i) neuroblast cells and spongioblast cells.

(i) The neuroblast cells develop into neurons or nerve cells and accumulate to form the mantle layer (middle layer) of neural tube.

(ii) The spongioblast cells develop into four types of neuroglia cells. The neuroglia cells have extremely thin fibrous processes and act as a packing material.

The spongioblast cells which remain near the neural canal and also some original columnar cells of neural tube form tall cells. These tall cells are called ependymal cells and the layer formed by them is called ependymal layer. These border the neural canal.

In adult the ependymal cells are pyramidal with their bases directed towards the central cavity and the tips produced into filaments which lie amongst the nerve cells of the brain and spinal cord.

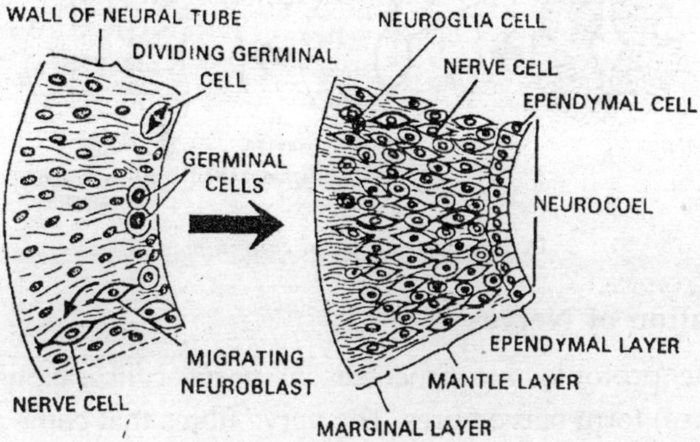

Development of nerve cells (After Balinsky).

From Cells of Neural Crest : The neural crest cells migrate to various places and develop into the following — (i) ganglia of dorsal root of spinal nerves, (ii) parts of ganglia of cranial nerves (other parts of these ganglia are formed from the ectodermal thickenings called placodes), (iii) ganglia of autonomic nervous system, (iv) nerve net in the wall of intestine, (v) pigment cells, visceral skeleton, parts of subcutaneous connective tissue, medulla of adrenal gland, etc.

The part of spinal cord from the central canal to the outer boundary of the mantle contains numerous neurons and neuroglia and develops into gray matter of spinal cord. Outside the mantle lies the marginal layer of cord. It contains processes of neuroglia, neurons and ependymal cells and forms the white matter of the spinal cord.

The spinal ganglia are formed from the neural crest. Some cells of the neural crest migrate from their site to the sides of the spinal cord and aggregate as to form spinal ganglia. The main part of the cells in spinal ganglia differentiate, as nerve cells and their long processes grow out as axon. These connect the neurons to peripheral organs.

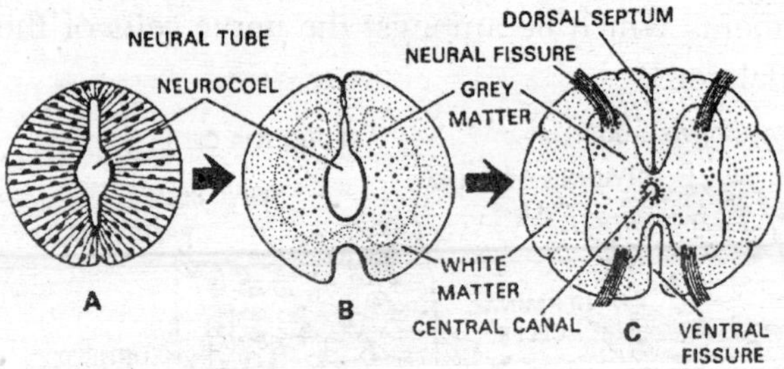

Development of spinal cord in man

Formation of Nerves

The protoplasmic processes of nerve cells (axons and dentrites) form nerve fibres. The nerve fibres that come out of the brain, spinal cord or ganglia in the form of bundles form the nerves. The presumptive nerve cell body sends out an amoeboid process. The protoplasm flows into the process causing it to move ahead forming nerve fibre. Special cells called Schwann cells then flatten out and wrap themselves around the fibre like an insulation. The free ends of these fibres keep on extending till they reach among the cells of various organs.

The first fibres to penetrate into the surrounding tissues are called pioneer fibres. These are followed by others which apply themselves to the pioneer fibre and form a cable. In case of olfactory nerve cells, ear ganglia cells and retinal nerve cells, the nerve fibres come to the brain from these organs.

Induction for the Differentiation of Central Nervous System: The roof of archenteron, the prechordal plate, induces formation and differentiation of neural plate and neural tube. The anterior part of the prechordal plate induces the differentiation of forebrain and eyes. It is called archencephalic inductor. In most posterior part of archenteron roof induces the formation of hindbrain and associated structures (the deuterencephalon inductor) and the most posterior part of archenteron roof induces the formation of spinal cord and muscle (spino-caudal inductor)

Development of Eye

The development of eye begins during late neural stage soon after the differentiation of primary brain vesicles.

Formation of Optic Cup : The rudiments of eye project out as a pair of sac-like protrusions from the lateral walls of prosencephalon. These are called optic vesicles. When fully formed, these become constricted from the prosencephalon. The narrow connection between the optic vesicle and brain is called optic stalk. It forms the basis for the development of optic nerve.

The optic vesicles grow outward until they almost touch the epidermis. Soon after the outer-wall of optic vesicle flattend and then invaginates. Thus the optic vesicle changes into a double-walled optic cup. The entire optic cup has nervous origin. The invaginated thick layer (inner one) develops into neurosensory retina of the eye, while the external thin layer develops into the pigmented coat of retina, called the tapetum nigrum. The cells of inner wall multiply rapidly and change into nerve cells (ganglionic cell), glial cells or Muller fibres and rods and cones. The cavity of the optic cup is the future posterior chamber of eye. The rim of the optic cup later develops into the edge of pupil.

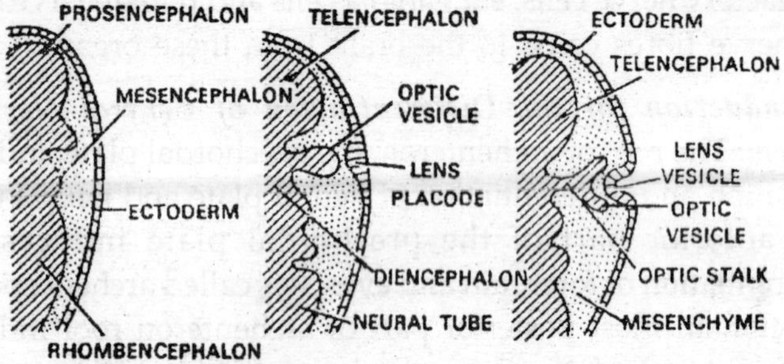

Development of optic vesicle in human embryo.

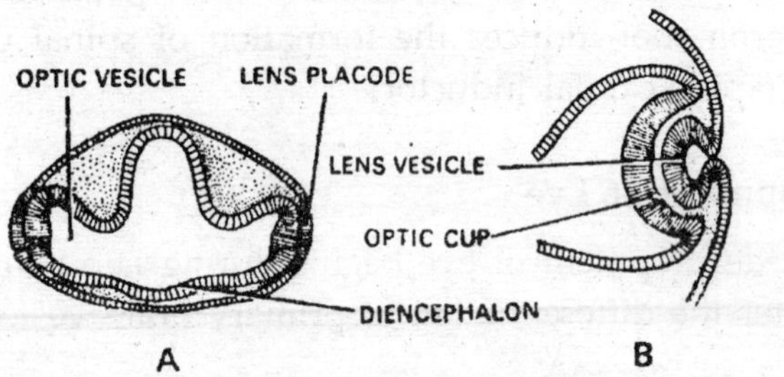

Development of optic cup and lens.

The opening of optic cup is very large at first. Soon its rim bends inward and converges reducing the opening of the pupil. The rim of the optic cup surrounding the pupil becomes the iris. Later on, larger amount of pigment is deposited in the outer epithelial layer of iris. A groove extends along the ventral side of optic cup. It is choroid fissure. It extends to the middle of optic stalk. It serves for the entry of blood vessel and mesenchyme cells into the posterior chamber of eye. These cells and blood vessel develop into the vitreous body.

Development of Lens

Formation of Lens Placode : The lens rudiment develops in the epidermis on the lateral side of head. Its differentiation is initiated by the optic vesicle. When lateral surface of growing optic vesicle comes in contact with the epidermis it gives off a stimulus of some kind, which causes the epidermal cells to elongate, forming a thick disc-shaped thickening. This is called lens placode or lens rudiment. The lens placode curves inwards into a cup and finally separates from the ectoderm. The free edges of the cup fuse to form a globular hollow lens vesicle. The lens vesicle comes to lie in the cavity of the optic cup. (ii) Cytodifferentiation of Lens — The cells on the inner side of the lens vesicle elongate, become columnar and are finally transformed into long fibres. Their nuclei degenerate and cytoplasm becomes hard and transparent making it refractile. A part of the lens epithelium remains unchanged. It covers the sphere of fibres. The junction between the unchanged lens epithelium and mass of lens fibre represents the growing point of the lens. Here, lens epithelial cells are transformed into lens fibres adding to the growth of lens.

There is a direct relation between the development of optic cup and lens. The optic vesicle induces the formation of lens placode, which in turn, induces the optic vesicle to invaginate.

When lens is formed the free margin of optic cup touches the edge of lens and grows in front forming iris. Thus lens hangs in the opening of optic cup.

Development of Cornea

The mesenchyme between the lens and the lens ectoderm forms a transparent fibrous covering the cornea. It gets joined with the free margin of celerotic coat. The ectodermal cells covering cornea form an extremely thin, transparent membrane. This is known as conjuctiva of the eyeball. In adult this becomes continuous with the inner lining of upper and lower eyelids.

The space between the lens vesicle and the overlying presumptive anterior epithelium of cornea represents the anterior chamber. It contains cellular material called anterior vitreous body.

Development of Choroid and Sclerotic Coats : When the

optic cup and lens are forming the mesenchyme cells appear all around these structures. The inner layer of these mesenchyme cells gives rise to a network of blood vessels surrounding the pigmented retinal epithelium and is called the choroid layer. The outer layer of mesenchyme cells forms a fibrous capsule the sclerotic coat around the eye. Some mesenchyme cells form a thin capsule around the lens. This is called the lens capsule.

Ciliary Body : The circular band all around the iris is the ciliary body. It is formed by a part of the rim of the optic cup and the mesenchymal cells. The mesenchymal cells differentiate into smooth muscle fibres of the ciliary body. These get arranged radially and circularly. Some of them get attached to the lens capsule through zonal fibres.

Eye Lids : The ectoderm of the lens placode region left after forming the lens changes into conjunctiva. The ectoderm from above and below the original lens placode region grows out as two folds. These folds grow over the conjunctiva and come to touch each other forming a complete layer of ectoderm over the conjunctiva. At a later stage these folds separate along the line of fusion to form the regular upper and lower eyelids.

Development of Olfactory Organ

The nose rudiments are determined at late gastrula stage, but these appear as two distinct thickenings only after the closure of neural tube. The epidermis on the head, ventrolateral to the forebrain thickens into two circular patches to form the olfactory placodes. Each placode then invaginates into a cup-like structure, called nasal sac or olfactory sac. The rims of sac grow outward so that the sac becomes a horse-shoe-shaped structure. In man and other mammals the two sacs with their rims approach each other. Finally, they come to lie side by side in front of mouth. The rims of the sacs form the wall of nostrils and nasal septum, while the cells of roof and sides of the olfactory sacs form the olfactory epithelium. Its cells differentiate into olfactory neurons and supporting cells. Later, the olfactory neurons give out protoplasmic processes that form the olfactory nerve. The olfactory nerve joins the olfactory sac with the olfactory lobe of the brain. The openings of the nasal sacs form the external nares or nostrils and the openings of extensions of nasal sacs into pharynx as internal nares.

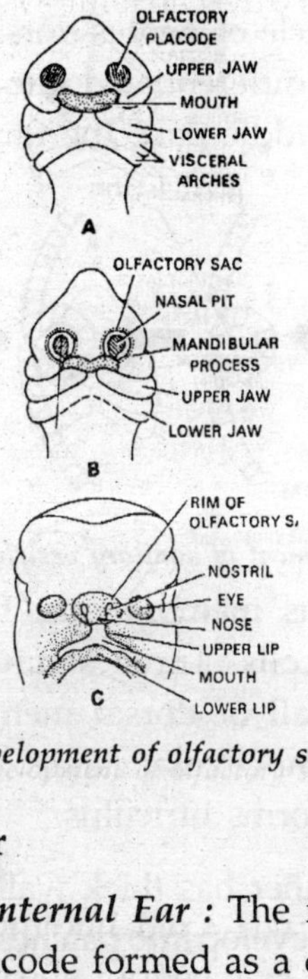

Development of olfactory sacs

Development of Ear

Development of Internal Ear : The internal ear develops from the auditory placode formed as a circular thickening in the ectoderm near the side of rhombencephalon. In human embryo it develops about the third week after fertilization. The auditory placode invaginates to form a cup-like structure with a wide opening on the surface. The rim of the cup grows making the opening narrower. Ultimately, the edges fuse and an auditory visicle is formed, which finally separates from the ectoderm.

In frog, the auditory placode is formed from the neuroectoderm. Therefore, the auditory cup does not open to the surface at any time. In bony fishes, the auditory vesicle arises as a solid mass of cells which later develops a cavity.

Formation of Membranous Labyrinth : From the auditory-vesicle arises a short blind tube which develops into endolyphatic duct.

The auditory vesicle elongates dorsoventrally and due to unequal growth gets differentiated into two sacs, joined by a narrow cylindrical middle part, the utriculo-saccular duct.

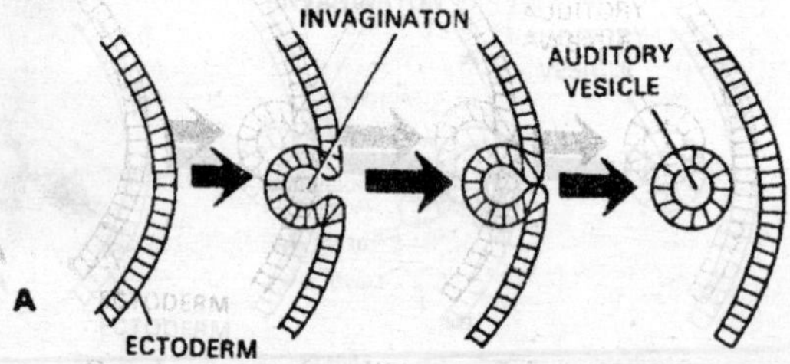

Development of auditory vesicle in man

The dorsal part is membranous. Its wall is formed of flattened epithelial cells. Three semi-circular outpushings develop from the wall of dorsal membranous part. These develop into three semi-circular canals. The remaining part of the dorsal chamber forms utriculus.

The ventral chamber has thick wall formed of columnar cells. At places these develop into patches of second epithelium. These sensory patches are called maculae of the internal ear. The ventral sac develops into the sacculus. A cochlear tube bulges out from the wall of sacculus. It develops into a spiral having 2,1/2 turns. The cochlear duct remains connected with the sacculus by a narrow duct, called ductus reunions. A hollow outgrowth of the sacculus forms the rudiment of lagena in frog but is not formed in man.

The semi-circular canals, utriculus, sacculus, ductus endolymphaticus and cochlea, etc. all are filled with endolymph. The wall of membranous labyrinth is very thin. It is formed of a single layer of flattened epithelial cells, covered by a thin fibrous layer of connective tissue. The surrounding mesenchyme cells give rise to cartilaginous ear capsule or otic capsule. This protects the membranous labyrinth. Later on it becomes bony and is called bony labyrinth. The space between the bony labyrinth and membranous labyrinth is filled with perilymph.

At two places the bony labyrinth remains membranous. At one place the membrane is oval and other one round. The former is called oval window (fenestra ovalis) and gets connected to the stapes, the bony piece of the middle ear. The round membrane is called the round window (fenestra rotunda). It faces the cavity of the middle ear. The bony labyrinth gets embedded in the petrous part of the temporal bone.

In fishes and amphibia, the utriculus and sacculus are formed in the same fashion but cochlea is not formed. In reptiles and birds a short tubular lagena develops instead of cochlea.

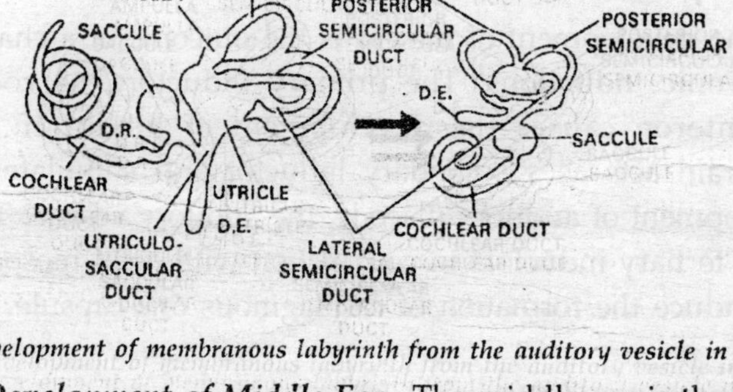

Development of membranous labyrinth from the auditory vesicle in man

Development of Middle Ear : The middle ear is the space containing ear ossicles (in mammals) or columella (in amphibians, reptiles and birds) and its openings is covered with tympanic membrane. The middle ear is formed from the first pharyngeal pouch, which is formed as an out- pocketing of the endoderm of pharynx and grows towards the first pharyngeal groove. The cavity of the pharyngeal pouch forms the cavity of middle ear and the mesenchyme present between the pharyngeal pouch and pharyngeal groove develops into three ear ossicles — the malleus, incus and stapes.

Initially the pharyngeal pouch is a wide space. It gradually narrows into a tube. It opens into the pharynx at one end by a narrow eustachian tube. Its opening to the exterior is covered by tympanic membrane. Its cavity is connected with the internal ear by oval window and round window.

Development of External Ear : The tubular external auditory meatus is formed by the first pharyngeal groove; the tympanic membrane from the ectoderm of the first ectodermal groove and endoderm of the first pharyngeal pouch and the pinna is formed from the mesenchyme and ectoderm from a region near the first pharyngeal groove. The mesenchyme forms the fibro-cartilage, connective tissue, blood vessels of the pinna and the ectoderm forms the skin epidermis of the pinna.

Auditory Induction

The development of the ear is the outcome of a chain of embryonic inductions. The primary inductor, the roof of archenteron causes the development of hindbrain. The hindbrain acts as a secondary inductor and stimulates the development of auditory placode, the auditory vesicle. These act as tertiary inductors in conjunction with head mesoderm and induce the formation of cartilaginous otic capsule.

Development of Skin

The epidermis part is formed from the embryonic ectoderm and dermis from the mesenchyme.

Development of Epidermis

In human embryo, the skin is formed of a single layer of cuboidal ectodermal cells. These divide by mitosis to form two layers. The upper layer of cells forms the periderm or epitrichium and the lower layer forms ectoderm. Periderm is lost during development. By the end of second month, the ectoderm cells multiply and form 2-3 layers of cells. The basal layer of ectoderm cells is called stratum germinativum or stratum basale. Its cells continue to divide adding layers towards the outer side. Its cells are columnar. The new layers formed get differentiated in distinct layers of different types of cells. The epidermis in adult human being gets differentiated into following layers —

Ectoderm

Stratum Germinativum or Stratum Basale : It lies on the basal lamina and is formed of single layer of columnar cells. These divide very fast.

Stratum Spinosum : The cells of this layer have spinous protoplasmic processes. That is why this layer is called stratum spinosum.

Stratum Granulosum : The cells of this layer have keratohyalin granules. The cells are arranged in 3-4 layers.

Stratum Lucidum : This is a layer of dying cells. The cells are without nuclei and their cytoplasm contains a substance called eleiden (a modified keratohyalin).

Stratum Corneum : It is a thick layer of dead cells. The cells contain protein keratin and are greatly pressed. These are continuously sloughed off from the surface of epidermis.

Development of Dermis

The dermis is formed from the mesenchyme, originally derived from the mesoderm. In human embryo, some cells of dermatomes also join the mesenchyme. The mesenchymal cells form the connective tissue, blood vessels, pigment cells, etc. of the dermis. The nerve and nerve endings are extensions of peripheral nerves coming towards the skin.

Development of Circulatory System

Development of Heart : The heart in all vertebrates initially develops in a somewhat similar fashion. Let us study the development of heart in frog. The first rudiment of heart develops after the neurulation in the region beneath the pharynx from the mesenchyme and mesoderm.

Origin of Endocardium : The endocardium or inner lining of heart develops from the endocardial cells. These are derived either from the splanchnic mesoderm or are the remnants of the invaginating mesodermal cells of the ventral lip of blastopore. The endocardinal cells form a thin and loose sheet in the space between the pharynx and developing pericardium. Finally, these cells get organised to form a tube, the endocardial heart tube and the layer of endocardinal cells is the endocardium.

Origin of Pericardium : Simultaneously, under the inductive influence of archenteron, the free edges of lateral plate mesoderm converge towards the middle in the mesoderm-free zone just beneath the pharynx and the endocardium. The mesenchyme cells proliferate from the ingrowing tips of lateral plate mesoderm and get arranged into a longitudinal sheet of compact mesenchyme. Soon a pair of coelomic spaces appear within this mesenchyme sheet one on either side of the middle line. These spaces are called anterior coelomic spaces. These separate the mesenchyme sheet into two layers corresponding to the somatic and splanchnic layers of mesoderm.

On further development the paired coelomic spaces converge mesially and fuse together in the middle line below the pharynx encircling the endocardial tube. This is called the pericardial cavity. The outer somatic layer gives rise to pericardial membrane or pericardium, while the inner layer that corresponds to the splanchnic mesoderm forms the epimyocardium. The epimyocardium lies opposed to the endocardial tube. The epimyocardium now hangs from the remaining splanchnic mesoderm into the pericardium by a septum formed by the fusion of mesoderm above the epimyocardium. The septum is called dorsal mesocardium. It disappears a little later. The epimyocardium cells form a thin membranous outer coat, the epicardium and a thick muscular inner coat, the myocardium. The myocardium forms the muscles of the cardiac wall.

The somatic and splanchnic mesoderms of heart region join the somatic and splanchnic layers of lateral plate mesoderm, and the pericardial cavity becomes confluent with the body coelom. At a later stage a septum is laid down transversely between the pericardium and body coelom, completely separating them as independent cavities. This is called septum transversum.

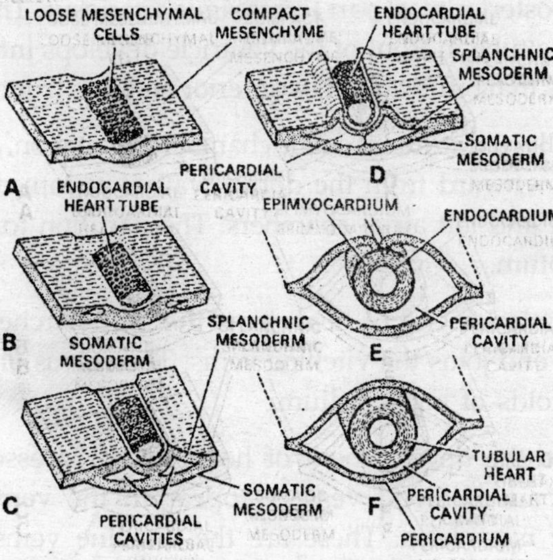

Formation of endocardial heart tube and the pericardium in frog embryo.

Differentiation of Heart : The heart thus formed is a straight tube, situated longitudinally in the middle line below the pharynx and surrounded by the pericardium on all the sides. Its wall is formed of three layers—outer epicardium, mesial myocardium and inner endocardium. The myocardium grows in thickness.

The tubular heart elongates rapidly in antero-posterior direction. The small size of pericardial cavity and the anterior and posterior attachments do not permit its increase in antero-posterior direction. The increase in size causes the originally straight tube to curve and fold forming S-shaped coiled tube. The anterior part is folded ventrally and posteriorly and the posterior part becomes folded dorsally and anteriorly.

At the same time different regions of the tube grow differently in thickness and constrictions appear demarcating different presumptive chambers of the adult heart. The bottom part of the loop with thick wall forms the ventricle. The posterior part of the tube above the ventricle forms thin-walled atrium, and the posterior most part forms sinus arteriosus. The anterior part of the tube in front of the ventricle develops into bulbous arteriosus that bifurcates at its anterior end into truncus aortae.

Initially, the atrium is single chambered. Later on, a partition grows downward from the dorsal wall of atrium dividing it into right and left atrial chambers. The partition forms inter-atrial septum.

The anterior end of heart joins the aortic arches and the posterior end joins the vitelline veins. The valves of the heart arise as folds of endocardium.

Before the development of heart has progressed to this stage a pair of blood vessels appear in the ventro-lateral splanchic mesoderm. These are the vitelline veins and are derived by the separation of yolk endoderm and ventral mesoderm. The two vitelline veins are connected with the sinus venosus. Further growth and enlargement results in more pronounced curvatures and foldings. Ventricle becomes folded caudally and ventrally to the atrium. Truncus arterious becomes partially subdivided by a vertical and longitudinal septum giving rise to paired aortae. Even prior to that a longitudinal sheet of endocardium grows down from the roof of atrial chamber and forms inter-atrial septum. This divides the atrium into right and left auricles. The sinus venosus comes to lie dorsally and opens into the right auricle. The left auricle gets connected with the pulmonary veins. With further changes in form and growth in size the heart of the adult frog is formed.

The heart is the first organ to start functioning, because it has to circulate blood which brings nourishment from the endodermal cells to other parts of the embryo.

11

Germinal Layers

As a result of gastrulation, the three primary germ layers or the embryonic layers become distinctly organized. These are ectoderm, mesoderm and endoderm. All the organs of the embryo are formed from these layers. The development of various organs is called organogenesis.

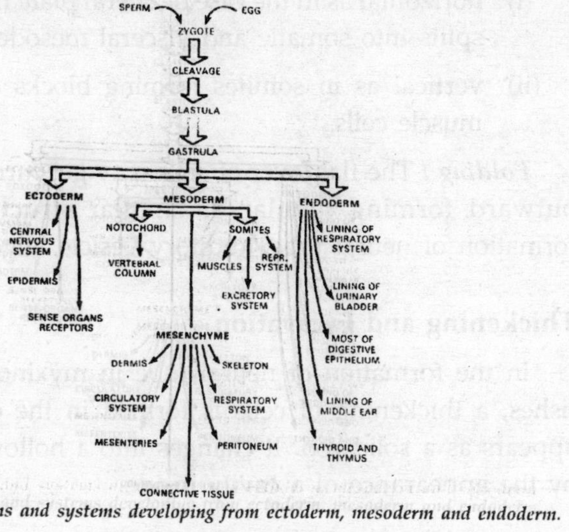

Summary of the organs and systems developing from ectoderm, mesoderm and endoderm.

Tubulation : In the first phase of organogenesis, the germinal layers get subdivided into groups of cells, the primary organ rudiments. The process of separation of primary organ rudiments is called tubulation. In the second phase the primary organ rudiments further subdivide forming secondary organ rudiments that differentiate into specific organs of the larva or adult.

Method of Organ Formation

Local Thickenings : Local thickenings in the germ layer are formed by the accumulation of cells. The cells may be derived either by increased mitosis in the cells of localised area or by the migration from the neighbouring regions. The thickenings may be of continuous type as in the formation of neural plate or discontinuous type as in the formation of hair germs, or placodes for scale or feather papilla.

Hair Follicle

Separation of Layers : This is separation of a multi-cellular layer into two or more layers. The split may be :

(i) horizontal as in the case of lateral plate mesoderm that splits into somatic and visceral mesoderm, and

(ii) vertical as in somites forming blocks or bundles of muscle cells.

Folding : The flat layer of cells may get turned inward or outward forming tubular or circular structures such as formation of neural tube, auditory vesicle, digestive glands.

Thickening and Excavation

In the formation of neural tube in myxinoids and bony fishes, a thickening of cells is formed in the ectoderm that appears as a solid rod. It changes into a hollow neural tube by the appearance of a cavity inside.

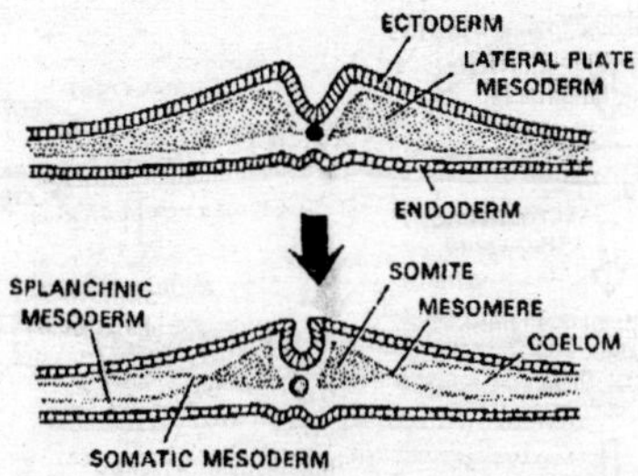

Splitting of lateral plate mesoderm into somatic and visceral layers by splitting.

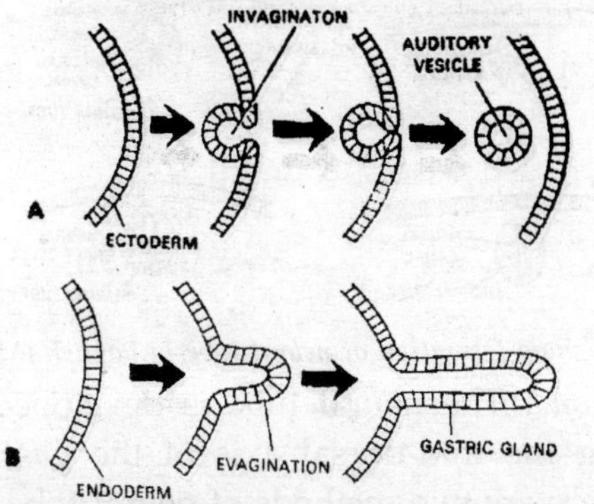

Splitting of lateral plate mesoderm into somatic and visceral layers by splitting.

Fusion : In amphibians, reptiles, birds and mammals the neural tube is formed by the fusion of neural ridges.

Mesenchyme Formation

The mesenchyme is formed from the cells of mesoderm. Some cells get detached from the mesoderm become amoeboid. These cells aggregate into sheets, form epithelium or endothelium and get associated with other tissues or structures forming bone, cartilage, blood vessels, smooth muscles of the alimentary canal or the peritoneal covering.

Neurogenesis (Development of Nervous System) : Neurogenesis is the formation of neural tube and its further differentiation into brain, spinal cord and different sense organs.

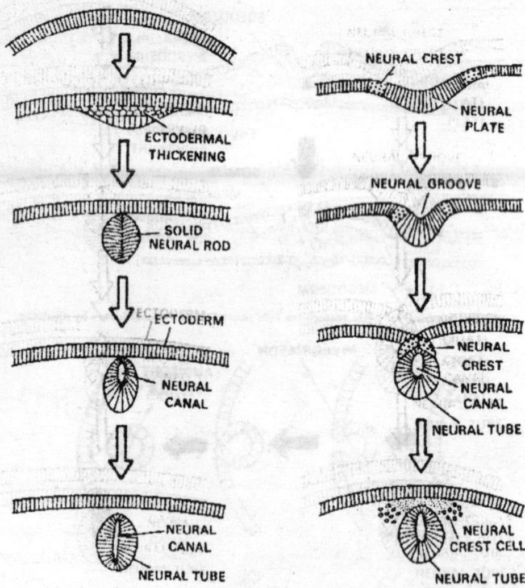

Diagram to show formation of neural tube in hagfish (Myxine)

Neuralisation : The neural tube is developed from the ectoderm along the mid-dorsal axis of the gastrula in all vertebrates. There are two methods of neural tube formation:

Thickened Keel Method : In cyclostomes and fishes, during neurula stage, the neural plate material becomes aggregated into an elongated ridge or rod of cells along the mid-dorsal axis of the embryo. The keel separates from the rest of the ectoderm and sinks below. Eventually, it becomes hollow forming the neural tube.

Neural Fold Method : In amphibians, reptiles, birds and mammals the neural plate formation begins by the division or accumulation of cells in the region of neuro-ectoderm. The ectodermal cells immediately in front of the blastopore (or in front of primitive streak in chick and mammals) begin to divide rapidly forming a thick plate of ectoderm. The division extends forward along the entire dorsal line. Soon the margins of neural plate elevate and its centre gets depressed forming a shallow neural groove. Later on the margins of neural groove meet dorsally in middle-line completing the formation of neural tube. Subsequently, it separates from the parent ectodorm.

- **A. Ectoderm or (Neuroectoderm)**
  - **1. Somatic Ectoderm** – Epidermis, epidermal derivatives (scales, feathers, hair, nail, claws, glands etc); olfactory organs, lens of eyes, auditory vesicles (labyrinth), ant.pituitary, lining of stomodaeum and proctodeum.
  - **2. Neural crest** – Ganglia; sensory nerves; branchial skeleton, adrenal medulla, pigment cells.
  - **3. Neural tube** – Brain, spinal cord, cranial and spinal motor nerves, retina, optic nerve and posterior pituitary.
- **B. Mesoderm (Chorda mesoderm)**
  - **1. Notochord** – Persists as a rod in *Amphiaxus;* in others replaced by vertebral column.
  - **2. Epimere**
    - **(a) Dermatome** – Dermis
    - **(b) Sclerotome** – Vertebral column
    - **(c) Myotome** – Skeletal muscles and appendicular skeleton.
  - **3. Mesomere**
    - (a) Excretory organs
    - (b) Reproductive organs
  - **4. Hypomere**
    - **(a) Somatic layer** – Parietal peritoneum
    - **(b) Splanchnic layer** – Visceral peritoneum, mesenterics, heart, blood cells, blood vessels, gonads, muscles of viscera.
    - **(c)Coelom** – Body cavity.
- **C. Endoerm (Archenteron)** – Lining of degistive tract, liver, pancreas, respiratory system, bladder, endocrine galnds (tyroid, parathyroid, thymus); lining of vagina, urethra, reproductive glands, auditory the tube and cavity of middle ear.

The anterior part of the neural tube differentiates as brain and the posterior part forms the spinal cord.

Neural Crest Cells : After the completion of neural tube and of epidermal layer a few cells are left between the two. These form strip along the crest of the neural folds and are called neural crest cells. During development, these form ganglionic cells, pigment cells, mesoderm of the head and branchial area of the adult.

Neural Induction or Initiation of Neurulation : The formation of neural tube is stimulated by the chordamesodermal cells present in the underlying roof of archenteron. These are called primary organizers or neural inductors. The neural inductor (the chorda-mesoderm) imposes regional specificity or the neural plate. Its anterior part induces formation of brain and head organs and is called head inductor. Its posterior part induces the differentiation of trunk organs and tail buds and is called spinocaudal inductor or trunk inductor.

Notogenesis and Mesogenesis

The development of notochord from chordamesoderm is called notogenesis, and the separation of mesoderm as mesogenesis. The cells of the middle line in the roof of archenteron round off to form the notochord. It lies just below the developing neural tube.

On the sides of notochord, the mesoderm spreads out in the form of sheet. It grows down on either side of the gut and meet in the mid-ventral line. The mesodermal sheet splits into two layers, the outer layer near the ectoderm is called somatic mesoderm and the inner layer applied to endoderm is the splanchnic mesoderm. The space between the two is the coelom. At the same time, the sheet gets subdivided horizontally into three distinct regions : (i) the dorsal-most segment flanking the neural tube and notochord is the epimere, (ii) the middle segment mesomere, and (iii) the ventral segment flanking the gut is hypomere.

The lateral wall of epimere is called dermatome. It forms the dermis part of the skin. Its dorsal median wall is called sclerotome. It forms vertebrae. The ventro-median wall is the myotome that forms the skeletal muscles and appendicular skeleton. The mesomere gives rise to excretory and reproductive organs.

12

The Gastrulation

The events which transform a blastula into a gastrula are collectively called gastrulation. According to McEwen (1923) gastrulation refers to the formation of the primordial gastric or gut cavity called the archenteron. In addition to the formation of gastrular cavity, the process also involves the development of two of the three primordial germ layers, referred to as the ectoderm (epiblast) and endoderm (hypoblast). The third layer called mesoderm (mesoblast) is derived from one or the other or both of the two layers; the endoderm is the inner layer; and the mesoderm is the middle layer.

Lankester (1875) and Hubrecht (1906) were of the opinion that the gastrulation is a process during which the single layered blastula is converted into a two-layered (e.g., Amphioxus) or three-layered (e.g., most vertebrates) embryonic stage called gastrula.

During gastrulation, the cells are recognized and rearranged. This arrangement of cells is brought about by very complex but coordinated movements and shifting of positions of large masses of cells. According to Balinsky(1970) "The process of gastrulation involves displacement of parts of the early embryo. As a result the endodermal and mesodermal organ rudiments are removed from the surface of the embryo, where the presumptive material for these rudiments is to be found in the blastula-stage. These are then brought into the interior of the embryo, where the respective organs are found in the differentiated animal. Concomitantly, the single layer of cells, called blastoderm, gives rise to three germinal layers - the ectoderm, the endoderm and the mesoderm".

Prominent Features of Gastrulation

The process of gastrulation is basically characterized by following events :

1. A rearrangement of the cells of the embryo takes place by means of formative or morphogenetic movements.
2. The pace of cellular division is slowed down.
3. Growth, if any, is trifling.
4. The rate of oxidation is intensified and the type of metabolism changes.
5. The nuclei become more active in governing the activities of the embryonic cells.
6. The influence of the paternal chromosomes becomes clear during gastrulation.
7. New kinds of proteins, that were formerly not present in the egg, begin to be synthesized.

General Processes Involved in Gastrulation: Morphogenetic Movements : Gastrulation is essentially a process of movement of parts of the embryo. As a result of these movements new structural elements e.g., the archenteron, the neural tube and the notochord, are created in place of the simple layer of cells found in the blastula. The cell movements during gastrulation create new shapes, new forms in the embryo. They have been, therefore, designated as the morphogenetic movements.

Morphogenesis: (Greek *morphe, shepe; genesis,* production) literally means the origin and development of new form. The gastrulation movements are irreversible in nature i.e., each part remains in the position into which it has been brought by the preceding movement.

In the majority of animals, the regions of the blastula which will give rise to the germ layers are already determined on its *surface,* as revealed by studies of organ-forming zones. Therefore, gastrulation must involve an interiorisation of the endoderm — and mesoderm-forming zones. Interiorisation of the endoderm-forming regions occurs first, by *either or both* of two general processes : (1) epiboly, and (2) emboly.

Epiboly : The term epiboly is derived from Greek meaning 'throwing on' or 'extending upon'. This morphogenetic movement involves overgrowth of the ectoderm-forming regions around the endoderm-forming regions. Epiboly is characterized by a rapid proliferation of cells in the animal half and concomitant spreading of this enlarging sheet of cells over the vegetal half. It merely involves the gradual growth of the blastoporal lip over the yolk, or the yolk-filled vegetal cells. The movement takes place not due to any actual process of stretching, but on account of active cell division in the overgrowing layers. This activity is most intense in the region of the blastoporal lip. The epibolic movement is enhanced by surface tension changes which produce a crawling of the cellular rim over the yolk.

Epiboly of ectodermal blastomeres (epidermal and neural areas) has been observed most typically in the development of eggs possessing abundant yolk. In the rounded blastulae *of amphibians,* the prospective ectodermal cells spread over the inwardly moving presumptive notochordal, mesodermal and endodermal blastomeres. In flattened blastulae of *teleost fishes, reptiles* and *birds,* epibolic movements take place in the form of antero-posterior extension, associated with migration and expansion of the ectodermal blastomeres on the peripheral region.

Emboly **:** The term emboly is also derived from Greek meaning 'throw in' or 'thrust in'. This morphogenetic movement involves in growth of the endoderm forming-regions under the ectoderm-forming regions. Stating simply, it is the movement of chorda-mesodermal and endodermal blastomeres from the external surface of the blastula to the interior of the embryo. The inward formative movement of prospective chordamesodermal and endodermal blastomeres in different groups of vertebrates may occur by following methods :

Invagination: The simplest method of gastrulation is invagination. The movements *of in folding"* or *"inward bending"* of the endoderm and mesoderm are known as invagination. In this process, the vegetal half of the blastula is pushed in or invaginated until it almost touches the animal half opposite to it. Thus a simple spherical body becomes converted into a double-walled cup, as if one side of the wall of an elastic hollow ball had been pushed in by an external force. The original blastocoel becomes virtually obliterated and the cavity arising through the invagination is called the primary gut or archenteron. The opening leading from this cavity to the exterior is called the blastopore. The blastopore, being the opening leading into the primary gut, has been likened to the mouth. Its rims, therefore, are usually referred to as the lips of the blastopore. As such, we may distinguish the *dorsal lip,* the *ventral lip* and *lateral lips* of the blastopore, respectively.

The archenteron is lined by the original vegetal cells which give rise to endoderm and mesoderm. The part of the gastrula that remains on the surface becomes ectoderm.

Involution or Inflection: The term involution means a *"turning in"* or *"rolling under"* of chorda-mesodermal cells along the blastoporal lip. It is very common among the vertebrates and is often accompanied with invagination. The blastocoel is greatly reduced egg that gastrulate by involution. At some point on the edge of the blastoderm the dividing cells begin to be turned over the blastoporal rim, *i.e. involuted* in the blastocoel. As a result, the cells located on the external margin of the blastoporal lip, roll over the lip and are brought to the inside edge of the lip just beneath the ectodermal blastomeres. These inturned cells then constitute the hypoblast (chorda-mesoderm) while those which remain without are epiblast (ectoderm). The involution is most active on the dorsal lip of the blastopore.

Infiltration: This process involves the *"inwandering"* or infiltration of cells from the blastoderm into the blastocoel lying beneath. This space may be largely filled with yolk, e.g., chick, while in mammals the amount of yolk is not much. In any case the cells originating in this way soon spread out to form a continuous layer called hypoblast. The cavity which formerly represented blastocoel, now becomes the *archenteron.*

Delamination: Gastrulation by delamination takes place most typically in mammals and to some extent in amphibians and birds. The process consists simply the separation of, *splitting off* of the cells from a pre-existing layer. These cells then unite together to form the hypoblast.

Concrescence: There is a gradual drawing together of the blastoporal lips during epiboly with the result that the blastopore is continuously diminished in size. However, in the course of this procedure, there is no thickening of the lips as their circumference decreases. This fact may be explained by assuming that much of the material which blastoporal lips contain is required to form the germ layers. It is thought, therefore, that during the course of gastrulation two sides of the blastoporal ring *"flow"* together at a certain point upon the margin of the blastoderm. This movement is, therefore, designated as confluence or concrescence. According to this theory, it was believed that each side of the blastoporal ring forms a lateral half of the axial structure of the embryo. This theory was applied specifically to telolecithal eggs with large quantity of yolk.

Convergence: This refers to the movement of groups of cells from each entire posterior half of the blastoderm toward the median line forming the axial structure of the embryo.

Ingression: It is the *"inward migration"* of mesendoderm-forming cells from the external layer of the blastula or blastodisc into the blastocoel. Gastrulation by invagination was described by Pasteels (1945) in reptiles, birds and eutherian mammals.

Extension or elongation: It refers to the extension of cellular masses in the antero-posterior axis during gastrulation. The elongation of the presumptive neural plate, and of the notochordal, mesodermal and endodermal materials after they gather up beneath the neural plate, are examples of extension. Extension or elongation is a prominent procedure during gastrulation of all chordates.

Constriction: This term is used with reference to the convergence of cell areas which results in the gradual closure of blastapore. It occurs in frog's egg during gastrulation and is due to a narrowing of the marginal zone and a pull of the dorsal lip.

Significance of Gastrulation

1. Gastrulation brings the presumptive structures from a position on the external surface of the blastula into their definitive positions in the embryo.
2. It is necessary for the morphogenesis of nervous system.

Growth : Growth is the developmental increase in mass. It results due to synthex of new protoplasm which includes both the cytoplasm and nucleus of cells. Besides, protoplasmic products such as the fibres of connective tissue and the matrix of bone and cartilage are also responsible for growth. Increase in mass is usually accompanied by cell division. Cell multiplication continues throughout the development and to a variable degree, throughout the life of the individual. Thus, cell multiplication is a distinguishing characteristic of growth.

Differentiation : The increasing diversification of form and function in an organism is called differentiation. It refers to the events by which cells or other parts of an organism become different from one another and also different from their previous state. The differentiation may be of three types :

(i) morphological,

(ii) behavioural, and

(iii) chemical differentiation.

Morphological Differentiation: During multiplication, individual cells and groups of cells differentiate structurally from other cells. For example, *nerve cells* and *epidermal cells* which start from a common point in generalized ectoderm, develop diagnostic features of size, shape and internal organization.

Behavioural Differentiation: Although all cells possess common basic characteristics, such as irritability and metabolism, yet special functional responsibilities are laid upon these general properties. For example, nerve cells conduct neural in pulses, muscles function to contract, epithelium serves to protect, skeletal elements provide support, and so on.

Chemical Differentiation: It is based on enzymes. Enzymes direct the synthesis of the organic compounds that provide the cell its uniqueness. Cell constituents such as carbohydrates, lipids, and organic acids are synthesized under the influence of enzymes. Therefore, a given battery of enzymes will operate the pattern of these organic compounds. For example, as the various vertebrate eggs undergo cleavage and progressively become converted to blastula, gastrula, and definitive embryo; individual cells, and areas of cells in each case become biochemically different from the other. It results in the formation of a different and distinct adult from a particular egg.

Major Events during Gastrulation

(i) There is rearrangement of cells due to morphogenetic movements of the cells of blastoderm.

(ii) The three primary germ layers get differentiated.

(iii) The cleavage rate is slowed down.

(iv) Growth if any is insignificant.

(v) Oxidation becomes intensified, so oxygen consumption increases and the nature of metabolism changes.

(vi) Nuclei become physiologically active and control activities of embryonic cells. The influence of paternal chromosomes on the embryo becomes evident.

(vii) Synthesis of new kinds of proteins begins.

Gastrulation in Amphioxus (with Isolecithal and Holoblastic Eggs) : In isolecithal egg (as in *Amphioxus*), gastrulation is essentially an inpocketing of blastula. This results in the formation of a double- layered cup from a single-layered hollow sphere much as one might push in a rubber ball with a thumb.

In *Amphioxus*, blastula is ball-like with a large blastocoel surrouned by a single layer of columnar cells. At the onset of gastrulation, the blastoderm at the vegetal pole becomes flat. It gradually bends inwards till the embryo assumes the appearance of a double-walled cup. Its external layer is the presumptive ectoderm and the inner layer is formed of the presumptive endoderm and elements of notochord and mesoderm.

The cavity formed by invagination is called archenteron or primitive gut. Its opening is called blastopore and the embryo at this stage is gastrula.

As a result of invagination, the presumptive endoderm, mesoderm and notochord are shifted from the surface to the interior of the embryo. The blastocoel is gradually obliterated till the two layers come in contact. By the completion of gastrulation, the lateral horns of mesodermal crescent converge and come to lie on either side of the presumptive notochord.

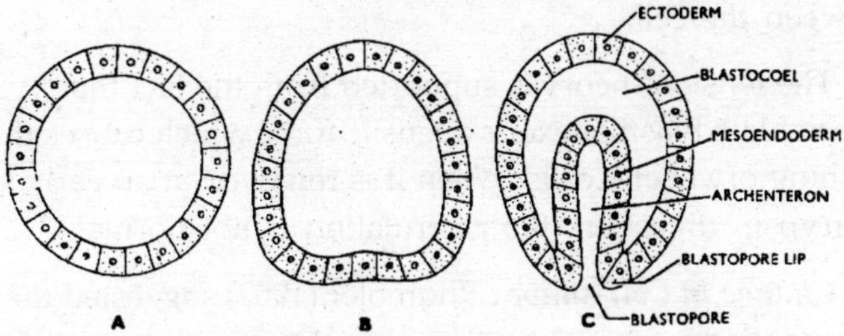

Gastrulation in Amphioxus by invagination (After Conklin, 1932).

Physiology of Invagination

Pressure of Dividing Cells : The early interpretation was based on the concept that a lateral pressure develops among the cells of blastoderm due to increase in their number. This pressure acts in the plane of polar axis of the egg and causes invagination of cells.

Moore (1941) conducted experiments on echinoderm embryos to test this concept. He found that the isolated cell plates from vegetal pole undergo invagination, though there are no cells to exert pressure. This indicates that invagination is not caused due to the pressure of dividing cells.

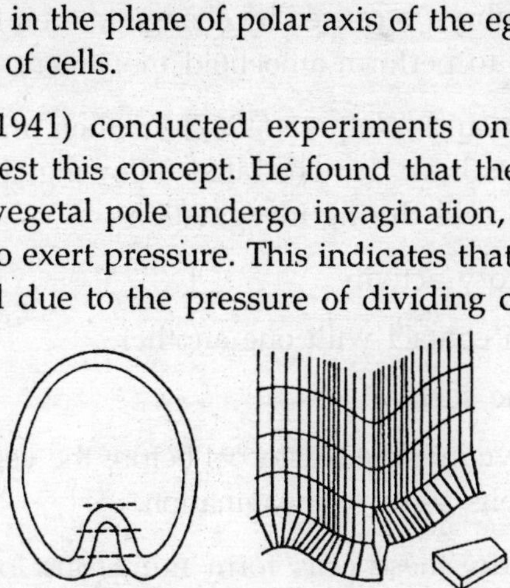

Diagram to represent Moore's experiment on isolated plates from vegetal region. A- A normally invaginated gastrula. B- An isolated piece from vegetal plate undergoing invagination.

Tension Theory : Moore's experiments indicated that the forces producing invagination in isolated plate of vegetal cells to form a comparatively small gastrula, exist in the endodermal plate. These forces act in the plane of vegetal plate and are disposed from the centre outward in the form of a radial gradient. The pocketing is caused by the differential cohesion between the cells.

The tension theory is supported from the fact that hyaline layer of late blastula exerts a tensile force which causes the in-pushing of vegetal cells. When it is removed at an early stage by trypsin digestion, the gastrulation is not normal.

Change in Cell-shape : Rhumbler (1902) suggested that the invagination is caused by change in the shape of vegetal cells. Butschli (1915) and Spek (1940) described a differential swelling between the outside and inside of endodermal layer. The differential swelling is caused by special arrangement of lyophilic and lyophobic colloids in the cells of endoderm.

Holtfreter also advocated that the inward migration of cells of the embryo is caused by change in their shape, which enables them to perform amoeboid movement.

Gustafson and Wolpert (1967) in their microcinemato graphic studies have demonstrated following changes in the mesenchymal cells during invagination—

(i) pulsatory activity,

(ii) loosen contact with one another,

(iii) hyaline surface.

These move into the blastocoel before the vegetal plate as a whole exhibits signs of invagination.

Once inside, these cells form numerous long and thin temporary pseudopodial outgrowths, which attach to the inner surface of gastrular ectoderm. Their contraction pulls the tip of archenteron into the blastocoel.

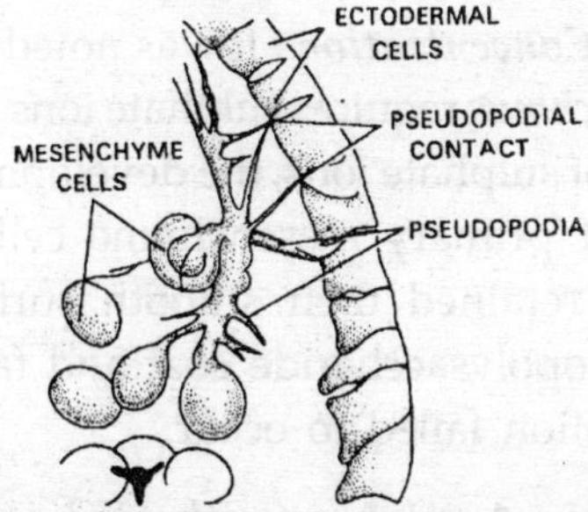

The pseudopodial attachment of primary mesenchymal cells to the ectodermal wall in sea urchin embryo (Alter Gustafson 1967).

The cells of vegetal plate continue to maintain contact with the inwardly-migrating mesenchyme cells and also with the hyaline surface layer, but have reduced mutual contacts with each other. Therefore, these cells become pearshaped with rounded inner ends which exhibit pulsatory activity indicating that these are being pulled in by the invaginating mesenchyme cells.

Fibrilisation Theory : Waddington (1940) suggested that the tonofibrils that pass through cell boundaries produce the effect necessary for invagination. Definite evidence in favour of this theory is not as yet available. Microphotographs of invaginating mesenchyme cells by Tilney, Gibbilens and Porter have, however, shown large number of microtubules which are distributed parallel to the long axis of pseudopodia of mesenchyme cells. When these pseudopodia fuse, their microtubules become aligned parallel to the long axis of the cell. These influence the development of filopodia from the primary mesenchyme cells.

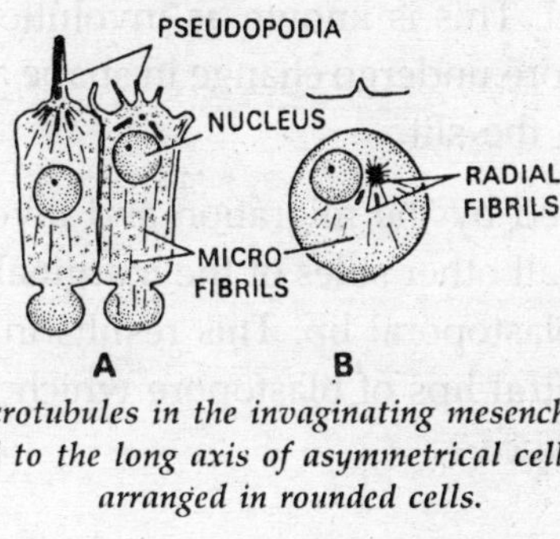

Distribution of microtubules in the invaginating mesenchyme cells. These are arranged parallel to the long axis of asymmetrical cells, but are radially arranged in rounded cells.

Sulphate Ion Concentration : It was noted that the embryo of sea urchin, *Lytechinus* requires sulphate ions for invagination. In sea water free of sulphate ions, the development was normal upto the stage of primary mesenchyme cell migration. But after that, these retained their smooth surface; lacked the sulphonated mucopolysaccharide coat and failed to migrate. As such invagination failed to occur.

Gastrulation in Amphibia (with moderately telolecithal holoblastic eggs) : In the eggs of amphibians, certain fishes and the jawless vertebrates, the flattening and inward bending of vegetal region as in *Amphioxus* cannot occur because the vegetal wall of blastula is far too thick, is overladen with yolk and is rather passive. In them, gastrulation is brought about by the processes of invagination, involution and epiboly occurring simultaneously.

The onset of gastrulation is marked by the appearance of an infolding on the border-line of vegetal region and marginal zone exactly below the gray crescent area. The infolding forms a narrow groove. It marks the beginning of archenteron and its opening represents the beginning of blastopore. The fold above the groove represents the dorsal lip of developing blastopore.

Involution : The cells of prospective chorda-mesoderm (mesenchyme cells present along the posterior margin of grey-crescent) start rolling inward along the dorsal lip of blastopore into the blastocoel. This is known as involution. The cells at the rim of blastopore undergo change in shape and this causes them to sink into the slit.

This is followed by the migration and involution of new micromeres from all other sides of the marginal zone towards and around the blastoporal lip. This results in the formation of lateral and ventral lips of blastopore which finally assume a circular appearance.

Epiboly : Meanwhile, the more active micromeres of the animal half that represent the future ectoderm, divide rapidly and gradually spread over the macromeres of vegetal hemisphere and gradually push the blastopore towards the vegetal pole. Eventually the circular blastopore gradually moves downward and gradually diminishes in size. In the end it can be seen as a small closed circle with a few macromeres jutting out of it in the form of yolk plug.

Invagination : Along with the epibolic growth of micromeres, the macromeres of presumptive endoderm of the vegetal region stream inward, increasing the archenteron. Their insinking is known as invagination.

During invagination, the surface cells of the dorsal lip of blastopore become elongated and flask-shaped as they approach the blastopore. This process continues until bulk of each cell has moved completely inside.

Electron micrographs of invaginating cells show that their inner ends are produced into long microvilli that interdigitate with the adjacent cells, through which these cells are attached to the archenteron surface. Though, the inner ends of these cells have loose cohesion with the adjacent cells. Their outer ends are firmly attached together and to the surface coat. This tight coherence of cells is responsible for the continuation of invagination.

Primary Germ Layers : Once inside, the chorda-mesoderm and endoderm elements move to their final positions. The endoderm cells come to occupy the floor and sides of the archenteron, while the roof is formed of prechordal plate. It is formed of the material of notochord and mesoderm. This forms a continuous-sheet, called chorda-mesodermal mantle which finally gets constricted off the archenteron and comes to lie between the ectoderm and endoderm. Its lateral ends grow down between the ectoderm and free margin of endoderm.

Integration of Gastrulation

Various theories have been put forward to account for the orderly integrated movements of cells responsible for amphibian gastrulation. According to Holtfreter (1943) these movements are associated with the following basic facts:

(i) all the cells respond to changes in their environment,

(ii) cells have different kinetic behaviour and

(iii) in the embryo cells with different kinetic behaviour are grouped together in local patches and finally the cell coat which is an integral part of egg surface, influences the behaviour of cells.

Holtfreter has summed up the role of cells and surface coats as follows:

(i) The shape of individual cells reflects the direction of their movement.

(ii) Invagination is associated with the temporary transformation of constituent cells into flask-shaped cells.

(iii) The boundaries of the inner cells are not continuous so that each cell is a descrete unit, interconnected with its neighbours only by slender processes.

(iv) All peripheral cells are firmly held together by a common surface coat of plasticity.

(v) The elastic cell coat produces tension on the egg surface.

When the cells enter the phase of morphogenetic movement by the origin of epibolic and invagination activities within them, the cell coat acts as a supercellular agency to coordinate their activities in the following two manners—

(a) it regiments the amoeboid activities of the invaginating cells, so that their collective effect is able to produce pulling force;

(b) it transmits the gliding movement of cells to adjacent regions.

The significance of cell coat has been demostrated by Holtfreter by the following experiments —

Experiment 1 **:** When endodermal cells covered with surface coat are placed on a mass of uncoated endoderm cells of the deeper layer, the coated cells spread over the uncoated cells.

Experiment 2 **:** In contrast, when a mass of uncoated endoderm cells is placed on uncoated endoderm substrate, it becomes incorporated.

Experiment 3 **:** If a mass of blastoporal cells partly covered with external coat is grafted to the endoderm substrate, the graft invaginates and forms a blastopore, with bottle cells adhering to the coated area.

Gastrulation in Birds (with Highly Telolecithal, Meroblastic Eggs) **:** Gastrulation in highly telolecithal eggs (birds, reptiles and fishes) is greatly modified due to exceptionally large amount of yolk. The excessive yolk prevents the formation of blastopore, though an area homologous with the blastopore can be identified.

The blastodisc of chick blastula is differentiated in area pellucida and area opaca. In area pellucida the blastoderm is formed of an outer layer, the epiblast and an inner layer, the hypoblast. The hypoblast is separated from the underlying yolk by a subgerminal cavity. The epiblast and hypoblast are separated by blastocoel. The epiblast has mixed blastomeres for ectoderm, mesoderm and endoderm while hypoblast represents the presumptive endoderm only. The process of gastrulation and embryo formation is confined to area pellucida (embryonal area) and is closely related to the formation of primitive streak whose long axis establishes the antero-posterior axis of the embryo.

Pregastrular Movements

A series of morphogenetic movements of the cells from epiblast bring the presumptive areas of blastoderm to their definitive positions. These are —

1. The growth of blastoderm margins over the yolk to form yolk-sac. These growth movements are unrelated to the formative movements.
2. *Forward Movement of Hypoblast Cells* : The hypoblast cells from the posterior end of area pellucida flow in a 'fountain-like fashion' and spread out towards anterior and lateral edges of the blastodisc.
3. *Formation of Primitive Streak :* At about 6-7 hours after fertilization, the cells of lateral platemesoderm begin to converge at the posterior edge of area pellucida in the middle line. The cell aggregate forms a thickening and marks the future caudal end of the embryo. By the addition of more and more cells the thickening becomes more demarcated and lengthens in cephalo-caudal axis.

This is primitive streak. By 16 hours after incubation, the primitive streak is fully formed. It is differentiated into — (i) A narrow median furrow extending along the middle-line of primitive streak—the primitive groove. (ii) The thickened sides of the streak form the primitive ridges. (iii) The thickened caphalic end of the streak represents Hensen's node or primitive knot.

Morphogenetic Movements

The morphogenetic movements leading to the formation of primitive streak include movement of cells from the epiblast towards the posterior median end of area pellucida and their convergence in the middle-line. The cells from the lateral and antero lateral parts of the epiblast swing in a curve backward and inward during primitive steak formation.

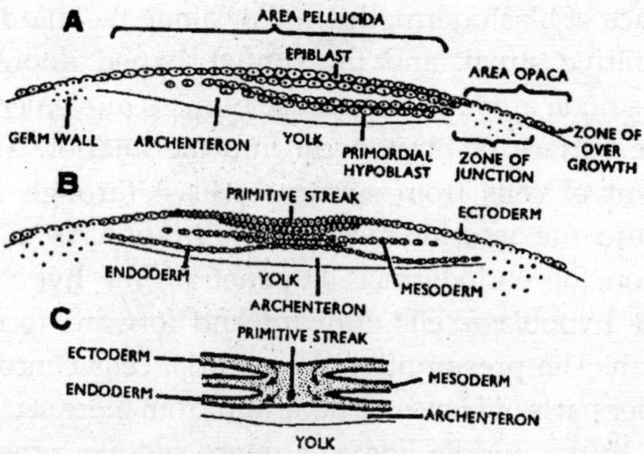

Diagram showing gastrular movements in chick —in Section.

The primitive sreak is the symbolic homologue of the blastopore, that could not be formed because of impeding effect of enormous yolk. Therefore, the movement of cells towards the thickened area is comparable to epibolic movements of cells towards amphibian blastopore. The equivalence of these structures with amphibian gastrula are as follows- (i) Primitive streak = dorsolateral margins of amphibian blastopore. (ii) Hensen's node = dosal lip of blastopore.

The primitive streak has bipolarity. Its anterior half comprises of elements of presumptive endoderm and mesoderm both, while the posterior half forms the extra-embryonic mesoderm.

Gastrular Movements

These include migration of cells of mesoderm and endoderm from the primitive streak. In the primitive streak region, the cells from the blastoderm detach, become amoeboid and move singly downward the hypoblast. This type of gastrular movements are called immigration. This is followed by the arrival of new cells from epiblast to the primitive streak, so that entire epiblast and the primitive streak are masses of moving cells.

Thus in birds process of invagination is different from both *Amphioxus* and amphibians. The formation of depression on the surface of blastoderm, the furrow along the middle-line of the primitive streak and the funnel-shaped depression in Hensen's node are formed because of mass movement of cells from the surface of blastoderm into the interior. This mass movement of cells from surface epiblast through primitive streak into the interior is called infiltration.As a result of infiltration the endoderm cells penetrate the hypoblast and push the hypoblast cells outward and forward forming the endoderm. The presumptive notochordal cells concentrate in the deeper parts of Hensen's node and from there start moving forward in the middle line as a dense rod-like process. This is known as head process or notochordal process. This marks the beginning of notochord. The presumptive mesoderm cells from primitive streak sink in and migrate laterally between the epiblast and hypoblast. These form the mesoblast. The mesoblast cells retain junctional contact with the cells of primitive streak. At this stage, the chick embryo consists of upper layer of ectoderm, middle layer of chorda-mesoderm and inner layer of endoderm. The presumptive notochordal tissue underlies the median embryonic axis with mesoderm on either side.

Gastrulation in Mammals

The small alecithal eggs of mammals are almost certainly derived from large yolky meroblastic eggs like those of reptiles and birds. The process comparable to gastrulation is completed by cell-segregation and delamination. The cells of inner cell mass or the embryonic knob, nearest to the blastocoel split off to form the endoderm. This is known as delamination. The endoderm cells spread rapidly and line the blastocyst as a relatively large sac. Its cavity is known as yolk-sac cavity or the gastrocoel. In the posterior half of the blastoderm a short primitive streak develops as a thickening of the embryonic ectoderm. Mesoderm is formed from the cells moving sideways from the streak between ectoderm and endoderm. Notochord also develops from the primitive streak.

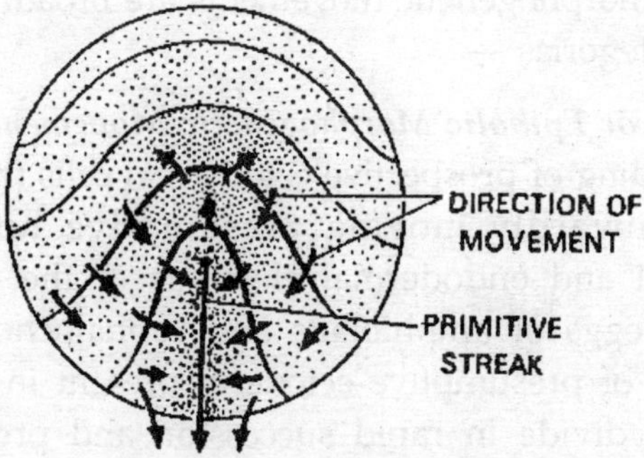

Movements of the epiblast cells during the formation of primitive steak (After Wetzel, 1929).

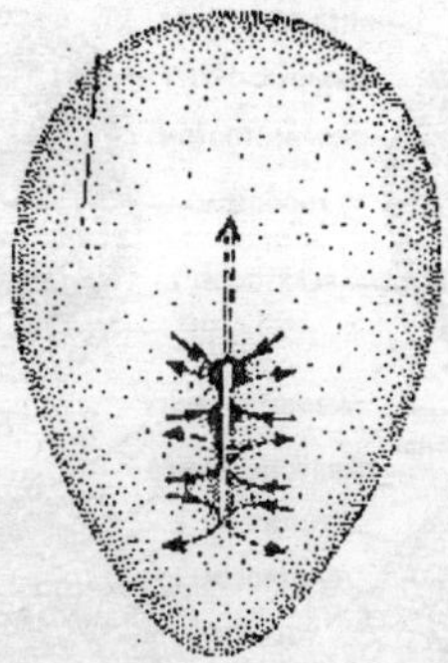

Diagram showing morphogenetic movements during gastrulation. Solid arrows indicate movement of cells in epiblast while broken line arrows on the right show immigration of cells from primitive streak into the interior Based on Rosenquist 1966).

Formative Movements or Morphogenetic Movements : The migration of cells of organ-specific areas from the surface of blastula to their prospective positions is the most important event of gastrulation. These movements of cells are described as formative movements or morphogenetic movements, because such movements help in morphogenesis (development of a particular structural pattern). The morphogenetic movements occur during blastulation, gastrulation and neurulation stages. The morphogenetic movements that occur during embryogenesis are of irreversible nature, while those of adult are reversible.

All the morphogenetic movements are broadly separated into two categories —

Epiboly or Epibolic Morphogenetic Movements : Epiboly is the spreading of prospective ectodermal cells (micromeres) over the inwardly moving presumptive notochordal, mesodermal and endodermal elements of the embryo. In holoblastic eggs of amphibians and cephalochordates, the micromeres of presumptive ectoderm present in the animal hemisphere divide in rapid succession and produce large number of cells which migrate downward and spread over the macromeres of the presumptive endoderm.

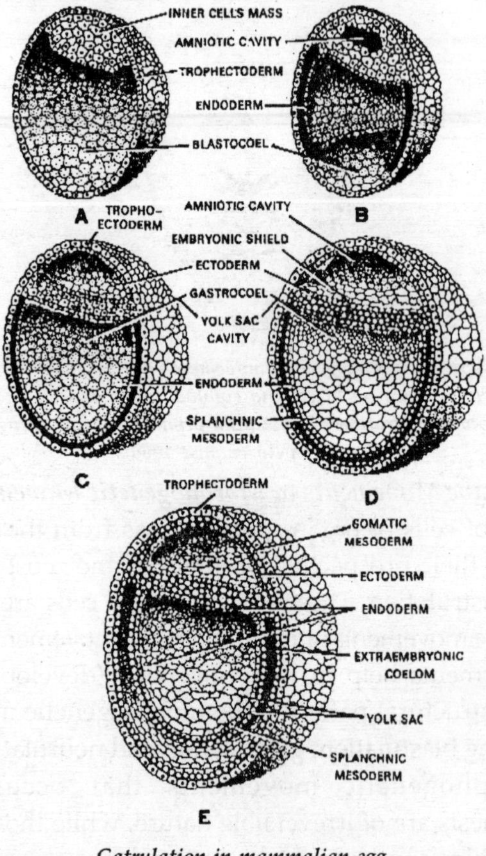

Gatrulation in mammalian egg

In flattened blastula of reptiles, birds and teleosts the epibolic movements are represented by antero-posterior extension and expansion of blastomeres associated with peripheral migration during the formation of primitive streak and the separation of germ layers.

Emboly or Embolic Morphogenetic Movements : Embolic movements are concerned with the inward migration of prospective chorda-mesodermal and endodermal blastomeres from the surface of blastula and their extension along antero-posterior axis of the developing embryo. The tendency of inward migration of specific cells is inherent and involves changes in the morphology of cells. These embolic movements are different in different animals and are as follows —

Invagination : It is the insinking or infolding of a layer of cells (prospective endoderm) to form archenteron. This process occurs in unmodified form in microlecithal egg as in *Amphioxus*, and Ascidian. In higher chordates with macrolecithal eggs, the process is greatly altered and augmented by other means. (ii) Involution — it is turning in or inward rotation of cells of mesoderm and endoderm from the surface of blastula inside over the edge of blastopore. In frogs and amphibians (moderately telolecithal eggs), the dividing micromeres (the yolk-free cells) which had started spreading over the yolky macromeres from all sides, now begin to turn inside over the blastoporal rim at one point. The inturned cells form chorda-mesoderm. The edge of blastoderm at which this inflection takes place is known as blastoporal lip.

Infiltration or Ingression : In reptiles, birds and fishes, gastrulation is brought about by infiltration or ingression. The cells or groups of cells from the epiblast detach and move downward into the blastocoel and arrange themselves into distinct layers, the mesoderm and the endoderm. Loutrup (1974) has described two types of ingressions —

(a) Multipolar ingression implies the movement of randomly distributed cells from their original positions into the blastocoel. The ingression of cells may be either because of paratangential cell division or by primary delamination. Multipolar ingression occurs at the time of segregation of two primary germ layers in reptiles and birds.

(b) Unipolar ingression occurs only in one region which is always located around the vegetal region. It is involved in the segregation of germinal layers in the flagellated blastulae of Porifera and Cnidaria. In amphibians, the segregation of mesoderm takes place.

Delamination : In mammals, gastrula is formed by the separation of splitting off of the cells from pre-existing layer of mass into the blastocoel. The separated cells arrange themselves below the trophoblast to form the hypoblast. The blastopore is not formed.

Accessory Processes

Three important processes always occur alongwith either of the processes described. These are:

Concrescence or Convergence : As process of epiboly continues, it gradually draws the two lips of blastopore towards the middle line leading to the convergence of those areas towards the middle-line which will form the axial structures in the embryo (such as neural tube, notochord). This movement of areas is called convergence or concrescence.

Divergence : It is opposite to convergence. After the cells have involuted over the blastoporal lip, they migrate and diverge to occupy their future positions inside the developing embryo, as for example, the movement of lateral plate mesoderm, ventral mesoderm in frog and the extraembryonic mesoderm in reptiles, birds and mammals.

Extension : It is the elongation of the entire embryo in antero-posterior axis.

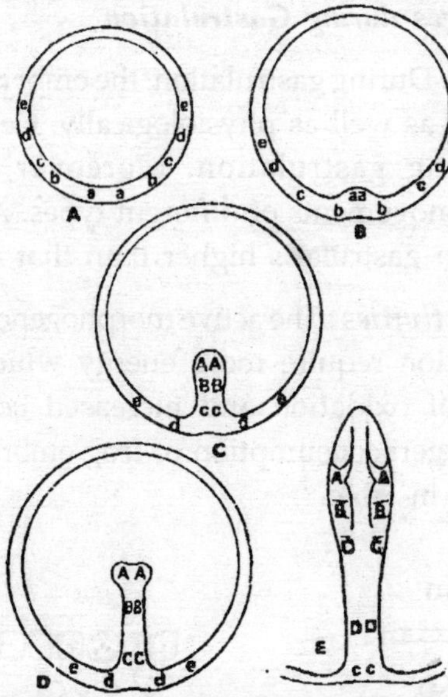

Diagrams showing the formation of an embryo by confluence (Concrescence). A—germ ring before the formation of embryo is indicated. (The latters a-e represent symmetrical portions of the germ ring); B—beginning of confluence; C—embryo forming (AA, BB, represent regions of the embryo formed out of the materials of the germ ring at aa, bb); D and E—later stages in the formation of the embryo (The germ ring regions cc and dd have been differentiated into the embryonic regions, CC, DD). (After McEwen, 1949).

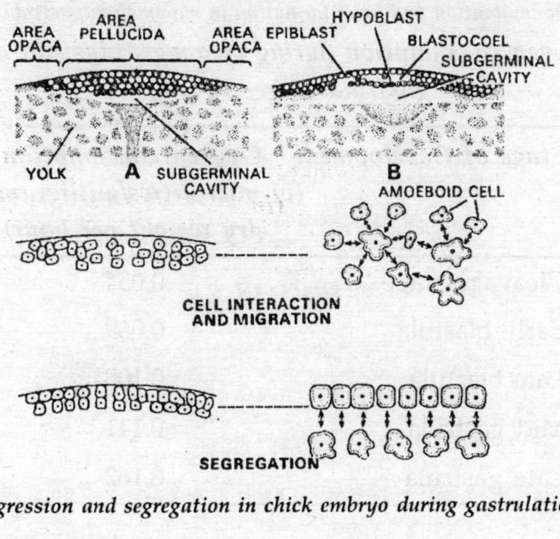

Ingression and segregation in chick embryo during gastrulation.

Chemical Changes during Gastrulation

Metabolism: During gastrulation, the embryo is very active morphologically as well as physiologically. Cell-division still continues during gastrulation. Moreover, cells exhibit morphogenetic movements of different types. As a result, the metabolic rate in gastrula is higher than that of blastula.

Catabolic Activities: The active morphogenetic movements during gastrulation require more energy which leads to an increased rate of oxidation and increased consumption of oxygen. The oxygen consumption of frog embryo in different stages is shown in table.

Layer Formation

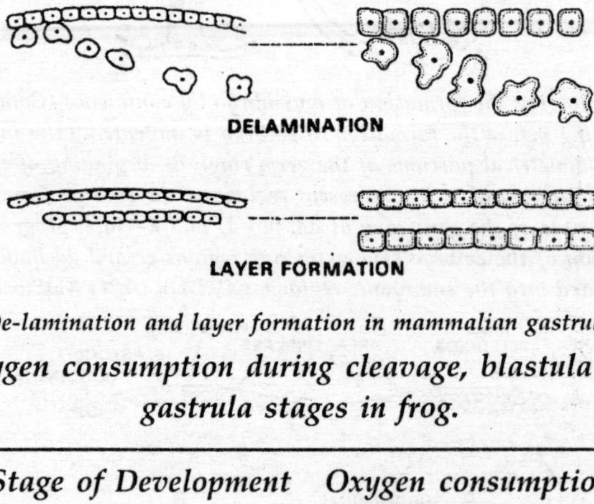

De-lamination and layer formation in mammalian gastrula.

Oxygen consumption during cleavage, blastula and gastrula stages in frog.

S.No.	*Stage of Development*	*Oxygen consumption (in microlitres/milligram of dry weight per hour)*
1.	Cleavage stage	0.054
2.	Early blastula	0.069
3.	Late blastula	0.108
4.	Mid gastrula	0.141
5.	Late gastrula	0.162

The food reserve utilized for oxidation and release of energy in the form of ATP are glycogen and yolk. In frog embryo it has been observed that:

(i) the amount of glycogen reduces considerably in the invaginating cells of dorsal lip of blastopore;

(ii) the highest consumption and breakdown of glycogen is at the animal pole on the dorsal side and it is lowest at the vegetal pole

Under electron microscope, the breakdown of yolk platelets has shown following steps :

(i) The amorphous or granular peripheral layer gets dissolved. This layer is formed of proteins and considerable quantity of RNA. The dissolved material enters the cytoplasm and is made available for different synthetic activities. The dissolution of peripheral layer occurs at different times in different parts of the embryo. For example, during early gastrula the solubilization occurs in the invaginating chorda-mesoderm cells; whereas in the gastrula it takes place in the cells of epidermis that exhibits movement.

(ii) The crystalline core or the main body of yolk-platelets gets dissolved in later stages.

Anabolic activities-Protein synthesis and systhesis of nucleic acids are the anabolic activities in gastrula.

Protein Synthesis : During gastrulation there is sharp increase in protein turnover. By measuring the uptake of radioactive precursors, Tiedmann and Tiedmann (1954) have recorded five-fold increase in protein synthesis in *Triturus* embryo between early gastrula and late tail bud stage when gastrulation is completed and organ rudiments are formed. The increase in protein synthesis is three-fold in the gastrula of sea urchin.

The raw material required for protein synthesis is availed from the protein yolk contained in the eggs of most animals.

The proteins synthesized during gastrulation are markedly different from those present during cleavage and blastula stages. The new proteins are synthesized under the instructions of parental genes which become active only during gastrulation.

In sea urchins and amphibians, the gastrulae possess antigen-proteins, capable of initiating the formation of antibodies. Such antigen proteins are not present before gastrula stage.

Synthesis of Nucleic Acids : Division of cells by mitosis continues throughout gastrulation. Therefore, there is continuous replication of DNA for the duplication of chromosomes during each mitosis.

During gastrulation the rate of transcription of new mRNA and tRNA molecules increases greatly for the synthesis of new kinds of proteins. The increase is more than ten fold within one hour in the frog, *Xenopus laevis.*

Gene Activity during Gastrulation

It has been observed that the enucleated fragments of sea urchin eggs undergo cleavage but fail to undergo gastrulation. During cleavage, the duplication of chromosomes at each cell division is controlled by the proteins already present in the egg cytoplasm. On the onset of gastrulation, the genes present in the chromosomes produce large quantities of RNAs of different types.

Their production can be demonstrated and measured by using radio actively labelled uridine which is taken up into the synthesis of RNA molecules. Presence of mRNA, tRNA and rRNA can be detected in gastrula indicating the activity of genes present.

Experimental Evidences to Indicate the Involvement of Parental Genes in the Control of Development : Hybridization experiment between closely-related species provide convincing evidence that parental genes exercise influence on the development.

Evidences from Andromerogones : When the enucleated egg of one species is fertilized with the sperm of another species, the embryo is called hybrid andromerogone and its development is known as androgenesis. The andromerogones are actually haploid. These fail to complete the development. The andromerogones of *R. pipes* and *R. capito* develop normally upto the gastrulation stage by the end at early neurula stage or in some cases the hybrid dies during gastrulation.

Evidences from Hybridization: The crosses between related species producing viable hybrids illustrate the influence of the nucleus. In two species of sea urchin, *Dendraster eccentricus* and *Strongylocentrotus franciscanus* differing in rate of cleavage, are crossed, the cleavage of hybrid has the maternal rate of cleavage. But the character of the larva are clearly intermediate between two parents. In some special cases, the influence of sperm nucleus has been discovered as early as the beginning of gastrulation. In a cross between sea urchins, *Lytechinus* and *Cidars,* the influence of paternal genes can be seen in early gastrula. In *Lytechinus,* the mesenchyme cells produced from micromeres migrate into the blastocoel slightly earlier than the beginning of invagination of archenteron. On the other hand in *Cidaris,* the mesenchyme cells do not separate from the epithelium after the archenteron begins to invaginate. When *Cidaris* eggs are fertilized by *Lytechinus* sperm, the early stages of development upto gastrula proceed exactly as in maternal species. But the mesenchyme cells begin to separate just as the invagination of archenteron begins.

Therefore, the stage at which the mesenchyme cells migrate into the blastocoel is intermediate between the two species. It proves that the paternal nucleus has manifested its influence at the beginning of gastrulation.

Immunological Method : Direct evidence that in hybrids the paternal chromosomes cause the synthesis of proteins of their own species from the beginning of gastrulation onward has been obtained from immunological experiments. The enucleated eggs of sea urchin *Paracentrotus lividus* were fertilized with the sperm of *Psammechinus microtuberculatus*. The blood serum immunity against proteins of *Psammechinus microtuberculatus* shows no traces of these specific antigens characteristic of *Psammechinus*. However, twenty- four hours after fertilization, the hybrid embryos in early gastrula stage show the presence of specific paternal antigens. From the above experiment it is evident that these antigens were not present in the egg cytoplasm. These antigens are new proteins that have been synthesized under the influence of sperm chromosomes (Harding, Harding and Perelman, 1954).

The increase in the amount of different types of ribonucleic acids is a clear indication that the new molecules of RNA are synthesized to bring about the synthesis of new proteins. In crosses between distantly-related species, the development arrests at the gastrula stage or later because of incompatibility between the foreign paternal nucleus and the maternal cytoplasm.

Significance of Gastrulation

1. Gastrulation is an important and very significant stage in the development. It brings the presumptive organ rudiments from the external surface of the blastula to their prospective normal positions, which will develop into the organs of the adult. Once the presumptive organ rudiments have reached their future position in the gastrula, these induce the development of different organ systems.

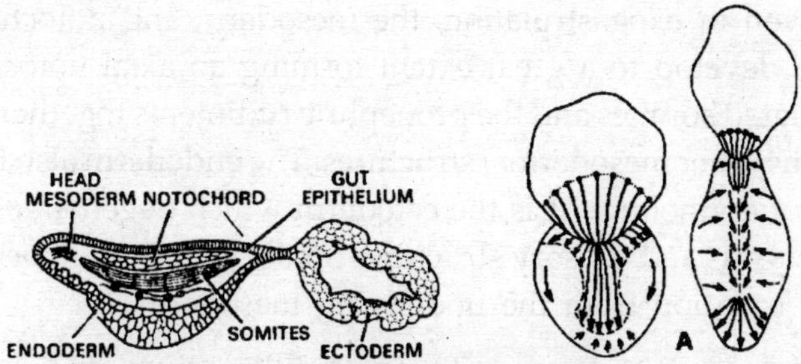

Differentiation in an exogastrulated amphibian embryo.

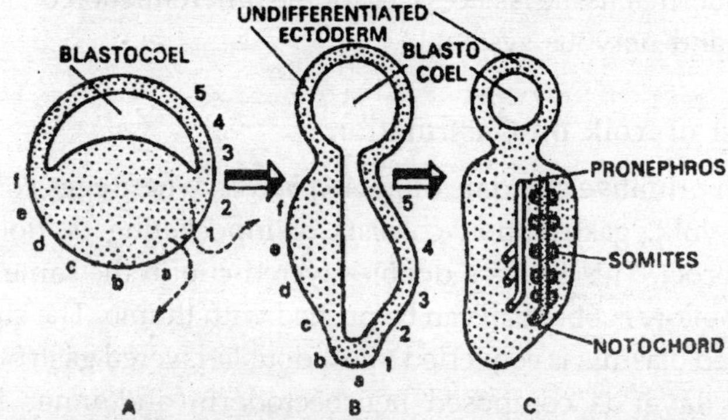

Exo-gastrulation Results.

A—Section of early gastrula along a with the regions above and below the dorsal lip indicated by numbers and letters. The doted lines and arrows indicate the movement of regions 1 to 5 and a to f.

B—The presumptive notochordal somites and endoderm fail to move interior to gastrula and ectoderm fail to form nervous system.

C—Pronephros notochord and somites form in remaining tissues. (After Bodemer, 1968)

2. Gastrulation is necessary for the formation of central nervous system. This can be demonstrated by the occurrence of exogastrulae of frog and other amphibians. If the protective surface coat is removed from the egg surface by keeping the fertilized eggs in hypertonic saline solution, the embryo developed is an exogastrula. In an exogastrula the archenteron is everted, the endoderm encloses the chorda-mesoderm tissue, while the ectoderm becomes isolated as an empty, crumpled envelop from rest of the tissue.

Even in exogastrulation, the mesoderm and notochordal tissue develop to a great extent forming an axial notochord, associated somites and the pronephric rudiments together with various other mesodermal structures. The endoderm also forms the gut epithelium. It is the ectoderm which degenerates and no nervous and sensory structures are formed from it, because of its isolation from the underlying mesoderm.

The exogastrulation indicates that the presence of chorda-mesodermal tissue is necessary for the differentiation of neural tube and nervous system.

Effect of Yolk on Gastrulation

In primitive chordates, like *Amphioxus,* where eggs contain little yolk, gastrulation consists of inpocketing of floor of blastocoel. This forms a double-layered cup in the same way as a hollow rubber ball can be pushed with thumb. The single-layered blastula is converted into a double-layered gastrula. Its outer layer is composed neuroectoderm and inner layer endoderm.

In large yolky eggs, the inert yolk precludes the simple inpocketing as in *Amphioxus.* In frog with moderately teloecithal eggs, initial steps in gastrulation resemble those of isolecithal eggs. The formation of blastoporal groove by invagination is homologous to invagination occurring during gastrulation in isolecithal eggs, the presence of large yolky cells in the vegetal hemisphere modifies the gastrulation to some extent.

In highly telolecithal eggs of reptiles and birds even this invagination of cells is not possible. Gastrulation occurs as the elaboration of three germ layers as sheets upon an enormous sphere of passive yolk mass. This is achieved by mass migration of cells as seen in chick gastrulation.

13

The Blastulation

The series of cell divisions that transform a single cell—the fertilized egg into a multicellular embryonic stage *blastula* is called cleavage or segmentations. The mitotic divisions during this phase are called *cleavage divisions* and the resulting daughter cells are known as *blastomeres.*

Characteristics of Cleavage

The cleavage takes place in the beginning of development and is characterized by following events :

(1) All divisions are mitotic and occur consecutively.

(2) During cleavage, there is no growth in the resulting blastomeres. This results into cells of continuously diminishing size.

(3) The general shape of the embryo does not change, except, for the formation of a cavity among the cleaving cells. This is called the blastocoel.

(4) Cytoplasmic substances transform into nuclear

substance, but qualitative changes in the chemical composition of the egg are very few.

(5) A great increase in the synthesis of DNA takes place because it is needed for duplication of chromosomes.

(6) The ratio of nucleus to cytoplasm is very low at the beginning of cleavage, but at the end it is brought to the level found in ordinary somatic cells.

(7) During cleavage oxygen consumption is greatly increased.

(8) The constituent parts of ooplasm remain unaltered during cleavage.

The Planes of Cleavage

The cleavage is initiated by the appearance of a constriction or groove called cleavage furrow. The cleavage furrows may divide the egg from different angles or planes. There are four important planes of cleavage. They are as follows :

Meridional Plane: When cleavage furrow bisects both the poles of the egg, passing through the animals vegetal axis, the plane of cleavage is called *meridional plane.* Examples are, I and II cleavage furrows of frog ; I cleavage furrow of chick.

Vertical Plane: This plane of cleavage is a furrow which passes from the animal pole to the vegetal pole, but it does not pass through the median axis of the egg. Instead, it is oriented towards one side of the axis. Example : III cleavage furrows of Amia *calva, Lepidosteus osseus* and chick.

Fquatorial Plane: This plane of cleavage bisects the egg at right angles to the median axis and halfway between the animal and vegetal poles. Examples : I cleavage plane of eggs of higher mammals.

Transverse Latitudinal or Horizontal Plane: The transverse plane resembles the equatorial plane, but it passes either above (towards the animal pole) or below (towards the vegetal pole) the equator of the egg. Examples : III cleavage plane of Amphioxus and frog.

Patterns of Cleavage

During segmentation, the cleavage furrows are not formed at random but are oriented in a particular manner with reference to the main (animal-vegetal) axis of the egg. The orientation of successive cleavage furrows with respect to each other and to the main axis of the egg is, however, unlike in different species. As such, various patterns of cleavage are found among animals. Based upon symmetry, four patterns of cleavage have been recognized. They are : radial, biradial, spiral and bilateral.

Radial Cleavage: In this cleavage pattern, divisions take place in such a manner that all the blastomeres are placed in a radially symmetrical fashion around the polar axis. When such an egg is viewed from the poles, the blastomeres seem to be arranged in a radially symmetric form. Example : sponges, coelenterates, sea-urchin, sea-cucumber, *Amphioxus*.

Biradial Cleavage: This pattern of cleavage is found in ctenophores like Beroe. Four blastomeres arise by the usual two meridional cleavages. The third cleavage plane is vertical resulting in the formation of a curved plate of 8 cells arranged in two rows of 4 each. In these rows, the central cells are larger than the end ones.

Spiral Cleavage: The spiral cleavage is diagonal to the polar-axis. In this type, the spindles for the third cleavage, instead of being erect, are oriented diagonally so that the resulting upper tier of cells is displaced sidewise. The upper 4 cells are placed over the junctions between the four lower cells. The upper smaller cells are called micro and lower larger cells are known as macromeres. The spiral cleavage results due to oblique positions of the mitotic spindles. This type of cleavage is called the spiral type because the four spindles during the third cleavage are arranged in a sort of spiral.

The turn of the spiral as seen from the animal pole may be in clockwise direction (dextral) or in a counter clockwise direction (sinistral). Moreover, the spindles are alternately tilted obliquely to the dextral and sinistral directions, so that successive generations of blastomeres are oriented in a twisted fashion.

This pattern of cleavage characterises the eggs of annelids, molluscs, nemerteans and some of the planarians.

Bilateral Cleavage: In this pattern of cleavage, the blastomeres are so arranged that the right and left sides becomes distinct. This cleavage pattern is dependent upon differences in the size of the blastomeres. In this case, two of the first four blastomeres may be larger than the other two, thus establishing a plane of bilateral symmetry in the developing embryo. Subsequent cleavages may make the bilateral arrangement of the blastomeres still more obvious. Examples are nematodes, cephalopod molluscs, some echinoderms and tunicates.

Determinate and Indeterminate Cleavage : Eggs of mollusks annelids, flatworms, nematodes, ctenophores, and ascidians undergo determinate cleavage in which definite blastomeres give rise to specific parts of the embryo. A special type of bilateral cleavage in *Ascaris* is an example of determinate cleavage. The first division produces two unequal cells : a slightly larger cell AB and a smaller cell Pr. In the second division, the two cells divided in mutually perpendicular planes with the result that the blastomeres in the four-cell stage are arranged in the form of a letter T. The transverse shaft of the T is made up of blastomeres A and B which are descendants of the cell AB. The vertical shaft is made up of the derivatives of blastomere Pr. These cells are designated as EMST and P2. EMST is abbreviation for *Endoderm, Mesoderm* and *Stomodaeum* which indicates the destiny of this cell. The P2 cell soon shifts towards the B cell and the blastomeres are arranged in a rhomboid figure.

The indeterminate or regulative cleavage occurs in the eggs of echinoderm, balanoglossids, coelenterates, and amphibians. In this type, the cleavage pattern bears no definite relation to the embryo. If a first cleavage blastomere from the embryo of a sea-urchin, an amphibian or a mammal is isolated, it can change its usual destiny and could develop into a perfect, though small, embryo. Likewise, when two fertilized eggs are made to stick together, they produce a single giant embryo.

Effect of Yolk on Cleavage

Yolk is a mechanically inert material, which when present in large quantities, may interfere physically with the subdivisions of an egg during cleavage. It retards the progress of the furrow to divide the cytoplasm following nuclear division. During cleavage, the chromosomes and the achromatic spindle are generally shifted into the more protoplasmic portions and away from the yolky areas of the egg. Consequently, the protoplasmic portions divided into smaller cells than the yolky areas. Besides, they divided more frequently.

The cleavage involves mitosis. Mitosis is characterized by the movements of cell components viz., the chromosomes, achromatic figure, mitochondria etc. The activity of these components along the equator of the maternal cell leads to the ultimate separation of the daughter cell. The yolk granules or platelets are passively distributed between the daughter blastomeres during these movements. When yolk becomes abundant, it tends to retard and even inhibit the movement of the concerned cell components. Hence the process of cleavage slows down. The yolk in the uncleaved egg is generally more concentrated toward the vegetal pole of the egg than the animal pole. Therefore, the cleavage is most retarded at the vegetal pole of the egg and here the blastomeres are larger in size.

Frog's egg provides a good example of the effect of the yolk on cleavage. The first cleavage furrow is meridional but it does not appear simultaneously all around the circumference of the egg. At first it is seen only at the animal pole of the egg where the amount of yolk is less. It then gradually prolongs along the meridians of the egg.

Passing through the yolk-laden cytoplasm or deutoplasm, it eventually reaches the vegetal pole. This divides the egg into two first blastomeres. The same process is repeated during the second Meridional cleavage which takes place at right angles to the first. During the third cleavage; when the plane of division is Latitudinal, the cleavage furrow appears simultaneously all over the circumference of the egg because it meets with an equal resistance from yolk at all sites. There is a greater accumulation of yolk at the vegetal pole of telolecithal egg. This interferes with the cell division at this pole and as a result the cleavage here becomes inhibited more and more.

The pattern of cleavage is determined considerably by the amount of yolk in the egg. *Isolecithal* and *telolecithal eggs* undergo complete or holoblastic cleavage. In this type, the cell membranes formed during cleavage cut completely through the egg, including the yolk. In *centrolecithal* and *discoidal eggs,* the cleavage is incomplete or meroblastic. Such eggs contain so much yolk that only a small amount of cytoplasm with nucleus undergoes segmentation.

Types of Cleavage

The major types of cleavage have been distinguished on the basis of the amount and distribution of yolk in the egg. They are : *(i)* holoblastic, and *(ii)* meroblastic cleavage.

Total or Holoblastic Cleavage: In total or complete cleavage, the entire egg divides by each cleavage furrow. It is of two types :

(i) *Equal Holoblastic Cleavage:* When the daughter blastomeres are approximately of the same size, the total cleavage is called equal holoblastic cleavage. It occurs in *microlecithal* and *isolecithal eggs, e.g.*, sponges, echinoderms, lower chordates - tunicates, Amphioxus, marsupials and eutherian mammals.

(ii) *Unequal Holoblastic Cleavage:* If the daughter blastomeres are unequal in size, the complete division of the egg is referred to as unequal holoblastic cleavage. This is the case with the *mesolecithal* and *telolecithal eggs* of cyclostomes, elasmobranch fishes, Dipnoi, amphibia and cephalopod molluscs. In these eggs the third cleavage gives rise to four small and four large blastomeres. The smaller blastomeres are called micromeres and the larger ones macro or megameres.

Partial or Meroblastic Cleavage: In partial, incomplete or meroblastic cleavage, the division furrows divide only a small amount of active cytoplasm on the periphery of egg or at the animal pole, and most of the yolky portion of egg remains undivided. This cleavage takes place in *macro-* or*polylecithal* eggs, and may be of the following two types :

(i) *Superficial Cleavage:* This type of incomplete cleavage is found in *centrolecithal eggs, e.g.*, insects and many other arthropods. At the beginning of cleavage the nucleus (synkaryon) located in the centre of the yolk divides repeatedly. Then the daughter nuclei start moving away from the centre of the egg. Each nucleus remains surrounded by a small portion of the original central cytoplasm. When the nuclei reach the surface of the egg, the cytoplasm surrounding them fuses with the Superficial layer of cytoplasm. Later the cytoplasm becomes subdivided, by furrows going inward from the surface. In this way, a layer of superficial or peripheral cells surrounds an undivided central yolk mass.

(ii) *Discoidal Cleavage:* In the large, yolky *macrolecithal* eggs of elasmobranchs, bony fishes, birds, reptiles and egg-laying mammals, the cleavage remains restricted to a disc-shaped area of active cytoplasm, the *blastodisc,* at the animal pole. The remaining yolk-filled part of the egg shows no division. Such incomplete cleavage is called discoidal and results in a disk of cells resting upon the undivided yolk.

Morula : Morula is the late cleavage stage before the blastocoel has appeared. The blastomeres in a morula tend to assume a spherical shape. Their mutual pressure flattens the surfaces of the blastomeres in contact with each other, but the free surfaces of each blastomere remain spherical. The solid mass of blastomeres appears to be like a mulberry. On account of this superficial similarity, the embryo in this stage is called a morula (Latin for *mulberry).*

Blastula : At the end of cleavage, the embryo consists of a *hollow sphere of cells* in holoblastic types, and a *layer of cells* over yolk in meroblastic types. This developmental stage is called a blastula. The layer of cells is known as the blastoderm and the cavity is the blastocoel. At first, the blastocoel may be represented, just by narrow crevices between the blastomeres, but it gradually increases as the cleavage goes on. The blastocoel may be identified in the 8-cell stage as the space enclosed by the two quartets of blastomeres.

Blastulation : The development of blastula is called blastulation. The types of blastulae greatly varies among different animals depending upon various factors such as the egg size, the amount and distribution of yolk, and the rate and pattern of cleavage. The various types of blastulae can be classified into four types :

(i) stereoblastula,

(ii) coeloblastula,

(iii) *periblastula,* and

(iv) *discoblastula.*

Holoblastically Formed Blastulae

In holoblastic embryos, the blastula is either solid (stereoblastula) or hollow (coeloblastula).

Stereoblastula: This type of blastula is composed of densely-packed but larger sized and relatively small number of cells. Blastocoelic space in the centre is very small or virtually absent. The blastomeres in a stereoblastula may reach from the surface to the centre ; or separate blastomeres may occupy the interior. Examples : Insects, some worms *(e.g., Nereis)* and some mollusks *(e.g., Crepidula).*

Coeloblastula: This type of blastula consist of one or several layers of cells arranged around a large blastocoel. It is of two types :

(a) *Adequal :* The cells of the blastoderm are of about the same size throughout. The blastocoel is centrally placed, *e.g.,* echinoderms.

(b) *Inequal :* The wall of the vegetal half is thicker than that of the animal half. The blastocoel is reduced in volume and distinctly eccentric, i.e., displaced towards the animal pole, *e.g., Amphioxus,* amphibians.

Meroblastically Formed Blastulae

The blastula stage consists of a layer of cells over yolk.

Periblastula: This type of blastula is found in insects and some arthropods having centriolecithal eggs with a superficial cleavage. In such blastulae, there is no cavity comparable to the blastocoel. It consists of a single layer of epithelial cells, the blastoderm which envelopes the mass of uncleaved yolk. Birds and reptiles corresponds to the blastocoel of amphibians and fishes. The space between the hypoblast and the yolk is designated as the subgerminal cavity.

The cavity in birds and reptiles is formed only under the central part of the blastoderm. No cavity is formed under the layer of blastomeres in the periphery of the blastodisc. The disc is thus subdivided into two parts :

(i) the more transparent central part called the area pellucida and,

(ii) the opaque peripheral part, the area opaca. Area pellucida is transparent because of the presence of the cavity under the layer of blastomeres.

The peripheral area looks opaque as the blastomeres rest directly on the yolk and there is no cavity underneath.

Discoblastula: It is found in sharks, bony fishes, reptiles, birds and prototherian mammals. In these animals, eggs are highly telolecithal. They undergo discoidal cleavage which results in the formation of a blastodisc on top of the undivided yolk. The disc consists of several layers of cells.

In a *bony fish* or a *shark,* cleavage is restricted to the cap of cytoplasm on the animal pole of the egg where formation of blastoderm takes place. Therefore, the blastoderm assumes the shape of a disc called blastodisc lying on the animal pole. The blastodisc is more or less convex. It encloses, between itself and the uncleaved residue of the egg, a cavity representing the blastocoel.

In *reptiles* and *birds* blastocoel forms by a lifting away of some of the cells of blastoderm. The cells are incorporated into a superficial layer, called the epiblast. A small number of cells remain underneath the superficial layer, forming a thin flat epithelium, called the hypoblast.

The Cleavage

Within few hours of fertilization, the fertilized egg undergoes a series of repeated mitotic cell divisions, which occur in rapid succession to produce an increase in the number of cells without any addition to its volume. This phase of repeated divisions of the egg is known as cleavage or segmentation. The cleavage can be defined as *'the process of progressive subdivision of the zygote by mitotic cell divisions into an increasing number of cells of progressively decreasing size.*

Historical : The cleavage was first observed by Swammerdam in 1738 in frog's egg. In 1780 SPALLANZANI described first two cleavage planes of toad's egg. The first attempt to describe cleavage in the eggs of rabbit was made in 1839, of fish in 1842 and of bird in 1847.

Special Features of Cleavage

(i) Cleavage begins immediately after the nuclear fusion of the two gametes. The egg provides sufficient energy and the substances needed for cell division.

(ii) The divisions continue till the reserves are exhausted and the average size of the daughter cells (blastomeres) reaches the characteristic size of the differentiated somatic cells of parent organisms. The number of successive divisions, therefore, depends upon the size of the egg in relation to that of the typical somatic cell.

(iii) The resultant cells are called blastomeres (Gr., *blastos,* germ + *meros,* parts).

(iv) The volume as well as the general shape of the embryo does not change during cleavage.

(v) No growth occurs during cleavage.

(vi) The reserve food material (yolk and glycogen, etc.) is converted into amino acids, monosaccharides, lipid molecules and the enzymes that are required for cell division. The nucleus and nuclear membrane, spindle fibres, etc. are all synthesized from these small molecules.

(vii) The pace or rhythm of cleavage is determined by the cytoplasm rather than by the nucleus.

(viii) The ratio of nucleus to cytoplasm is very low at the beginning of cleavage. It gradually increases during cleavage and at the end it is brought to the same level as is found in the ordinary somatic cells.

(ix) The constituent parts of the egg cytoplasm, on the whole remain in the same positions as in the egg at the beginning of cleavage. However, some cytoplasmic regional specialization takes place leading to cytodifferentiation later on.

(x) During early cleavage mitosis follows mitosis with very short interphase that is essentially required for chromatin replication.

(xi) As a result of cleavage, the zygote changes into a hollow ball of numerous small cells with a surface layer and enclosing a central space, the blastocoel.

Peculiarities of Cell Division in Cleavage : The cleavage divisions differ from the normal mitotic divisions in the following aspects:

1. In mitosis, the daughter cells grow and reach the size of mature cell and then only divide again. Thus the cells maintain an average size in all types of tissues. As the blastomeres do not increase in size during cleavage with each division the resulting blastomeres are half the original size.
2. Due to the absence of the growth phase, the interphase is very short.
3. The nuclei of the early cleavage cells are comparatively larger than those of the ordinary somatic cells. The nuclear-cytoplasmic ratio is very low in comparison to that found in the somatic cells. For example, in a mature sea urchin egg before fertilization the ratio of volume of the nucleus/volume of cytoplasm is 1/550 (Brachet, 1950), while at the end of cleavage (in blastula stage) the same ratio is 1/6.

Rate of Cleavage : The rate of cleavage varies in different species. It is inversely proportionate to the duration of interphase. The inter-cleavage interval is about 20 minutes in goldfish, about an hour in frog and 10-12 hours in mouse.

The cleavage rate is rapid during early development and is synchronous, but it becomes very slow and asynchronous by the completion of blastula. Depending upon the duration of intermitotic interval, the cleavage period has been separated into three phases: (i) early phase with rapid cleavage, (ii) late phase with an intermitotic period of noticeable length and (iii) terminal phase with a very long intermitotic period.

The progressive increase of intermitotic interphase results due to gradual exhaustion of a specific substance present in the cytoplasm of the fertilized egg. Lovtrup, (1974) Mazia, (1961) suggested that this substance can be the protein of the mitotic apparatus (the TP monomeres).

The rate of cleavage is determined by the cytoplasm. It is also affected by changes in temperature, oxygen and carbondioxide concentration. The excess of CO_2 inhibits cleavage.

Chemical Changes during Cleavage

Following substances are synthesized during cleavage period:

Synthesis of DNA: With every division of blastomeres the number of daughter cells and their nuclei is doubled. The doubling of nuclei is accomplished by the replication of nuclear substance, the DNA. The egg cytoplasm contains an enzyme the ribonucleotide reductase which converts ribo-nucleotides of the egg cytoplasm into deoxyribonucleotides that join to form new DNA molecules.

Synthesis of Ribonucleic Acid: The synthesis of RNA during cleavage is limited. The nucleolus is absent in the dividing blastomeres indicating the complete absence of ribosomal RNA synthesis. Ribosomal RNA available for protein synthesis is the one that was produced in the ova during orogenesis under the influence of maternal genes. However, very little mRNA and tRNA are synthesized during this period. Their synthesis increases considerably in the later stages of cleavage.

Protein Synthesis: Protein synthesis is initiated after fertilization and continues throughout the cleavage period. The first proteins of the embryo are synthesized from the templates present in the unfertilized eggs. The proteins synthesized are mostly those that are required in the cell division. The nucleo-histone proteins are used in chromosome replication. The protein tubulin is used in the formation of microtubules of the fibres of archromatic mitotic spindle. The proteins in the form of enzyme ribonucleotide reductase is helpful in the conversion of riboncleotides into deoxyribonucleotides.

Planes of Cleavage

Each cleavage of the dividing zygote is marked by a cleavage furrow. Usually the first cleavage furrow is vertical and passes through the main axis of the egg. It bisects the egg into two equal blastomeres. The second cleavage furrow is also vertical but at right angles to the first one. The third cleavage furrow is horizontal or parallel to the equator. Four different cleavage planes have been recognised. These are:

Meridional Plane: When cleavage furrow passes through the polar axis of the egg and bisects both the animal and vegetal poles through the middle, the plane of cleavage is called meridional (i.e. passing through meridian). Example — *Amphioxus*, frog and *Lepidosteus*.

Vertical Plane : The vertical cleavage furrow passes through the animal and vegetal pole but not through the median axis. The cleavage furrow passes either to the right or left of the axis, as for example, third cleavage furrow in eggs of *Amia, Calva, Lepidosteus* and chick.

Equatorial Plane : The cleavage furrow is horizontal and is laid down in the equatorial plane at right angles to the main axis between the animal and vegetal poles (through the equator of egg). Example- — the first cleavage plane of eggs of higher mammals and fifth cleavage plane of egg of *Ambystoma maculatum.*

Latitudinal Plane : The cleavage furrows of the latitudinal division are laid down transversely or horizontally not on the equator but on either side of it. Example—third cleavage planes in the eggs of *Amphioxus.*

Determination of Plane of Cleavage : The plane of cleavage is determined by the position of mitotic spindle in the dividing zygote or its blastomeres, because the cleavage furrow passes through the cell in a plane perpendicular to the long axis of the mitotic spindle. The position and direction of mitotic spindle is determined by the factors present in the cytoplasm. The spindle formation proceeds independently despite the number of mitotic divisions. This was demonstrated by HORSTADIUS. He delayed the first cleavage in the fertilized egg until the time the third cleavage of egg normally occurs; the spindle formed parallel to the animal-vegetal axis instead of perpendicular to it as in normal first division.

In almost all eggs and blastomeres, the mitotic spindle is formed approximately in the geometric centre of the yolk-free area of cytoplasm and in majority of cases, the spindle is formed nearer to the animal pole. Any increase in the yolk distribution causes a more eccentric spindle formation. Factors other than yolk distribution also affect the location of spindle.

In fact, the cleavage plane is fixed soon after fertilization during the first few minutes. The control factors are located in the egg cortex, which is more rigid.

Patterns of Cleavage : The. repeated cleavage furrows produce a number of blastomeres which exhibit a specific pattern of arrangement. The following types of cleavage patterns have been specific pattern of arrangement. The following types of cleavage patterns have been studied in different animals.

Radial Cleavage Pattern: In radial cleavage the successive cleavage furrows cut straight through the egg, at right angles to one another so that the resultant blastomeres appear to be arranged radially. All those eggs which have holoblastic cleavage, exhibit radial cleavage. Example—*Synapta* eggs.

In *Synapta,* the first cleavage furrow is meridional, the second cleavage furrow is vertical but at right angles to the first one. The third cleavage furrow is equatorial and at right angles to the polar axis of the egg. The eight blastomeres produced this way are almost all equal in size and are arranged in two tiers of four each. These lie one above the other. These blastomeres exhibit radial symmetry.

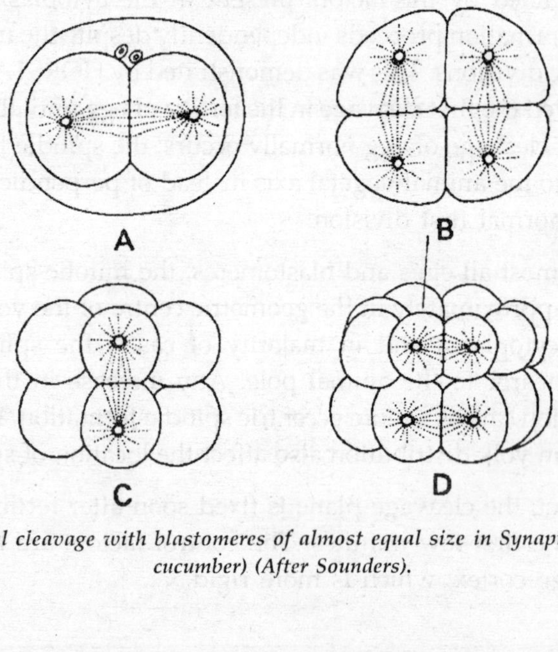

Radial cleavage with blastomeres of almost equal size in Synapta (sea cucumber) (After Sounders).

A slight deviation of radial cleavage is seen in sea-urchin and frog, where third cleavage is slightly above the equator. The blastomeres of the upper tier are smaller than those of lower tier. The small blastomeres of upper tier are called micromeres and the larger blastomeres of lower tier are macromeres.

Biradial Cleavage Pattern : When the cleavage furrows of first three divisions do not cut straight the axis of the egg and are not laid down at right angles to each other. Example—In the eggs of Ctenophora and Acoela.

Spiral Cleavage Pattern : It is a modification of the radial cleavage. In this, the mitotic spindles of the third cleavage in the four blastomeres are laid down obliquely and are arranged in a sort of spiral, so that the four blastomeres of upper tier do not lie over the corresponding blastomeres of lower tier but between them. This type of cleavage is known as spiral cleavage.

Spiral cleavage occurs in annelids, molluscs, nemertens and some of the planarians. The turn of spiral may be in a clockwise or counter-clockwise direction. Depending on this, the spiral cleavage may be divided into —

(i) Dextral or dextrotropic with clockwise spiral (*i.e.* right-hand spiral).

(ii) Sinistral or levotropic with counter-clockwise spiral (i.e. left-hand coiling).

Bilateral Cleavage : This is also a modified form of radial cleavage. The two of the four blastomeres are smaller than the other two and thus establish bilateral symmetry at the four cell-stage. The subsequent divisions make this bilateral symmetry more conspicuous. The bilateral cleavage is found in Tunicates and nematodes.

Determinate and Indeterminate Cleavage : Cleavage is classified as determinate and indeterminate, according to the developmental abilities of the egg cytoplasm.

Determinate Cleavage : In some animals *(Ascaris)* the blastomeres have a predetermined future *i.e.* definite blastomeres are determined to give rise to specific parts of the embryo. This type of cleavage is known as determinate cleavage. As a result of determinate cleavage a mosaic type of blastula is formed. This type of development is called mosaic development.

The determinate cleavage is seen in nematodes, annelids, molluscs and tunicates.

In *Ascaris,* the first cleavage is horizontal or transverse and divides the egg into two unequal blastomeres. The larger cell is designated as AB and small cell as P_1. These two blastomeres divide in mutually perpendicular planes, so that the blastomeres in four-cell stage are placed in the form of letter 'T'. The eight blastomeres formed by the third cleavage are arranged in a specific pattern, represented by A, a, B, b, C, c, MST and P3. The blastomeres A, B, and C give rise to skin, blastomere E to the endoderm of alimentary canal, blastomere MST gives rise to the mesoderm and stomodaeum and P3 to reproductive cells.

Indeterminate Cleavage : In indeterminate cleavage, the fate of blastomeres is not so rigidly sealed, but the blastomeres exhibit plasticity. For example, each of the two blastomeres of a zygote, if separated after the first cleavage, can produce one complete embryo. Similarly, when two fertilized eggs are made to cohere like two blastomeres at the two cell stages, will develop into a single giant embryo (tetraploid). Moreover, the dislocation of blastomeres of a blastula from one specific position to other is followed by readjustment and substitution so that a normal embryo is produced.

This type of early cleavage, in which the future of blastomeres is not predetermined, is known as indeterminate cleavage and this type of development is described as regulative development.

Influence of Yolk on the Nature of Cleavage : Yolk is nonliving component of the egg. It participates neither in cleavage nor in the formation of the embryo. It provides nourishment to the developing embryo.

Though, yolk is present in all the animal eggs, it may be scantly and evenly distributed in the cytoplasm (meiolecithal or isolecithal), more concentrated at one pole and less at the other pole (mediolecithal or telolecithal) or in large quantities and concentrated on one pole (megalecithal). The amount and pattern of distribution of yolk in the egg cytoplasm exerts a pronounced influence on the process of cleavage due to the following reasons-

(1) Mitosis involves the movement of various cell components like the chromosomes, part of the cytoplasm that constitutes the achromatic figure of the spindle, mitochondria and the surface layer of cytoplasm which helps in the formation of the cleavage furrow. During these movements, the yolk granules or platelets remain inert and are passively distributed to the daughter blastomeres. Thus the yolk retards and interferes with the process of cleavage. The cleavage occurs more rapidly in the active yolk-free cytoplasm than in the yolk-laden cytoplasm. Therefore, the blastomeres which are richer in yolk remain larger in size than those that have less yolk.

(2) With the increase of stored yolk, the amount of active cytoplasm gradually decreases in the eggs. The nucleus which is meridional (central) in position in microlecithal eggs is shifted to various positions in other types. In mesolecithal eggs, the nucleus from its original central position is displaced towards the animal pole that contains active cytoplasm. The displacement results in unequal cytokinesis and consequently unequal blastomeres.

Depending upon the distribution and amount of yolk, the following classification of cleavage has been introduced : —

Holoblastic Equal Cleavage (holos, whole; blastos, germs): In this type of cleavage, the cleavage furrows extend completely through the entire length of the egg and bisects it into equal or almost equal blastomeres. It occurs in aleacithal, mesolecithal and isolecithal eggs. The nucleus in these eggs occupies a central position. The first cleavage furrow is longitudinal or vertical beginning at the animal pole and extending to the vegetal pole, the second cleavage is also vertical but at right angles to the first two cleavage planes. The fourth cleavage has two vertical furrows starting at the animal pole at right angles to each other. The fifth cleavage includes two horizontal cleavage furrows, one in the animal half and the other in vegetal half. As a result 32 blastomeres are formed from the zygote and almost all of them are equal in size.

Example: Holoblastic equal cleavage occurs in the isolecithal eggs of *Amphioxus,* marsupials and placental mammals.

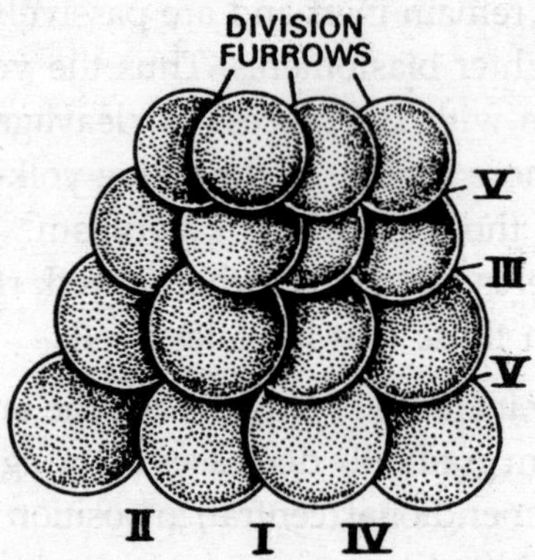

16 cells produced as a result of holoblastic equal cleavages in an isolecithal egg.

Holoblastic Unequal Cleavage : This type of cleavage occurs in the mesolecithal and telolecithal eggs where yolk is distributed along vegetal-animal axis. The yolk is sparse in the animal pole and gradually increases towards the vegetal pole.

The first and second cleavage furrows are laid down similar to those as in holoblastic equal cleavage. But the third cleavage furrow is not equatorial but towards the animals pole producing four small cells in the animal hemisphere, called micromeres and four large cells in the vegetal hemisphere, called macromeres or megameres. The fourth and fifth cleavage furrows are again similar to those of holoblastic equal cleavage.

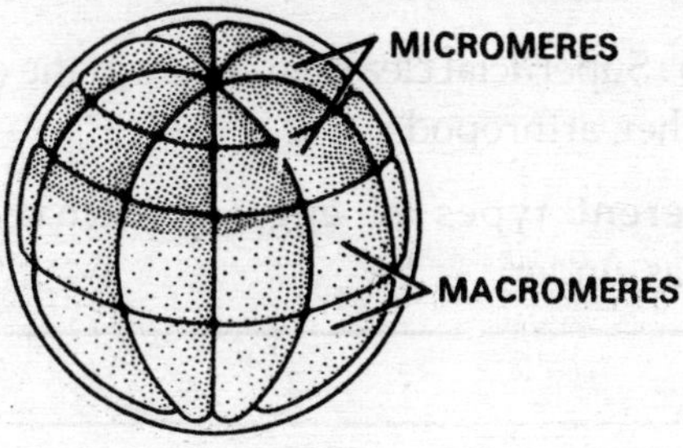

32-CELLED STAGE

A telolecithal egg of frog at 32-cell stage produced as a result of holoblastic unequal cleavage.

Example: Holoblastic unequal cleavage occurs in the eggs of frog, toad and certain fishes *(Amia, Lepidosteus)*.

Meroblastic or Discoidal Cleavage (Gr. meros, part): Meroblastic cleavage occurs in megalecithal or heavily telolecithal eggs, which have enormous amount of yolk. The active portion of egg is confined to a small cytoplasmic region at the animal pole, called the germinal disc or blastodisc. The cleavage furrows are restricted to the germinal disc; the yolk remains uncleaved. The first and second cleavage furrows are laid down radially at right angles in the germinal disc and divide it into four relatively equal but incomplete blastomeres. The remaining cleavage furrows are irregular. The early blastomeres are incomplete and are continuous with the underlying yolk.

Superficial Cleavage : This cleavage occurs in centrolecithal eggs. Here, the early divisions occur in the surface layer of the egg and cleavage furrows do not extend into the central yolk.

In centrolecithal eggs the zygote nucleus lies in the centre of the egg. It divides repeatedly without the division of the egg cytoplasm. As a result, a large number of nuclei are formed. These remain embedded in the undivided superficial layer of cytoplasm. The surface layer assumes syncytial appearance. The cytoplasm divides by furrows laid down from the surface towards inner side and separates into a large number of cells arranged around central yolk.

Examples : Superficial cleavage occurs in the eggs of insects and many other arthropods.

The different types of eggs and cleavages can be summarised as under:

Particulars	1	2	3
Amount and distribution of yolk:	Little and evenly distributed	Medium and much concentrated on one pole but less on the other pole	Much and concentrated on one pole only
Common name of egg type:	Yolk poor	Medium yolked	Yolk rich
Technical name of egg types and its meaning:	Microlecithal (Less yolk)	Mesolecithal (Medium yolk) or Telolecithal	Megalecithal (Large yolk)
Position of egg nucleus: Relative amount and position of active cytoplasm:	Near centre Much and distributed throughout the ovum	Near one pole Medium and present near the nucleus or animal pole	At one pole Very little and surrounds the nucleus
Types of cleavage:	Complete and nearly equal	Complete and unequal	Incomplete and unequal
Technical term for cleavage type:	Holoblastic equal	Holoblastic unequal	Meroblastic
Familiar examples:	*Amphioxus* and Man	Fishes, Frog and Toads	Reptiles and Birds

Principles of Cleavage

The cleavage of eggs of all the animals appears to be governed by certain principles. Following are some generalizations that have been put forward:

Sach's Law : Sach (1877) proposed that: *(i)* Cells tend to divide into equal daughter cells. *(ii)* The cleavage furrow of each new division tends to bisect the plane of preceding cleavage at right angles. *(iii)* Blastomeres tend to assume and maintain spheroidal shape.

Hertwig's Law : O. HERTWIG (1881) supplemented Sach's law with following generalization: *(i)* The archromatic mitotic spindle at each cleavage lies in the centre of the active protoplasm of the egg or blastomeres. This is evidenced from the following observations—(a) in microlecithal and isolecithal eggs, the spindle is located centrally and (b) in telolecithal eggs the spindle lies nearer the animal pole where active cytoplasm is present. *(ii)* The axis of mitotic spindle tends to coincide with the longitudinal axis of the yolk -free cytoplasm in which it lies. Therefore, the cleavage plane tends to cut this axis at right angles.

Balfour's Law: Balfour in 1885 suggested that the rate of cleavage is inversely proportional to the amount of yolk or deutoplasm. For example, in telolecithal eggs, the blastomeres in the yolk-free animal pole (*i.e.* the micromeres) divide faster than the macromeres that are present at the vegetal pole and contain yolk.

Pfluger's Law : The mitotic spindle always elongates in the direction of least resistance.

Products of Cleavage

Cleavage results in smaller cells, the blastomeres. By each cleavage the number of blastomeres multiplies in geometric progression in a typical doubling sequence producing 2,4,8,16 and 32 blastomeres. Only a few early cleavages are regular, the later divisions become entirely irregular.

Morula : During early cleavage the blastomeres maintain spherical shape like that of egg. But slightly later, these surfaces of blastomeres that remain in contact with one another become flattened because of compression. However, the free outer and inner surfaces continue to be spherical. As a result, the external surface of the developing embryo assumes a characteristic mulberry-like appearance. The embryo in this stage is called morula (L.*morum*-mulberry).

A true morula is absent in almost all the vertebrates because an incipient central cavity or blastocoel appears very soon in the early cleavage stages. A true morula is regarded to be a solid ball of cells as found in coelenterates. Some of the blastomeres form surface layer while others fill in the interior. The morula later on changes into a blastula.

Blastula : In majority of animals, the blastomeres produced as a result of repeated cleavage divisions are arranged in a single layer. A narrow space arises between the blastomeres in the form of crevices because of rounding of their inner ends. This cavity increases as the cleavage proceeds. It is known as blastocoel. The blastomeres get arranged in a single layer around the blastocoel. The layer thus formed is known as the blastoderm. The hollow spherical embryo at this stage is known as blastula. It has a central space, the blastocoel surrounded by a layer the blastoderm.

Mechanism of Blastula Formation (Blastulation) : The blastomeres produced as a result of cleavage tend to assume spherical shape like that of the egg due to the following reasons:

(i) These have viscous surface.

(ii) Any fluid or semifluid mass tends to assume spherical shape to reduce the free surface energy to a minimum.

(iii) The viscous surfaces tend to adhere to any adjacent surface that has similar physical and chemical properties.

(iv) When surface tension is high, a more or less spherical form is maintained. However, when it becomes low the surface becomes flattened.

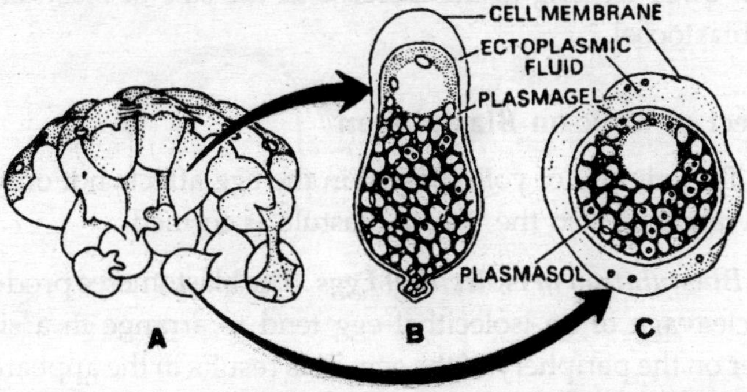

Possible mechanism of blastulation as given by Gustafson and Wolpert (From Berrill)

For the reasons cited above the free outer surfaces of blastomeres remain spherical, whereas the surfaces that lie in contact with one another become flat. As a result of the rounding of the cells a space appears in the centre and it is called the blastocoel. This gradually increases with the increase in the number of blastomeres.

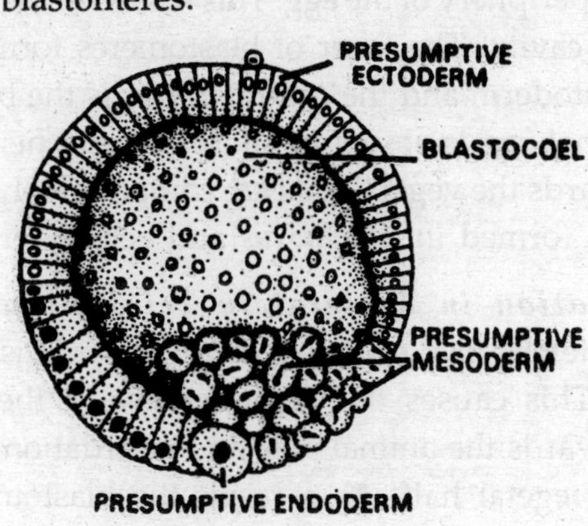

Diagram of blastula of Amphioxus.

Gustafson and Wolpert (1969) summarized the whole process as follows: The cells are firmly attached to the hyaline layer. At each cell-division the cells round up owing to increased tension in their own membrane, and their contact with each other is reduced. Since the plane of cleavage is radial, the elongating and constricting cells exert a tangential force upon each other leading to the increase in the size of blastula and its blastocoel.

Effect of Yolk on Blastulation

The amount of yolk present in the egg affects not only the cleavage but also the way a blastula is formed.

Blastulation in Isolecithal Eggs : The blastomeres produced by cleavage of an isolecithal egg tend to arrange in a single layer on the periphery of the egg. This results in the appearance of a central cavity. The layer of blastomeres forms the outer layer or blastoderm and the central cavity is the blastocoel. A true isolecithal egg is absent. The amount of yolk present in the egg affects not only the cleavage but also the way a blastula is formed.

Blastulation in Isolecithal Eggs : The blastomeres produced by cleavage of an isolecithal egg tend to arrange in a single layer on the periphery of the egg. This results in the appearance of a central cavity. The layer of blastomeres forms the outer layer or blastoderm and the central cavity is the blastocoel. A true isolecithal egg is absent in chordates and hence the cells present towards the vegetal pole are comparatively large. Such a blastula is formed in *Amphioxus* and echinoderms.

Blastulation in Moderately Telolecithal Eggs: In moderately telolecithal eggs (e.g. frog) the yolk is distributed unequally. This causes the displacement of the horizontal cleavage towards the animal pole and retardation of cleavage rate in the vegetal half. As a result the blastomeres in the vegetal half (macromeres) are much larger than those of the animal half (micromeres). Consequently, the blastocoel becomes eccentric, being displaced in the animal half. The small micromeres form the roof of the blastocoel, while the large macromeres form the floor. In such a blastula the roof of the blastocoel is no longer formed of a single layer but is made up of two or more layers of blastomeres. On the external surface of blastula, the blastoderm cells adhere to one another firmly.

Blastulation in Heavily Telolecithal Eggs: In heavily telolecithal or megalecithal eggs (found in reptiles, birds and fishes), the process of blastulation is restricted to the germinal disc only. As the cleavage progresses, the cells in the central part of the germinal disc become multilayered and get separated from the underlying yolk, while those present on the margins of germinal disc are continuous with the yolk. Due to the separation of cells from the yolk in the central part of the germinal disc, a clear space develops between the blastomeres and yolk. This is known as subgerminal cavity. Its floor is formed of yolk. The outer layer of blastomeres forming the roof of subgerminal cavity is called epiblast. A few blastomeres from the marginal region of the germinal disc migrate into the subgerminal cavity, where these get arranged into a thin layer over the yolk and form the roof of the subgerminal cavity. This layer is known as hypoblast and the cavity between epiblast and hypoblast is called the blastocoel.

Different Types of Blastulae

The different types of blastulae are recognized in different animal groups. These are as follows:

Coeloblastula: The blastula of echinoderms and *Amphioxus* is called coeloblastula. It is in the form of a hollow sphere. Its blastocoel is filled with mucopolysac charides. The blastoderm is formed of a single layer of cells.

Periblastula or Superficial Blastula : It is found in insect eggs. It is similar to coeloblastula except that the blastocoel is filled with yolk.

Discoblastula : It is found in reptiles, birds and fishes which have large yolky eggs. In such blastulae the floor of blastocoel is formed of yolk-sac, while the roof is formed of epiblast.

Amphiblastula : It is formed of two types of structurally-different blastomeres. As. for example, in Sycon the anterior half of blastula is formed of flagellated cells while the posterior half is formed of large- rounded granular cells or in amphibians where the two types of cells are micromeres and macromeres.

Blastocyst: It is found in mammals. During development in mammals, a solid ball of cells, called morula is formed. The cells of the outer peripheral layer of the morula are arranged more like an epithelium and form the trophoderm or trophoec toderm or the trophoblast. The cells inside the morula are irregularly shaped and form the inner cell mass. The cells of trophoderm stretch, flattened and also increase in number. This causes the appearance of a cavity within the morula, changing the embryo into blastula. This blastula is described as blastocyst. It consists of an inner cell mass attached to trophoectoderm on one side and separated from it on all other sides by the blastocoel.

14

The Parthenogenesis

In some animals an egg can develop without fertilization. This phenomenon is known as parthenogenesis or "virginal development" of an egg without fertilization. The term is derived from (Gr., *parthenos,* virgin : and *genesis,* origin). The individuals formed by parthenogenesis are called parthenotes.

Parthenogenesis is a regular natural phenomenon in a few groups of animals. Some animals reproduce exclusively by parthenogenesis. In some other species, parthenogenesis alternates with sexual reproduction. Parthenogenesis may be of two types :

(1) Natural parthenogenesis

(2) Artificial parthenogenesis.

Natural Parthenogenesis

Parthenogenesis occurs as a normal reproductive event in bees and other social insects, rotifers, water fleas and other Crustacea. It is known as *natural parthenogenesis* or obligatory parthenogenesis. The individuals may breed exclusively by parthenogenesis without any sexual reproduction. This type of natural parthenogenesis is called complete parthenogenesis. In this case only the females exist and the male individuals are unknown *(e.g. cladocerans)*. In many species parthenogenesis may alternate with sexual reproduction. This form of parthenogenesis is called incomplete or cyclical parthenogenesis.

Natural parthenogenesis is further classified into two types:

(A) Haploid parthenogenesis or arrhenotoky.

(B) Diploid parthenogenesis or thelytoky.

Haploid Parthenogenesis of Arrhenotoky

In a number of animals, the males arise from unfertilised eggs by parthenogenesis, and are therefore, haploid (ra). The females are diploid (2ra) as they arise from the fertilized eggs in the normal manner. This type of reproduction is termed the haploid parthenogenesis or arrhenotoky. The frequency of males in the population can be determined by the frequency with which unfertilised eggs are laid. Thus haploid parthenogenesis is not only a means of reproduction but is a method of sex determination also. Arrhenotoky occurs in 9 groups of animal kingdom. It occurs in *four orders* of *insecta, rotifers, arachnids, water fleas, lizards* and *birds*.

Haploid Parthenogenesis in Insects: *Hymenoptera* (bees, ants, wasps), *Homoptera* (scale insects, plant lice) *Coleoptera* (beetles, weevils) and *Thysanoptera* (thrips) are important orders which show the haploid parthenogenesis among insects.

In bees and wasps the males develop parthenogenetically and are haploid. Females are diploid because they arise from fertilized eggs. During spermatogenesis, the reduction division in male is omitted, therefore spermatozoa contain the haploid (n) number of chromosomes in the adult male. The female honeybee contains 32 chromosomes which represent the diploid number (2n). Oogenesis results in the formation of haploid *(n)* ova each with 16 chromosomes. The males, developing parthenogenetically from unfertilised eggs, therefore, possess 6 chromosomes only. The union of these sperms with ova results in the formation of a zygote with 32 chromosomes. It develops into a female.

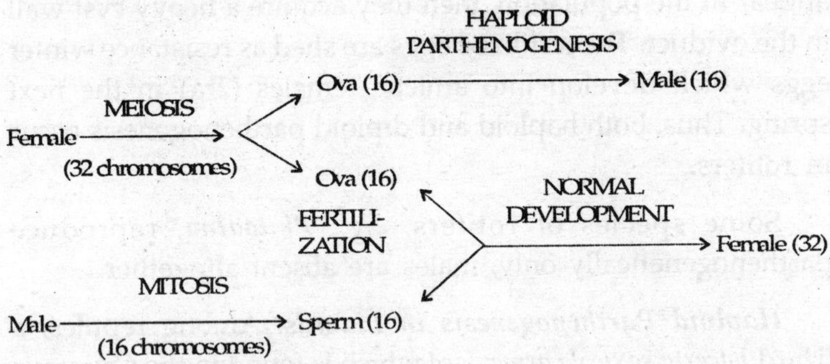

Haploid Parthenogenesis in Arachnids: In Arachnida haploid parthenogenesis is exhibited by *ticks* and *mites* only which belong to group Acarina. As in bees, the males are haploid and develop from unfertilised eggs, whereas the females are diploid arising from fertilized eggs. Male haploidy was demonstrated by Scharder (1923) in "red-spider" *Tetranyehus* and by Patau (1936) in *Pediculoides ventriconus.* Oppermann (1935). described male diploidy in one species of tick.

Haploid Parthenogenesis in Rotifers: Rotifers and water flees reproduce parthenogenetically during spring and summer. In bisexual forms, the eggs are of two kinds. Eggs maturing from diploid ovary nuclei undergo only one meiotic division and from only one polar body. As a result such eggs remain *diploid* and are called amictic eggs. They develop parthenogenetically into females. If environmental conditions remain favourable, as is usual in a pond during the spring and summer, female rotifers produce amictic eggs only. In this way, the population of females grows in pond.

In the event of sudden environmental changes, as during the fall months, diploid females give rise to *mictic eggs.* These undergo two normal meiotic divisions during their maturation and are hence smaller. Mictic eggs thus are *haploid.* If they are not fertilized, they develop parthenogenetically into males. Mictic eggs are fertilized by some of the males which now appear in the population, then they acquire a heavy cyst wall in the oviduct. The fertilized eggs are shed as resistance winter eggs which develop into amictic females (2ra) in the next spring. Thus, both haploid and diploid parthenogenesis occur in rotifers.

Some species of rotifers, *e.g., Philodina,* reproduce parthenogenetically only, males are absent altogether.

Haploid Parthenogenesis in Lizards: Among reptiles, a lizard *Lacerta saxicola armeniaca* which is found in the Caucasus region of the Soviet Union, population is propagated exclusively by parthenogenetic females. In this subspecies no males are found in nature. Although some embryos start developing as males, but they soon die in early stages.

Haploid Parthenogenesis in Birds: Spontaneous parthenogenesis has been observed in one species of the class, the *domestic turkey.* Some of the eggs isolated from males start developing, and a small number of embryos reaches the hatching stage. A few of these reach maturity and are males.

In *Rhabditis,* which is a roundworm, sperms do enter the eggs but they do not participate further in development. In fact, therefore, eggs remain unfertilised and they are said to develop parthenogenetically. This process is called gynogenesis or pseudofertilisation.

Diploid Parthenogenesis or Thelytoky

In some animals having natural parthenogenesis, *i.e.,* in the group of insects known as plant lice or aphids, the young individuals develop from the unfertilised diploid eggs. Such a condition is called diploid parthenogenesis. The diploid condition is retained either by omitting the reduction division or by the fusion of one of the polar bodies with the haploid ovum. Accordingly, diploid parthenogenesis is classified into two types namely, *ameiotic* and *meiotic thelytoky.*

Ameiotic Thelytoky: In some animals, during oogenesis the first meiotic division which is actually the reduction division is omitted and the primary oocyte directly undergoes second meiotic division which is equational or mitotic in nature. As a result the eggs are diploid and develop into new individuals without fertilization. Due to the absence of meiosis this type of parthenogenesis is known as ameiotic or apomictic parthenogenesis. It occurs in *Trichoniscus* (Isopoda-Insecta), *Daphnia pulex* (Crustacea), *Campelona rufum* (mollusca), Weevils (Coleoptera—Insecta) and long-horned grasshoppers (Orthoptera—Insecta).

Thelytoky in Phylloxera: In Phylloxera, the males are deficient in one X-chromosome (2AX—X) than the female which possesses 2AX chromosomes. In summer, diploid stem mother reproduces into diploid females by parthenogenesis. In spring, these females develop into two types of eggs: (i) larger eggs with 2AX chromosomes which produce females, and *(ii)* smaller eggs with 2AX—X which produce males. Although diploid in respect to autosomes, these eggs lack one X-chromosome due to the loss of an X during oogenesis.

In winter, the females produce ova all of which are alike in having AX genotype, but the males produce two types of sperms : with AX, and A-chromosomes only. The A-sperms which do not possess X chromosomes abort out but those with AX chromosomes fertilize ova and result in the formation of zygote with 2AX chromosomes. The latter produce diploid females :

Larger eggs (2 AX) → Females —MEIOSIS→ Ova → AX (viable), AX (viable)

Smaller eggs (2 AX --X) Males —MEIOSIS→ Sperms → AX (viable), AX (viable)

Meiotic Thelytoky: Certain eggs develop by the usual process of oogenesis involving meiosis, but at some stage of reduction division some abnormality occurs which results in diplosis *i.e.,* doubling of the chromosomes. This type of diploid parthenogenesis is also known as automictic parthenogenesis. The diplosis occurs in any of the two ways namely, *restitution* and *auto-fertilization.*

Restitution: In this process, the first maturation division of the primary oocyte is incomplete. Karyokinesis (nuclear division) forms a nucleus of the secondary oocyte and a nucleus of the first polar body but it is not followed by cytokinesis (cytoplasmic division).

The chromosomes of both daughter nuclei arrange themselves on the equator and undergo second meiotic division. This results in the formation of a diploid ovum and a diploid polar body. The diploid ovum develops into embryo without fertilization. Insects of order *Hymenoptera* and *Lepidoptera* exhibit this type of parthenogenesis.

Auto-fertilization: In this process meiosis proceeds noımally upto the formation of secondary oocyte and second polar body, but the latter is not separated off from the ovum. Instead, its nucleus unites with that of the ovum and the diploid number of chromosomes is achieved. It gives rise to a parthenogenetic female. Auto-fertilization takes place in a small brachiopod crustacean, *Artemia salina,* found in saline water.

Artificial Parthenogenesis

In many animals it has been demonstrated that the ripe eggs can be incited to starts developing by certain treatments. This phenomenon is known as artificial parthenogenesis. It has been described to occur in Annelida, Mollusca, Echinodermata, Amphibia, Aves and some mammals.

Stimuli For Artificial Parthenogenesis: Parthenogenetic development of eggs may by induced artificially by various means :

(1) The unfertilised sea urchin eggs can be made to develop successfully by:

 (i) *Treating the eggs with various substances*: (a) hypertonic or hypotonic sea-water; (6) various salts, such as the chlorides, of K, Na, Ca, Mg, etc.; (c) weak organic acids — butyric acid, lactic acid, oleic acid and other fatty acids; (d) fat solvents—ether, toluene, alcohol, acetone and benzene ; and (e) urea and sucrose.

 (ii) *Temperature shocks: i.e.,* by transferring the eggs for a short while to cold (0° to 10°C) or warm (32°C) water.

 (iii) electric induction shocks.

 (iv) ultraviolet light, and

 (v) shaking the eggs in ordinary sea water.

O. Hertwig and R. Hertwig: demonstrated that ripe sea urchin eggs may be induced to develop parthenogenetically by treatment with chloroform or strychnine (R. Hertwig, 1896).

(2) An unfertilised frog egg can be induced to develop successfully by pricking the egg with a fine glass needle. Better results are obtained if the needle be smeared with blood or be contaminated by cells from other tissues. Constituent parts of cells may also be introduced into the egg with a micropipette.

Attempts have also been made to induce parthenogenetic development in the eggs of some mammals. In this field extensive investigations were undertaken by Pincus (1936) and associates.

Most of the experiments were done with rabbit's eggs. As a result of various treatments, eggs do start cleaving but the development is abnormal and does not proceed very far.

Significance of Parthenogenesis

Means of Reproduction: Parthenogenesis is a simple method of reproduction which ensures the continuity of race in the absence of sexual reproduction.

Rapid Multiplication: Parthenogenesis produces large number of individuals within a short span of time.

Elimination of Disadvantageous Characters: Parthenotes with unfavourable mutation are eliminated altogether from the population.

Persistence of Advantageous Characters: Sometimes useful characters appear in the parthenotes by mutations. Once formed, these mutations are retained as there is no genetic segregation in animals reproducing by parthenogenesis.

Sex Determination: Sex is determined by chromosomes, therefore, parthenogenesis is very useful in determining the frequency of males and females in a population.

Polyploidy: Parthenogenesis produces polyploidy.

Fertility: Parthenogenesis prevents sterility in the races.

Prevention of Wastage of Energy: Sexual reproduction involves mating which requires energy. Parthenogenesis does not involve mating. Hence, most of the energy can be stored and utilized for feeding and other vital activities.

Sexual Reproduction

The most widely distributed mode of propagation in animal kingdom is the sexual reproduction. The essential features of this method are:

1. Reduction in the chromosome number resulting in the formation of gametes; and
2. Fertilization or union of a male and a female gamete to form zygote which restores the diploid number of chromosomes similar to parents.

LOCT and certain other scientists observed that the fertilization is not essential and absolutely necessary for the development. In certain cases under certain conditions the unfertilised egg may be stimulated to develop without the aid of spermatozoon. Such cases of development are termed as parthenogenetic cases and the phenomenon is known as parthenogenesis (Gr. *partheno*, virgin + *genesis, origin)*. The individuals reproducing by this method are called parthenotes.

Sometimes, a sperm may stimulate an egg to develop without contributing its nucleus (i.e. the sperm enters the egg but its nucleus does not fuse with egg nucleus). Moreover, the developing embryo may attain the adulthood or the development may be arrested at any stage in between. Therefore, BEATTY (1967) has revised the definition of parthenogenesis as follows:

'Parthenogenesis *is the development of a female gamete into the embryo without any genetic contribution from the male gamete, with or without the attainment of adulthood.'*

Occurrence : Parthenogenesis occurs sporadically in a large number of plant groups, but it never seems to have become widely established in any of the major groups of animal kingdom. It frequently occurs in certain orders of insecta *e.g.* Hymenoptera (bees and wasps), Homoptera, Coleoptera (beetles), Rotifera and lower crustaceans. In some groups, parthenogenesis occurs as a regular feature and alternates with the sexual generation, whereas certain individuals propagate exclusively by parthenogenesis.

Artificial and Natural Parthenogenesis

Artificial or Induced Parthenogenesis : In many animals which usually reproduce sexually, the egg can be activated by artificial methods to start the development without fertilization. Such type of parthenogenesis is called artificial parthenogenesis. For example, eggs of sea urchin can be made to develop successfully if treated with weak salt solutions (chlorides of potassium, sodium, calcium and magnesium), weak organic acids, electric shocks or shaking them in sea water.

Even an unfertilised frog's egg can be induced to develop successfully by pricking the egg with a blood-smeared glass needle. Unconfirmed reports are available about the induction of parthenogenic development in mammals.

Natural or Obligatory Parthenogenesis : In many groups of invertebrates like aphids, phyllopods, rotifers and insects parthenogenesis occurs as a regular feature and is established as a natural phenomenon in the life-history. It is known as natural parthenogenesis or obligatory parthenogenesis.

The individuals may breed exclusively by parthenogenesis with no sexual generation; or might exhibit an alternation of a sexual and a parthenogenetic generation. Thus natural parthenogenesis may be complete or cyclical.

Complete Parthenogenesis : Individuals with complete parthenogenesis reproduce exclusively by parthenogenesis. In these forms males are unknown and population consists of females only. The females develop from the unfertilised diploid eggs. This is a highly specialized mode of reproduction, the occurrence of which has totally ruled out any possibility of exchange of genetic material and recombination of genes. It is found in aphids, phyllopods and rotifers.

Cyclic Parthenogenesis : In cyclical parthenogenesis sexual generation alternate with parthenogenetic generation. For example, in bees and wasps, some eggs develop without fertilization and produce males, while those eggs that are fertilized develop into females.

Natural parthenogenesis has been noticed in a few vertebrates also. For example, a lizard *Lacerta saxicola americana* reproduces exclusively by parthenogenesis and in this species only females are found in nature.

Haploid and Diploid Parthenogenesis : Whether the parthenogenesis is cyclical or complete it can be distinguished into two types on separate lines:

(A) Haploid or Arrhenotokous parthenogenesis.

(B) Diploid or Thelytokous parthenogenesis.

Arrhenotokous or Haploid Parthenogenesis

In haploid parthenogenesis, the haploid egg formed as a result of orogenesis develops into the embryo without fusing with the sperm. Therefore, the developing embryo and the adult are also haploid consisting of half the number of chromosomes as found in the species.

The ovum or egg is formed typically with one reduction division and putting out two polar bodies. These haploid individuals are male. The females, on the other hand, are diploid and develop from the fertilized egg in the normal manner. The haploid parthenogenesis, therefore, is not only a means of reproduction but is a method of sex determination also. The frequency of males in a population is determined by the frequency with which unfertilised eggs are laid.

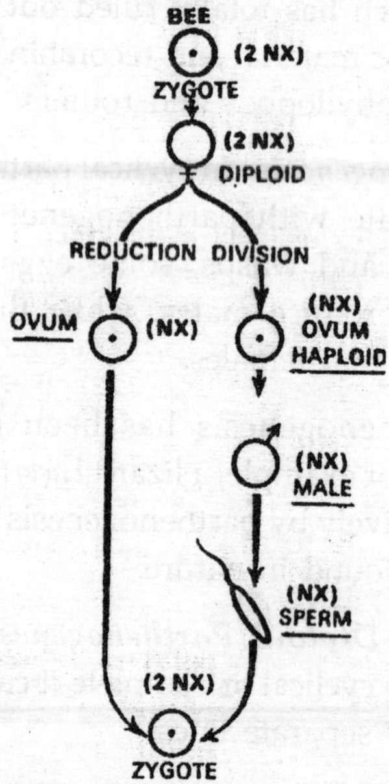

Life-cycle of Bee to illustrate haploid parthenogenesis.

The haploid parthenogenesis (haplo —diploidy) has been recorded in seven groups of animal kingdom where it has arisen independently in each group. It occurs in four orders of insecta, *i.e.* Hymenoptera, Homoptera, Coleoptera, Thysaneura and also arachnids and rotifers.

Haploid Parthenogenesis in Insecta

In insecta haplodiploidy has been observed in four groups. All the hymenopterous insects *(i.e.* bees and wasps) except a few which have become secondarily thelytokous, reproduce by haploid parthenogenesis.

In wasps and bees, the males develop parthenogenetically from the haploid eggs which are formed as a result of orogenesis *(i.e.* have already undergone the two phases of reduction division). Each such egg and, therefore, the individual developing from it both contain only half the somatic number of chromosomes. These haploid individuals are male. In hymenopterous type of sex- determining mechanism the females are diploid formed as a result of sexual reproduction by the fusion of gametes but the male is haploid and develops parthenogenetically from the haploid egg. In the formation of sperm from the testes of male no reduction division occurs. Each somatic cell of female honeybee possesses 32 chromosomes which might be represented as 2NX. The ova produced from the female will contain 16 chromosomes each, which might be designated by NX. The males developing from unfertilised eggs will naturally possess 16 chromosomes only which are passed as such to the sperms. The union of these sperms with ova results in the formation of zygote with 2NX number of chromosomes and develops into the female.

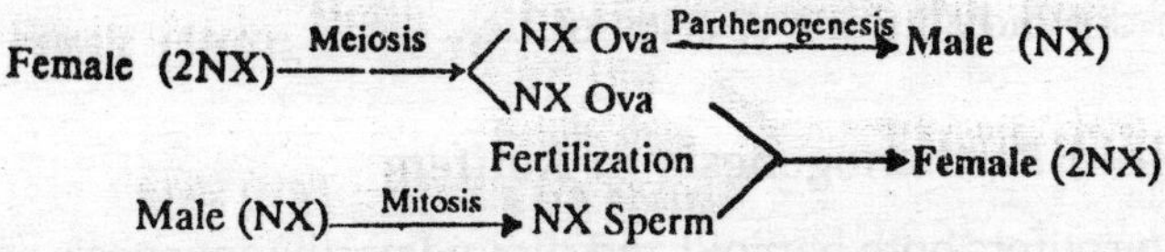

In connection with the origin of hymenopteran type of haploid parthenogenesis, Green Shield (1936) presumed that at the time of its origin, the males were diploid and females tetraploid. This has been supported by the presence of diploid tetraploid relation in primitive sandfly. Certain species of white flies (Homoptera, family Aleurodidae) also possess haploid males as reported by Schrader (1920) & Thomsen (1927). The haploid males of aleurodids undergo only first maturation division during spermatogenesis.

Although, Shull (1971), and DAVIDSON and Bald (1931) have observed the development of males from virgin female in *Anthothrips verbasi* and *Frankliniella insulasis* (Order Thysanoptera), occurrence of parthenogenesis in very much doubtful in Thysanoptera.

In Coleoptera, there is only one species exhibiting parthenogenetic mode of reproduction. In them the haploid males develop from the haploid eggs without fertilization. The sperm develop from the male without reduction division. Although, a vestigial aster is formed in the beginning but neither the nucleus nor cytoplasm divides. Thus first division is obliterated. The second division occurs normally and at the end only two sperms are formed from each spermatocyte.

Haploid Parthenogenesis in Arachnida

Parthenogenetic reproduction occurs only in ticks and mites, belonging to group Acarina. Here also the males are haploid and develop from the unfertilised eggs whereas, the females are diploid and sexual. SCHRADER (1923) has observed male haploidy in red spider *Tetranychus* and Patau (1935) in *Pediculoidas ventricusus,* but Oppermann (1935) has described male diploidy in one species of tick.

Haploid Parthenogenesis in Rotifers

In rotifers both haploid and diploid parthenogenesis occur. *Asplanchna amphora* is an example of haploid parthenogenesis, where the males are dwarf and develop from haploid eggs. In *Bolelloidoa* males are unknown and parthenogenesis is the only means of reproduction.

Diploid Parthenogenesis or Thelytoky

In diploid parthenogenesis the embryo develops from the diploid but unfertilised egg. The diploid number in the ovum is either retained by obliterating the reduction division or is secondarily restored by fusing with one of the polar bodies cast off during the process of maturation. Depending upon that the diploid parthenogenesis is distinguished into ameiotic and meiotic type of parthenogenesis.

Ameiotic Thelytoky

In normal process of orogenesis the first maturation division is a reduction division which results in halving the chromosome number. In ameiotic thelytoky the reduction division is completely suppressed. This means that in ameiotic thelytoky out of the two maturation divisions only the 2nd one *i.e.* mitotic division occurs at the time of egg formation. Thus the egg formed possesses the same diploid number as present in the oogonium. Due to the absence of meiosis this sort of parthenogenesis is known as ameiotic or apomictic parthenogenesis. It occurs in the following groups of animal kingdom.

Only one genus of Isopoda, *Trichoniscus, exhibits* parthenogenesis which is of heterogenic thelytoky. Here the diploid individuals occur both as males and females in equal numerosity and reproduce sexually. There are triploid females also, which develop ameiotically and reproduce in the same manner. At the time of gamete formation the three sets of chromosomes fail to pair so that the first maturation division does not occur. As a result of second maturation division only two eggs are formed from the oogonium each with diploid or somatic number of chromosomes.

Similarly, Mortimer (1936) has described the ameiotic parthenogenesis in *Daphniapulex,* Mattox (1937) in a fresh water mollusc, *Campelona rujum,* and Suomalalnen in weevils. In long-horned grasshopper, of course, no males have been observed and reproduction is of purely parthenogenetic nature. In all these cases only one polar body is discarded and no reduction division occurs.

Meiotic Thelytoky

In meiotic thelytoky the eggs are formed by the normal process of orogenesis *i.e.* the nucleus of oocyte undergoes two typical maturation divisions (first reduction and second mitotic). So the eggs possess haploid number of chromosomes. The reduction in chromosome number is compensated by diplosis *i.e.* doubling the chromosome number at some stage in the life-cycle. This type of diploid parthenogenesis is also known as automictic parthenogenesis. The diploid chromosome number is obtained and maintained by any one of the following methods:

By Restitution : In this process the first maturation division proceeds normally upto the movement of chromosomes to opposite poles, but after that the cytokinesis or division of the parent cell into two fails to occur, so that the cell now possesses chromosomes in quadruplicate. The process of chromosomal pairing and their separation with their distribution to daughter cells is known as restitution. Now, when this cell undergoes second maturation division (mitotic division), it produces two daughter cells each having $2n$ (diploid) number of chromosomes. Out of these two cells one is small and is known as polar body and the other bigger one as egg. This method of retaining the parental or somatic chromosomal configuration by partial omission of the reduction division is found in parthenogenetic Lepidoptera .

By Auto-fertilization : Another method of restoring the original or diploid or somatic chromosomal number is the fusion of any one of the two polar bodies with the ovum. This mutual fusion is known as auto-fertilization and is widely distributed among the parthenogenetic individuals.

The meiotic parthenogenesis is found to occur in a large number of animals belonging to different groups. In *Artemia salina,* a small branchiopod crustacean found in saline water with high salt concentration meiotic thelytoky is found to occur and the diploid number of chromosomes is maintained by auto-fertilization of the egg with second polar body. Parthenogenesis has been described as a regular feature in the life-history of several species of lepidopterous insects. In *Solenobia teriquetrella* three races have been found.

(i) Diploid bisexual race

(ii) Diploid thelytokous race

(iii) Tetraploid parthenogenetic race.

The primary oocyte in the parthenogenetic females (diploid or tetraploid) undergoes normal process of meiosis resulting in the formation of three polar bodies but after this all the four fuse in pairs together to restore the original somatic number.

In hymenopterous insects, although the arrhenotoky is of common occurrence but in certain forms like *Nemeritis conescеus* (a parasitic wasp) the diploid parthenogenesis occurs and the diploid number is restored by the process of restitution.

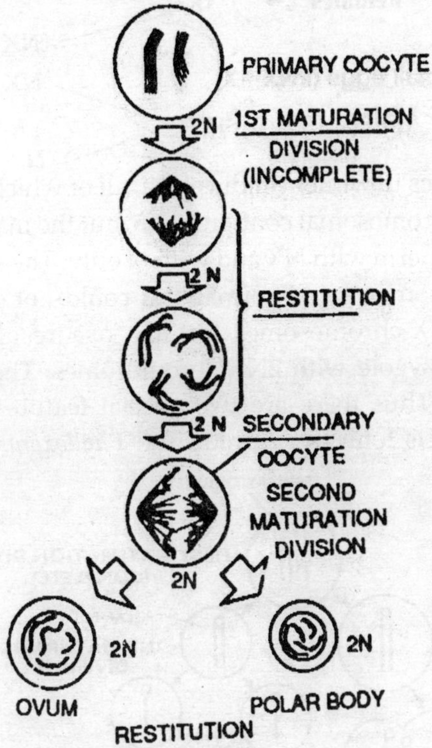

Origin of thelytoky by restitution

Thelytoky in Phylloxera and Aphids

In Aphids and *Phylloxera* the males possess one X-chromosomes less (*i.e.* 2NX-X) than the females which possess 2NX chromosomes. In winter and summer these develop two types of eggs- larger eggs with 2NX chromosomes are female producing, while the smaller eggs with 2NX-X are male producing. The larger eggs are diploid like summer eggs, and develop parthenogenetically into females, but the smaller eggs, although diploid in respect to autosomes, lack X-chromosome due to the loss of an X during maturation.

Thus:

Larger eggs (2NX)

Females → Ova → NX, NX

Small eggs (2NX – X)

Males → Sperm → NX, N

The females in winter produce ova, all of which are similar having NX-chromosomal configuration, but the males produce two types of sperm with NX and with N only. The sperms with no X-chromosomes are abnormal and could not survive. But those with NX-chromosomes fertilize ova resulting in the formation of zygote with 2NX chromosomes. These develop into females. Thus there are two special features of diploid parthenogenesis found in Aphids and *Phylloxera*.

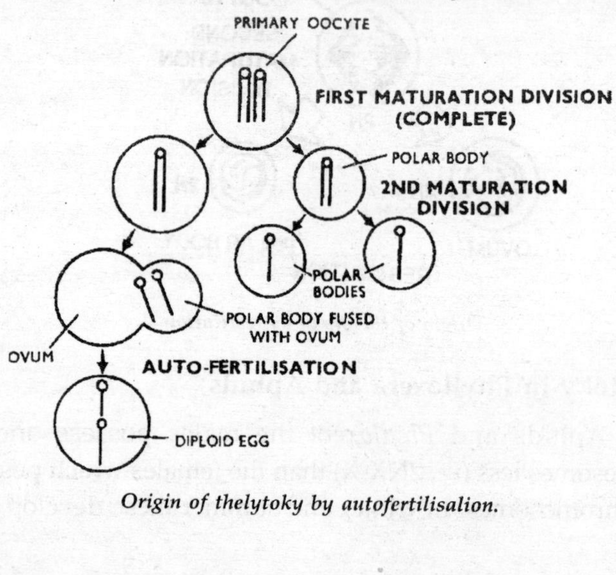

Origin of thelytoky by autofertilisalion.

Artificial Parthenogenesis

In certain group of animal kingdom parthenogenesis has been established as a natural phenomenon recurring regularly after every one or two sexual generations but in certain cases, the parthenogenesis is induced by the influence of external conditions *e.g.* diet, temperature and crowding, etc.

This is known as artificial parthenogenesis. It was first described erroneously by Boursier in 1847, when he observed that an unfertilised female silkmoth laid eggs on being kept in the sunlight. Apparently, this means that the eggs are activated by the warmth of the sunlight. In 1866, TichominoFF reported that the eggs could be artificially activated by being rubbed gently or by immersing in sulphuric acid for a short period.

In 1896 Richard Hertwig described the initiation of cleavage in sea urchin eggs immersed briefly in a dilute solution of strychnine. By now induced or artificially induced parthenotes rarely reach maturity. Mostly these develop upto the blastula or gastrula stage. Attempts are being made to induce mammalian eggs (rabbit) to develop parthenogenetically.

Stimulus for Artificial Parthenogenesis

A variety of agents can activate the eggs to develop, provided these damage cortical region. These may be:

1. *Physical Stimulus* : is provided by pricking the eggs slightly with a fine needle.
2. *Temperature* : Stimulus may be provided by temperature shocks.
3. *Chemical Stimulus:* The unfertilised eggs may be induced to divide by treating them with chemicals, such as butyric acid, lactic acid, oleic acid and a number of other fatty acids, a variety of fat solvents such as toluene, ether and acetone. Hypo or hypertonic sea

water and foreign blood serum, also initiate the egg to divide.

4. *Stimulus Provided by the Entry of Sperm* : Even the sperm from a totally different group, which does not contribute its nucleus to egg, can stimulate the egg of some different group. For example, when sperm from Annelids are made to enter the eggs of echinoaderms (Sea urchin) or the sea urchin eggs are fertilized with sperm of starfish, the nuclei of sperm and eggs do not fuse, but the eggs start dividing.

Advantages

1. *Means of Reproduction* : Parthenogenesis is a well extablished method of reproduction, even simpler and easier than the sexual method. It ensures the continuity of race when the sexual reproduction fails in the absence of fertilization.
2. *A Device for High Multiplication* : Aphids exhibit alternation of sexual and parthenogenetic generations (an example of cyclical parthenogenesis). These multiply very fast during parthenogenetic part of their life-cycle, indicating that it affords a rapid mode of multiplication.
3. *Establishment of Polyploid Generation:* It permits the establishment of triploid and aneuploid races having three or more sets of chromosomes. In these forms the three, four or more sets of chromosomes fail to pair during meiosis at the time of gamete formation, thus retarding the formation of gametes. This leads to sexual sterility. The parthenogenesis is thus a means for aneuploid individuals to propagate their own kind. The parthenogenesis has, therefore, been described by Darlington (1939) as an escape from sterility.

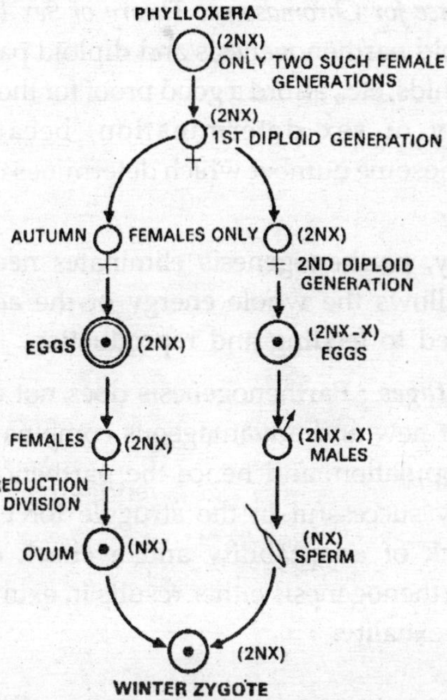

Life history of Phylloxera to illustrate diploid partherogenesis.

4. *Encouragement of Advantageous Combinations of Genes :* Parthenogenesis encourages combinations of characters of genes originated by mutation to remain as such because these are not liable to segregate by crossing over as there is no meiosis.

5. *Elimination of Disadvantageous Combinations of Genes :* All the mutagenic changes and their combinations are not useful to the organism. So natural selection in parthenogenetic forms will lead to the elimination of non-adaptive combinations of genes.

6. *Elimination of Variety in Population :* The offsprings developing parthenogenetically are more alike to and mostly the phenocopies of the parents, whereas a sexually-developed offspring will exibit marked differences from its parent, whereas eliminates variety in population.

7. *Evidence for Chromosomal Theory of Sex Determination* : Haploid parthenogenesis and diploid parthenogenesis of Aphids, etc., afford a good proof for the chromosomal theory of sex determination, because it is the chromosome number which determines the sex in these forms.
8. Finally, parthenogenesis eliminates need for mating and allows the whole energy of the adult life to be devoted to feeding and reproduction.

Disadvantages : Parthenogenesis does not encourage the appearance of new and advantageous combinations of genes within the population, and hence the parthenogenetic forms are frequently successful in the struggle for existence. This results in lack of adaptability and a check on evolution. Therefore, parthenogenesis either results in extinction or leads to return to sexuality.

15

Embryogenesis

The Essence of Life is Change : The change is more characteri-stically exhibited during the transformation of an apparently structureless blob of jelly (the egg fertilized or unfertilized) into a new highly complex multi-cellular organism (plant or animal). This is known as development. It involves three fundamental processes:

(i) increase in cell numbers by cell division (cleavage).

(ii) the differentiation of cells into tissues (cell differentiation and tissue formation).

(iii) the arrangement of these cells and tissues to form parts and organs (organogeny).

Embryogenesis and Blastogenesis

The study of all these sequential orderly processes comprises developmental biology or embryology. In other words embryology can be defined as the study of ontogenetic development (i.e. development of individual). The ontogenetic development may include embryogenesis (development of the embryo or new organism from fertilized egg, i.e., zygote) or blastogenesis (the development of new individual from some portion of parental body or the asexual reproductive bodies like bud, fragment, gemmule, etc.).

Thus, the embryology or developmental biology includes more than the study of the development of egg. It is also concerned with the asexual development of the embryo from structures other than egg and also with the regeneration of lost or damaged parts and repair of defects.

Embryology and Developmental Biology : The literal meaning of embryology is the study of embryos, where embryo denotes the juvenile stage, either within the egg shell, egg membranes or in the mother's womb. However, as discussed above the developmental processes also embrace changes in the post-embryonic or larval and even adult period. For this reason, presently the usage of term developmental biology is preferred.

Ontogenetic and Phylogenetic Development : The term 'development' is used with two different meanings. Ontogenetic development is the development of an individual. It involves transformation of fertilized egg into a new adult. Phylogenetic development involves gradual historical transformation of forms of life, starting with simple forms leading to the present diversity existing in the present-day forms. It is also referred to as evolutionary development.

Historical Review

Descriptive and Comparative Embryology : The correct interpretation of developmental phenomena rests on the cell theory, put forth by Matthias Jacob Schleiden and Theodor Schwann in the year 1838-39. Prior to this many observations in embryology were erroneous and even grotesque. Anaximander (660 B.C.) was the first Western philosopher who proposed the idea that 'living creatures arose from the moist element' as it was evaporated by the sun. Empedocles, the Greek philosopher, suggested that foetus arose partly from male and partly from female semen. Aristotle (384-322 B.C.) wrote 'The Treatise on Embryology'. He described the ontogenetic development of chick and many other animals and elaborated a kind of classification of animals based on their mode of reproduction and development. He postulated that human embryo develops out of mother's menstrual blood.

Harvey (1651) and Malpighi (1672) presented description of different stages in the development of chick as seen with simple lenses. Graaf (1672) described the ovarian follicles. Hamm and Leeuwenhoek (1677) first observed sperm of man and other mammals. Bonnet (1745) discovered that eggs of some of the insects could develop parthenogenetically. Pander (1817) reported three germ-layers from which the different parts of chick embryo are developed. Von Baer (1827) observed mammalian egg. However, the significance of egg and sperm was not understood for long.

To explain various embryological riddles, some important contributions are discussed under the following heads:

Preformation Theory

In mid seventeenth century, the Dutch scientist Swammerdam (1637-80) proposed that the sex cells (either ovum or sperm) contain preformed embryo or a more or less perfect miniature of the adult. In case of man, this miniature organism was called homunculus. The development process involves the growth and unfolding of the miniature into the adult. This theory was supported by Malpighi (1628-1694). Haller (1708-77); Bonnet (1720-93) and Spallanzani (1729-99). This group of scientists who believed that miniature organism was present in the egg were called ovists. According to these ovists every ovum in the ovary of a female contained a tiny miniature of the adult, which by proper stimulus from the seminal fluid, developed into the adult. Some ovist advocated extreme form of preformation theory, which they named encasement or emboitment theory. It holds that the miniatures of successive generations of individual organism preexisted one inside and the other in the germ cells of mother.

Another group of scientists believed that the preformed miniature organism is present in the head of sperm. These were called spermists. They described sperm as the seeds and egg as the soil in which seed was planted. Hartsoeker (1656-1725) gave an illustrated diagram of man's sperm with homunculus.

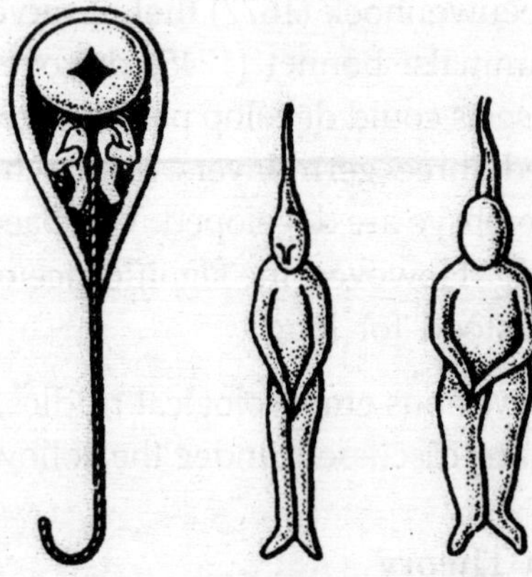

The human sperm cells with homunculus as drawn by Hartsoeker. 1694.

Epigenetic Theory

Casper Friedrich Wolf (1759) in volume entitled *'Theoria Generationis'* described that in chick egg, there is no pre-formed minieture chick. He advocated that the future embryonic regions of an egg are formed of granules or globules or vesicles. During development, these gradually organise into rudiments which can be called the germinal layers. This method of progressive development from simpler to more complex organization through the utilization of building units is called epigenesis.

The theory was supported by Johan Friedrich Haeckel (1781-1833).

The theory of epigenesis is accepted even today but in a different form. With great advances in the field of cytology and genetics, it is known that the genetic constitution of an organism is fixed by heredity in the fertilized egg from which the organism develops in specific lines.

Baer's Law

Karl Earnst Von Baer (1792-1876) who is called 'The father of modern embryology' contributed immensely to the field of embryology. He proposed 'germ layer theory', and Baer's law. Baer's law proposes that *'more general features that are common to all the members of a group of animals, develop earlier than the more special features which distinguish the various members of the group.'* For example, in the development of different groups of vertebrates, the vertebrate features (viz. notochard, spinal cord, brain and segmental muscles) develop earlier than the distinguishing features of various classes like hair in mammals, feathers in birds and scales in reptiles.

Recapitulation Theory and Exogenetic Law : In the light of evolutionary theory, Muller and Haeckel (1864) reinterpretted Baer's law and called it Recapitulation theory. It implies that *"the embryo of any species undergoes or repeats in its development the evolutionary or phylogenetic history of its race.* Haeckel worded it as follows *'ontogeny recapitulates phylogeny'*. Ontogeny refers to the development of an individual while phylogeny is the evolutionary history of the group.

However, repetition is not complete. The modified version of recapitulation theory, the biogenetic law states that *'ontogeny is a shortened and modified recapitulation of phylogeny'*, i.e., during the development of an individual many steps of phylogeny of the group are ommitted, abbreviated and modified because the embryo has to compromise with the surroundings.

Following these discoveries, embryologists investigated the development of animals belonging to all major groups of animal kingdom in nineteenth century. So far the studies embraced only two aspects, descriptive and comparative embryology.

Experimental Embryology

During late 19th and early 20th century, weismann (1883), Roux (1888), Driesh (1891), Endres (1895), Spemann (1901-1903) and Morgan (1905) made experimental and analytical approach and founded a new branch of embryology—the experimental embryology. These established following theories-

Mosaic Theory

Wilhelm Roux (1950-1924), one of Haeckel's students asserted on the experimental approach for growth and differentiation. Based on the study of frog's egg he proposed that certain areas of the egg are predestined to develop into special regions, while the egg is in the ovary. He showed that in frog's egg the dark pigmented area of animal hemisphere is destined to develop chiefly into head region, while the vegetal hemisphere into posterior region. As cleavage proceeds more and more organ-specific areas are delineated on the surface of blastula. So the blastula in its final stage resembles a mosaic of blastomeres having different potencies for differentiation. This was called mosaic theory. It can be defined as follows:

'The ontogenetic development is the differentiation of cell from a more or less undifferentiated and homogeneous egg with simple prelocalization of material to greater differentiation and specialization of cells as development proceeds.'

Regulative Theory

German scientist Hans Driesch strongly opposed Roux mosaic theory. He conducted experiments on sea urchin egg in a fashion similar to ROUX. He separated the blastomeres at two cell stages and found that each half (blastomere)normally developed into a complete larva of somewhat smaller size. Blastomeres isolated at four-cell's stage also developed into whole embryos. From such experiments, he concluded that early cleavages of the egg are equational which divide the egg material equally, so that all the early blastomeres have equal potencies for development.

Their fate is determined by their position. However, in Sea urchin eggs, Driesch observed that development is regulative, since the fertilised egg exhibits distinct regions, each having a predetermined future.

Gradient Theory

The gradient concept was introduced by Boveri (1901), who postulated that the vegetal region of sea urchin egg influences the morphogenesis of animal region of the embryo and this influence gradually decreases towards the animal pole. C.M. Child (1940) and others proposed 'metabolic axial gradient theory' according to which there exists a gradient of the oxidative metabolism in the egg.

By using rate of reduction of vital dyes, particularly Janus green as an indicator of the rate of oxidative metabolism, CHILD demonstrated the differences in the rate of general metabolism in the ooplasm of the animal and vegetal hemispheres of the oocytes and the cleaving eggs of sea urchin and starfish. He proposed that there exists a gradual decrease in the rate of oxidative metabolism in the ooplasm from animal to the vegetal pole, which can be described as the metabolic axial gradient along the animal-vegetal axis.

Child's metabolic axial gradient theory was later modified by Horstadius (1955) and Runnstrom (1967). They proposed the existence of a double-gradient system to control the morphogenesis and differentiation during early development of sea urchin embryo. An animal gradient is maximum at the animal pole and is responsible for the formation of structures characteristic of that region. Similarly, the vegetal gradient, which is most intense at the vegetal pole, controls processes like invagination, formation of archenteron and mesenchyme. If the animal gradient is weakened or supressed, the vegetal gradient becomes preponderant and the embryo is vegetalised; and if the vegetal gradient is weakened, the animal gradient becomes preponderant and embryo becomes animalized. A normal development results only when two gradients are in correct equilibrium horstadius and Josefsson (1969) have shown the existence of specific animalizing and vegetalizing substances (such as tryptophan and nucleotide) in the mature fertilized eggs. The animalizing agents are presumed to promote synthesis of ribonucleic acid and proteins, while the vegetalizing agents inhibit the onset of these processes.

Spemann's Theory of Organizers

Spemann demonstrated the existence of interactions between the parts of developing embryo, which control the proper position and size of the various organs of the embryo. He conducted the following experiments-

(i) Between 1901 to 1912 Spemann demostrated the dependence of lens formation upon the presence of an optic vesicle. When epidermis of future lens region (prospective eye rudiment) was removed from the early embryo of grass frog and transplanted in the tail region, it failed to form a lens but developed into the epidermis of tail. Conversely, an optic vesicle transplanted under belly ectoderm formed a lens instead of belly skin.

(ii) In 1918 Spemann reported that small pieces of presumptive neural plate region and of skin ectoderm from early gastrula (salamander) when transplanted to some other part of gastrula, developed according to their new location. Conversely, when a piece from dorsal lip of blastopore of one embryo was transplanted in the epidermal region of other embryo, it was found to develop independently of the new surroundings and formed an additional neural plate, notochord and mesoderm. Spemann called this area as organizer. He got Nobel prize for this discovery in 1935. Based on this experiment and others Spemann et. al., gave the following definition for the embryonic organizer.

'When one embryonic tissue transmits a stimulus that influences another tissue to produce a structure that otherwise would not come into being, then the former tissue is called the inductor or organizer and its morphogenetic effect is called induction.

Summary of Major Events in the field of Developmental Biology during 19th Century

(i) Experiments involving separation and subsequent development of first cells (blastomeres) resulting from the division of fertilized eggs (in sea urchin and frog) by chemical and mechanical means by noted scientists. Wilhelm Roux, Hans Driesch and Theodor Boveri.

(ii) Cell lineage studies by E.B.Wilson and E.G. Conklin.

(iii) Culture of tissue cells in culture medium by Ross Harrison.

(iv) Grafting and Transplantation of Hans Spemann and W.H. Lewis.

(v) Regeneration mechanism by Hans Driesch, T.H.Morgan and C.M.Child.

(vi) Organizers and embryonic induction by Spemann and his students - Mangold and Holtfreter

(vii) Biochemical embryology by Needham.

Analytical Embryology

The foundation of analytical embryology was laid in 1919 by Morgan, T.H. and et. al. All the properties of any organism are determined by DNA, the hereditary material. This has brought the development directly into the realm of molecular domain. The recent work on embryology has a biochemical and biophysical approach. Methods such as chromatography, electrophoresis, ultra centrifugation, radioactive tracers and electron microscopy, scanning, etc. are at the disposal of modern embryologists. The modern embryologists aim to work on the principles and processes of development. This is called analytical embryology.

Methods in the Study of Embryonic Development : Over the years many methods have been devised for studying various aspects of embryonic development. These range from the examination of entire embryos with the naked eye or simple lenses to extremely sophisticated molecular probes.

Direct Observation of Living Embryos : This was the earliest technique used in embryology. The living embroys are studied either with naked eye or with simple lenses. After the introduction of the microscope, gametes and small embryos were examined. The direct observation of living embryos provides an overall view of the embryo and impresses the observer with the dynamic and sweeping change occuring during embryonic development. These changes are studied through micro cinematography. It provides a moving picture of development.

Examination of Fixed Material : The embryo is fixed by using some chemicals. This arrests the process of development at a critical phase so that it can be examined at leisure. Formalin or glutaraldehyde are used as fixatives. The fixed embryonic tissue or the entire embryo is also used for preparing serial microscopic sections. From the study of these sections, the three-dimensional internal structure of an entire embryo can be reconstructed. Through scanning electron microscopy a three- dimensional view of entire embryos or parts of the embryos is seen.

Histochemical Methods

These methods are used to identify localized specific chemical substances or sites of chemical activity on morphological structures. The embryo or its tissue is rapidly frozen in liquid nitrogen and is sectioned with a special low temperature microtome called cryostat. The sections are placed on glass slide and subjected to specific chemical reaction. The reaction products are deposited as coloured products at the site of enzymatic activity.

Autoradiography : In autoradiography the precursors of macromolecules containing radioactivity-tagged atoms are introduced into the living biological system or into the embryo. The embryo or its part is placed in a solution containing radio actively labelled amino acid or a nitrogenous base (a precursor of a DNA or RNA). After a given period, the embryo is removed from the radioactive solution and is sectioned for microscopic examination. The tissue sections are covered with a photographic emulsion and kept in dark for several weeks. Radioactive emissions from the isotope, incorporated into the embryo through amino acid or nucleic acid impinge upon the photographic emulsion. It is then developed like a photographic film. The radioactively-labelled atoms deposit silver as tiny grains. This method of detecting pathway of readioactively-labelled markers is called autoradiography.

Autoradiographic technique has been a great help in localizing sites of nucleic acid and protein synthesis in embryo and in tracing the movements of cells from surface of blastula to their prospective areas.

Tracing Methods : Non-toxic markers are used to trace the cell movements in the developing embryo. The most common methods is the use of non-toxic vital dyes or vital stains. Nile blue sulfate or neutral red are applied to living cells. The movement of these stained cells can be followed during development and growth. Marking may also be carried out by placing finely-divided, physiologically inert carbon particles (such as blood charcoal) on a small groups of cells.

To identify the location of specific proteins in the specialized cells specific antibody to the protein is used. The antibodies are often combined with fluorescent dyes and then applied to the embryo. For long-term tracing of cells and cell lineage natural markers are used. Sex-chromatin and Japanese quail cells are used as marker grafts. The differences in nuclear size and morphology help in identifying the graft cells.

Microsurgical Techniques

Microsurgical techniques are used in the study of tissue interaction during embryonic development. The instruments used are micromanipulators for holding, the glass or tungsten needles and loops of baby hair for surgical removal of embryonic tissue, or micropipettes for the removal of nucleus from the zygote or ovum. The various microsurgical techniques are-

(i) Ablation or removal of part of an embryo by cauterization or by laser beams.

(ii) Explantation is excising a small sample of embryonic tissue and growing it in an artificial environment.

(iii) Transplantation is to graft the excised tissue of one embryo into the same embryo or some other embryo at some different location. Transplantation can be :

   (a) Autografting is transplanting the graft to some other side on the same embryo.

   (b) Heterografting is transplanting the graft from one embryo on to another embryo of some different species.

(c) Xenografting is transplanting the graft tissue on the embryo of some different order.

(d) Nuclear transplantation involves transplanting of nucleus from the adult tissue into an egg whose nucleus has been inactivated or removed. This technique was developed by Briggs and King in 1952.

Experiment : Gurdon (1962) transplanted the nucleus from the intestinal epithelium of a postembryonic frog *(Xenopus)* into the egg whose nucleus was inactivated by UV radiation. The adult frog developed from the egg shows that the nucleus of a highly specialized cell is still capable of guiding the development of an entire mature animal (totipoteny).

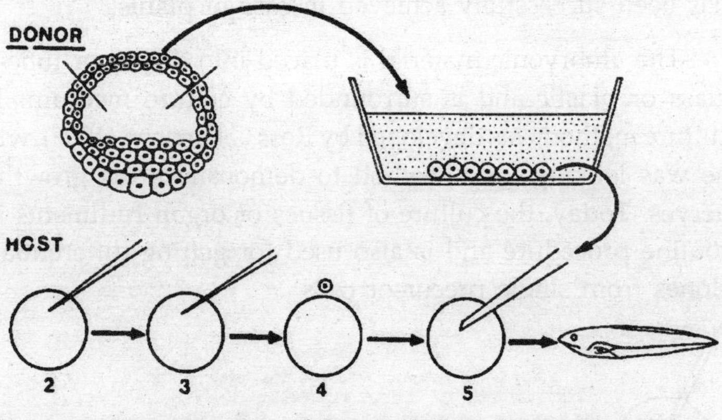

Diagrammatic representation of the procedure involved in the nuclear transplantation adopted by GURDON (1962)

(e) Embryo transfer is the transplantation of the fertilized egg or young embryo into the uterus of some other animal is called embryo transfer. Since then till date not less than 2,300 test tube babies have been born in Australia alone. The method has been successfully developed in India also.

Clinical application of embryo transfer resulted in the birth of first test tube baby in human beings. Two British reproductive biologists, Robert Edwards and Patrick Steptoe obtained an ovum from the ovary of a woman who had a blockage of uterine tube (which prevented the ovulated egg to reach uterus). This egg was fertilized *in vitro* with her husband's sperm. The embryo developed to the 8-cell stage in the culture medium inside the test tube and was then transplanted to the woman's uterine wall. The transplanted embryo developed into a normal baby girl.

Culture Techniques

It involves culturing or growing the components of embryos or even the whole embryos in culture medium. It may be cell-culture, tissue culture or whole embryo culture. Embryo culture has been successfully achieved in case of plants.

The embryonic material is placed into dishes or tubes of glass or plastic and is surrounded by culture medium. The culture method was developed by Ross G.harrison (1907), while he was looking for a method to demonstrate the growth of nerves. Today, the culture of tissues or organ rudiments is a routine procedure and is also used for getting differentiated clones from single precursor cells.

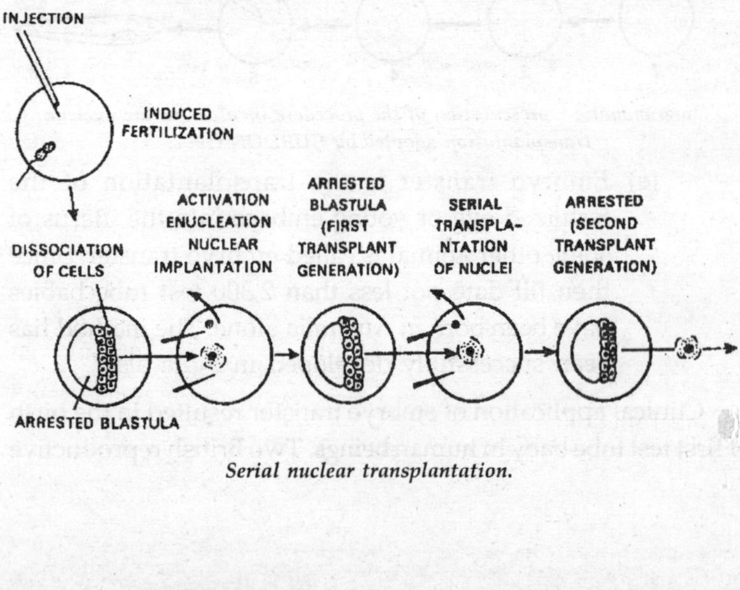

Serial nuclear transplantation.

Cellullar Dissociation and Aggregation : This is a new technique of studying growing tissue. It involves dissociation of the constituent cells of the growing tissue by using weak solution of certain protein digesting enzymes like trypsin. This breaks down the material responsible for adhesion between adjacent cells. The dissocated cells are throughly mixed and then grown in the tissue culture medium where they can move freely and re-associate.

Biochemical Techniques

The present-day biochemical techniques like chromatography, electrophoresis and spectrophotometry, etc., are used for the analysis of enzyme activity and in determining the metabolic properties of different embryonic tissues. Centrifugation of tissue homogenate is used to separate sub-cellular fractions or different classes of macromolecules.

Irradiation Techniques

X-rays, UV-rays are used to cause tissue injury or to inactivate a group of cells in a circumscribed area. Laser beams are another valuable tool in producing sharply-localized lesions in embryos.

Inhibitory Agents and Teratogens

Many chemicals are used to inhibit normal embryonic process. These result in abnormal development. Antibiotic actinomycin-D, a number of drugs, sleeping pills, pain killers are teratogenic agent or teratogens (causing abnormal development).

Genetic Markers (Use of Mutants) : Lethal or mutant strains of laboratory animals are used as genetic markers or as tracers. By determining when and where development first goes wrong in the mutant strain, it is possible to pinpoint the effects of specific genes in the developmental process.

Identification of specific isoenzymes by electrophoretic methods is another useful tracing technique.

Branches of Embryology

Descriptive Embryology : This field of embryology is associated with the mor-phological description of different embryonic stages in the ontogenetic development of individuals of different species. This involves the initial work of embryologists till 18th century.

Comparative Embryology: It embraces the comparative study of embryology of different animal groups.

Experimental Embryology : It involves all those studies that attempt to understand the various fundamental mechanisms in the development of different animals.

Chemical Embryology : This branch of embryology includes all those studies which employ various biochemical, biophysical and physiological techniques for understanding embryological events at molecular level.

Teratology : It is the branch of embryology concerned with the study of malfor mations or birth defects. The substances that cause birth defects are called teratogens.

Application of Developmental Biology : Developmental biology or embryology is most valuable science. Its importance can be discussed under following heads —

Scientific Significance

Ontogenetic Development : It helps in understanding the development of in dividual and also the general concept of ontogenetic development.

Phylogenetic Relationship : Comparative study of development of organisms belonging to different groups helps in assigning the phylogenetic relationship and systematic position of different animal and plant groups.

Evolutionary Significance : Study in developmental biology helps to explain the occurrence of vestigial structures. It explains the various phenomena pertaining to growth, differentiation and regeneration.

Medical Significance

Knowledge and understanding of developmental processes are important for human welfare in the following fields —

In Malformation : Abnormalities in structure or function of an organ or part may arise during development. These may be caused due to genetic defects, effect of drugs, viruses, hormones, etc. The type of abnormality produced depends more on the stage of development on which the effective agent acts.

Malignant Tumours : These are abnormal forms of tissue development. The nature and control of malignancy relates to the understanding of normal processes of growth and differentiation.

Ageing : Ageing process is one of the aspect of development. It requires proper understanding of cell, tissue and organismal growth throughout the lifespan.

Control of Reproduction and Development : The insight knowledge of reproduction has helped in controlling reproduction and development of humans and their livestock. This is being achieved by the use of hormones, sperm storage at low temperature and embryo transfer. It has led to the development of technique called 'test tube baby'.

Developmental biology holds out both a promise and a threat to human race.

Bibliography

Alcock, John : *Exploring Animal Behavior : Readings from American Scientist,* Sinauer, London, 1992.

Arbel, T. : *Annual Review of Genetics,* Oxford, New York, 1993.

Arey, L.B. : *Developmental Anatomy,* W.B. Saunders Company, London, 1954.

Austin, C.R. : *Ultra Structure of Fertilization,* Rinehart and Winston International, New York, 1968.

Balinsky, B.I. : *An Introduction to Embryology,* W.B. Saunders Company, London, 1920.

Benson, G. John and Bernard, E. : *The Well-Being of Farm Animals : Challenges and Solutions,* Blackwell, London, 2004.

Berill, N.J. : *Developmental Biology,* McGraw Hill Book Company, New York, 1971.

Black, Jonathan : *Biological Performance of Materials : Fundamentals of Biocompatibility,* Dekker, London, 1999.

Bodemer, C.W. : *Modern Embryology,* Rinehart and Winston International, New York, 1968.

Bolhuis, J.J. and Hogan, J.A. : *The Development of Animal Behaviour : A Reader,* Blackwell, London, 1999.

Bonner, J.T. : *Morphogenesis,* Oxford and IBH Publishing Company, Calcutta, 1965.

Bos, Cees J. : *Fungal Genetics : Principles and Practice,* Dekker, London, 1996.

Campbell, N.A. : *Biology : Concepts and Connections*, Oxford, New York, 1997.

Chaudhry, G. Rasul : *Biological Degradation and Bioremediation of Toxic Chemicals*, Dioscorides P., London, 1994.

Cooper, R. : *The Biology-Chemistry Interface : A Tribute to Koji Nakanishi*, Dekker, London, 1999.

Deen, Roger T. and Kelly, T. : *Atherosclerosis : Gene Expression, Cell Interactions and Oxidation*, Oxford, New York, 2000.

Dick, Stevan J. : *The Biological Universe : The Twentieth-Century Extraterrestrial Life Debate*, Cambridge, New York, 1999.

Dudley, Elizabeth C. : *The Unity of Evolutionary Biology : Proceedings of the Fourth International Congress*, Dioscorides Pub., London, 1991.

Ebert, J.D. and Sussex, I.M. : *Interacting Systems in Development*, Rinehart and Winston International, New York, 1970.

Ewen, R.S. : *Vertebrate Embryology*, Oxford and IBH Publishing Company, New Delhi, 1980.

Ferl, Robert J. : *Biology : The Realm of Life*, Harper Collins, London, 1996.

Fosberg, Dombois : *Vegetation of the Tropical Pacific Islands*, Springer, London, 1998.

Gould, Dr. E. : *Encyclopaedia of Mammals : A Comprehensive Illustrated Guide*, Academic Pub., London, 1998.

Gould, Laura : *Cats Are Not Peas : A Calico History of Genetics*, Copernicus, London, 1996.

Green, Ronald M. : *The Human Embryo Research Debates : Bioethics in the Vortex of Controversy*, Oxford, New York, 2001.

Gutmann, F. : *Charge Transfer Complexes in Biological Systems*, Dekker, London, 1997.

Helms, Doris R. : *Biology in the Laboratory*, Worth Pub., London, 1994.

Hunter, M.L. : *Fundamentals of Conservation Biology*, Blackwell, London, 1996.

Kardong : *Vertebrates*, McGraw-Hill, London, 2001.

Larket C.L., and A. Usprung : *Developmental Genetics*, Prentice-Hall of India Pvt. Ltd., New Delhi, 1974.

Linzey, Donald : *Vertebrate Biology : Biological Sciences*, McGraw-Hill, London, 2001.

Luettner, A.F. : *Fundamentals of Comparative Embryology*, The MacMillan Company, New York, 1949.

Martin, E.H. : *Developmental Behavior Genetics : Natural, Biometrical and Evolutionary Approaches*, Oxford, New York, 1990.

McGleenan, T. : *Genetics and Insurance*, BIOS, London, 1999.

Minkoff, Eli C. : *Biology Today : An Issues Approach*, McGraw-Hill, London, 1996.

Moody, Sally A. : *Cell Lineage and Fate Determination*, Academic Pub., London, 1999.

Nalbandov, A.V. : *Reproductive Physiology*, W.H. Freeman and Company, London, 1985.

Nelson, O.E. : *Comparative Embryology of the Vertebrates*, The Balkiston Company, New York, 1953.

Newell, Grove and Carthy : *Animal Biology*, University Tutorial Press Ltd., London, 1966.

Odell, W.D. and Moyer, D.L. : *Physiology of Reproduction*, St. Louis, Mosby, 1971.

Patten, B.M. : *Early Embryology of the Chick*, Tata McGraw-Hill Publishing Company Ltd., New Delhi, 1971.

Pedigo, Larry P. : *Entomology and Pest Management*, Prentice Hall, London, 1999.

Roodrich, E.S. : *Studies on the Structure and Development of Vertebrates*, The MacMillan Company, New York, 1958.

Rugh, Roberts : *A Laboratory Manual of Vertebrate Embryology*, Burgess Publishing Company, Bombay, 1962.

———— : *The Frog : Its Reproduction and Development*, Tata McGraw-Hill Publishing Company, New Delhi, 1972.

Russo, V.E.A. : *Development : Genetics, Epigenetics and Environmental Regulation*, Springer, London, 1999.

————: *Development : The Molecular Genetic Approach*, Springer, London, 1992.

Samuel, S. : *Biological Control of Crop Diseases*, Dekker, London, 2002.

Saunders, J.W. : *Pattern and Principles of Animal Development*, MacMillon Company, London, 1970.

Scheuer, P.J. : *Bio-Organic Marine Chemistry*, Springer, London, 1988.

————: *Biotechnology and Genetics in Fisheries and Aquaculture*, Blackwell, London, 2003.

Segel, Lee A. : *Biological Kinetics : Cambridge Studies in Mathematical Biology*, Cambridge, New York, 1991.

Shair, H.N. : *Developmental Psychobiology : New Methods and Changing Concepts*, Oxford, New York, 1991.

Singh, Bijay K. : *Plant Amino Acids : Biochemistry and Biotechnology*, Dekker, London, 1999.

————: *Practical Genetics for Aquaculture*, Blackwell, London, 2001.

Slafer, Gustavo A. : *Genetic Improvement of Field Crops*, Dekker, London, 1994.

Slater, P.J.B. : *Essentials of Animal Behaviour*, Oxford, New York, 1999.

Slickinger, R.A. : *Developmental Biology Dubuque*, MacMillan, London, 1966.

Spencer, J.F.T. : *Yeasts : Natural and Artificial Habitats*, Springer, London, 1997.

Spratt, N.T. : *Introduction to Cell Differentiation*, Van Nostrand Reinhold, New York, 1964.

Sreeman, W.H. and B. Bracegirdle : *An Atlas of Embryology*, Heinemann Educational Books, London, 1977.

Starr, C. : *Biology : The Unity and Diversity of Life*, Wadsworth, London, 1998.

Sussman, M. : *Animal Growth and Development*, Prentice Hall, New Delhi, 1958.

Taylor, D.J. : *Biological Science*, Oxford, New York, 1997.

Torrey, T.W. : *Morphogenesis of the Vertebrates*, John Wiley & Sons, London, 1971.

Townsend, R.R. : *Techniques in Glycobiology*, Dekker, London, 1997.

Trempy, J. : *Fundamental bacterial Genetics*, Blackwell, London, 2003.

Waddington, C.H. : *Principle of Development and Differentiation*, MacMillan, New York, 1966.

Walker, P.M.B. : *Chambers Biology Dictionary*, Chambers, London, 1989.

Wang, T.L. and Cuming, A. : *Embryogenesis : The Generation of a Plant-EPBS*, BIOS, London, 1996.

Weisz, Paul B. : *The Science of Biology*, McGraw-Hill Book Company, New York, 1971.

ENCYCLOPAEDIA OF
EMBRYOLOGY

ENCYCLOPAEDIA OF EMBRYOLOGY

(Vol. 2)

Dr. A. Tyagi

ANMOL PUBLICATIONS PVT. LTD.
NEW DELHI - 110 002 (INDIA)

ANMOL PUBLICATIONS PVT. LTD.
H.O.: 4374/4B, Ansari Road, Darya Ganj,
New Delhi-110 002 (India)
Ph.: 23261597, 23278000
B.O.: No. 1015, Ist Main Road, BSK IIIrd Stage
IIIrd Phase, IIIrd Block,
Bangalore - 560 085 (India)
Visit us at: www.anmolpublications.com

Encyclopaedia of Embryology

First Published, 2006

ISBN 81-261- 2676-0 (Set)

PRINTED IN INDIA

Published by J.L. Kumar for Anmol Publications Pvt. Ltd., New Delhi - 110 002 and Printed at **Arora** Offset Press, Delhi.

Contents

Preface

Literally, embryology is the study of embryos, where embryo denotes the juvenile stage, either within the egg-shell, egg membranes or in the mother's womb. In the development stage, the embryo undergoes a number of changes. The changes occur not only in the body of the larva but also in habit or behaviour also. It is due to these dramatic changes that embryology has now been termed 'Developmental Biology' preferably.

Metamorphosis, embryonic induction, embryonic nutrition, regeneration, cleavage, parthenogenesis (development of egg without fertilization), gametogenesis and fertilization are few of numerous other points of study under embryology.

Though a number of books on every subject are available in the market, there is being felt a dearth of such an encyclopaedia as may answer any queries regarding any of the points which come under embryology.

Present encyclopaedia may prove to be an appreciable step in this direction. Hopefully, this would cater to the maximum requirements of the bio-enthusiasts.

Editor

1

The Fertilization

Fertilization is the fusion of a male and female gamete, which, in animals, are the spermatozoon and the ovum respectively. It results in the formation of a zygote from which the body of the offspring is formed. Fertilization fundamentally performs two functions :

(1) It activates the egg to start developing.

(2) It injects a male haploid nucleus into the egg cytoplasm. The fusion of two haploid nuclei, one from the spermatozoon and the other from the ovum, restores the diploid state and introduces genetic variation in the new organism. The intermingling of the paternal and maternal hereditary characters in the offspring is known as amphimixis.

The process of fertilization has been studied mostly in marine invertebrates *e.g.*, sea urchins, echiuroids, polychaetes, and balanoglossids whose eggs are typically small, semi-transparent, and without much yolk. Among vertebrates, it has been extensively worked out in amphibians and mammals.

Site of Fertilization

Fertilization of the ova occurs either outside the body of maternal parent (external fertilization) or inside the oviducts of the female. In the latter case, the spermatozoa are delivered in the body of female by the insertion of a sexual appendage as in insects and mammals during copulation, or by mating as in birds (internal fertilization).

External Fertilization: In majority of aquatic animals, the sperms and ova are shed into the surrounding water where fertilization takes place. It is called external fertilization. Examples: *fishes, amphibians andechinoderms.* Delivery of large quantities of spermatozoa close to numbers of ripe eggs is a basic requirement of external fertilization. Since there are great developmental hazards in open waters, astronomical numbers of eggs as well as sperm are spawned during any one spawning period.

Internal Fertilization: In amniotes, the male introduces sperms into the female's genital tract where the fusion takes place. It is called internal fertilization. This mode of fertilization takes place in animals whose development is ovoviviparous (*e.g.,* certain lizards and snakes, scorpion, some fishes) or viviparous *(e.g.,* some fishes like *Mustelus,* marsupial and placental mammals, including man). Internal fertilization is the rule in those viviparous animals which lay eggs covered by hard shells *(e.g.,* insects, most reptiles, birds and egg-laying mammals). Animals in which internal fertilization takes place possess specialized sex organs for transmitting and receiving the sperms. In such forms the fertilization may occur either in the lower part of the oviduct *(e.g.,* Urodeles) ; in the upper part of oviduct *(e.g.,* salamanders, reptiles, apes and most mammals); or in the ovarian follicles *(e.g.,* viviparous fishes like *Gambusia affinis* and certain eutherian mammals such as *Ericulus).*

In terrestrial animals mature spermatozoa are generally stored in a physiological medium which is capable of maintaining their life and potential activity for days or even months. This medium is provided either in moisture-conserving capsules or in compartments of the male or female body from where the sperms are picked up, transferred or utilized in one way or the other. Yet even in mammals millions of spermatozoa must be ejaculated in order that some of them shall reach the upper end of a fallopian tube where one or more ripe eggs may be descending.

For example, during one mating amongst *humans*, about 350 million sperms are discharged, by the man into the vagina of the woman, but out of these very few reach the fallopian tube and only one succeeds in fertilizing the ovum present there.

Mechanism of Fertilization

The process of fertilization in animals is completed in 5 steps :

1. The meeting of gametes.
2. Barrier penetration.
3. Sperm and *egg* fusion : the acrosome reaction.
4. Activation of the ovum.
5. Migration of pronuclei and amphimixis.

Meeting of Gametes

Whether fertilization is external or internal, the first step is the encounter of spermatozoon and the ovum which is brought about by the swimming movements of the spermatozoa. The movements of the spermatozoa are entirely at random and they collide with the egg as a matter of pure chance. However, in all those vertebrates in which fertilization is internal, spermatozoa tend to be transported passively, from the site of deposition to the site of fertilization, but by the muscular contractions of the female genital tract.

Agglutination: In most animals it has been observed that in the presence of ripe eggs, the spermatozoa adhere to the surface of the egg and even to each other. The adhesion of spermatozoa to each other results in their clumping or agglutination.

Fertilizin-Antifertizin Reaction: The substance causing agglutination of spermatozoa was described by F.R. Lillie (1919). Lillie was the first to show that eggs produce a substance called fertilizin which combines with a substance termed antifertilizin present on the surface of spermatozoa. As a matter of fact, fertilizin is released in the surrounding water and, as a consequence of combining reaction with antifertilizin, most of the sperms agglutinate or clump together.

Chemically, fertilizin is a *glycoprotein* which consists of a number of amino acids and one or more monosaccharides (glucose, fucose, fructose or galactose). Depending upon their chemical composition, there are many types of fertilizins in different animals. The molecules of the fertilizins are quite large. Their molecular weight is about 300,000. The antifertilizins are *acid proteins* with a fairly smaller molecule (molecular weight 10,000).

The adhesion of the spermatozoon to the surface of the egg is brought about by linking of fertilizin molecules with antifertilizin molecules present on the surface of the spermatozoon. This phenomena establishes an initial bond which would later lead to the penetration of the sperm into the egg. This reaction is highly specific: fertilizin of one species of animal will not react with antifertilizin of another species. This is analogous to a lock-and-key effect, and serves as a barrier against cross breeding.

The reaction between fertilizin and antifertilizin is thus very similar to antigen-antibody reactions. It qualifies the spermatozoa to become fully capable of fertilizing an egg of the same species. Berill (1971) called it capacitation.

Barrier Penetration

The surface of the ripe egg is rarely naked (as in coelenterates). It is usually surrounded by egg membranes or follicle cells or both (as in mammals). The spermatozoan has to penetrate through these barriers before it can reach the interior of the egg. The mechanism of penetration is chemical. The egg envelopes are broken down by substances of an enzymatic nature known under the general name of sperm lysins released by the acrosome of the sperm cell (Colwin and Colwin, 1961).

In the case of eggs with very thick and resistant membranes *e.g.*, fishes and insects, the sperm penetrates through a special canal, the *micropyle* which is left in the egg membrane.

In mammals, the egg when released from the ovary, is commonly encased in a layer of cells of ovarian origin, termed the *corona radiata.* These cells are held together by a cementing substance known as hyaluronic acid. The spermatozoon has to pass through this barrier on its way to the egg. In order to do so, its acrosome produces an enzyme *hyaluronidase* which dissolves the cement and disperses the cells. The enzyme thus enables the spermatozoon to penetrate the corona radiata.

Sperm and Egg Fusion—The Acrosome Reaction : As the spermatozoon comes in contact with the egg, the acrosome of the sperm undergoes radical changes. Colwin and Colwin (1967) demonstrated the acrosome reaction clearly in the enteropneust *Saccoglossus.*

As the spermatozoon makes its initial contact with the egg envelope, the sperm plasma membrane and the acrosomal membrane rupture at the point of contact. The acrosomal membrane then joins with the plasma membrane around the margin of rupture so that the acrosomal granule is exposed to the surface of egg envelope. Now the peripheral part of the acrosome collapses and its lysins (enzymes) are extruded. The central part of the acrosome elongates and becomes transformed into a long thin tube known as the acrosomal tubule or filaments. The acrosomal tubule traverses the egg envelopes (jelly and vitelline membrane) and finally touches the egg plasma membrane. These two membranes now fuse at the point of contact. The pathway for the tubule is cleared by the action of the lysins.

Activation of the Ovum

The initial contact of the acrosomal tubule with the plasma membrane of the ovum triggers off a sequence of reactions that render the egg capable of starting on its way to develop into an embryo. In other words, it gets activated by coming out of its relatively quiescent state. The activation of ovum includes following events :

(a) Formation of fertilization cone.

(b) Cortical reaction and formation of fertilization membrane.

(c) Metabolic activation.

Formation of Fertilization Cone: Immediately after the fusion of the acrosomal tubule with the egg plasma membrane, the cytoplasm of the egg bulges upward at the point of contact as a conical projection called fertilization cone. (Colwin and Colwin, 1957). The fertilization cone gradually engulfs the sperm nucleus, middle piece, and tail. Now it begins to retract and carries the spermatozoon inward into the egg cytoplasm.

Cortical Reaction and Formation of Fertilization Membrane: The fertilization cone formation is followed by changes in the surface of the egg cytoplasm which are known under the general name of the cortical reaction. It is well studied in sea-urchin eggs. The events of cortical reaction in different groups of animals can be summarised as follows :

Sea-urchin

1. The colour of the egg surface changes gradually from yellow to white. The change begins to start from the point of attachment of the sperm and gradually spread all over the surface of the egg being the plasma membrane, is about 60 A thick. A layer of cortical granules is found beneath the plasma membrane.
2. Electron microscope reveals that the cortex of the unfertilized egg is bounded by two membranes. The outer one, called the vitelline membrane is about 30 A thick, whereas the inner one
3. The outer, vitelline membrane becomes lifted off from the plasma membrane. It undergoes an expansion, and gives rise to the *outer layer* of the fertilization membrane. The space between it and the surface of the egg is called perivitelline space.
4. The cortical granules swell and explode. They release three components :
   (a) *Lamellar and folded parts.* These are dark and dense bodies which unfold and subsequently fuse with the inner side of the already lifting fertilization membrane. The fertilization membrane thus becomes reinforced and becomes much thicker (upto 900 A).
   (b) *Globules.* These fuse together and form a new surface layer of the egg just outside the plasma membrane. This layer is called the hyaline layer. During cleavage it helps to keep the blastomeres intact.
   (c) *Liquid material.* The cortical granules contain muco-polysaccharides which absorb water and become liquified. This liquid releases into the perivitelline space and contributes to the perivitelline fluid. By further imbibition of water it assists in lifting the fertilization membrane still further.

Bony Fishes and Frog

In the eggs of these animals the cortical granules are broken down after sperm contact. Their contents become liquified and extruded on to the surface of the egg. The fluid fills the perivitelline space: (a) the space between the egg plasma membrane and vitelline membrane in frog ; and *(b)* the space between the egg plasma membrane and chorion in bony-fishes.

In frog the amount of perivitelline fluid increases swiftly, and the membrane is lifted from the surface of the egg.

The chorion in fishes become hardened or "tanned" after fertilization but no new membrane is formed as compared to the fertilization membrane of the sea-urchin.

Mammals

Eggs of all mammals do not possess cortical granules. When cortical granules are present as in human, hamster and the rabbit; these, release their contents into the space between the egg and zona pellucida (the perivitelline space) which are gradually dissolved. Therefore, no new membrane is formed around the egg at the time of fertilization.

Insects, Urodele Amphibians and some Mammals

(Rat and guinea pig) do not possess cortical granules. In these animals, morphological changes comparable to the cortical reaction of sea-urchin eggs do not occur at fertilization.

Metabolic Activation: The visible structural changes during fertilization are accompanied by alteration in the physiological properties of the egg substance. These include *(i)* changes in permeability of egg plasma membrane, *(ii)* ionic changes, *(iii)* respiration changes, *(iv)* change in the rate of protein synthesis, and *(v)* initiation of mitosis.

Migration of Pronuclei and Amphimixis (Union of Haploid Nuclei) : In the case of most vertebrate eggs, oogenesis comes to a standstill after the first meiotic division and is resumed only following sperm penetration. Entrance of spermatozoon serves to act as a stimulus which causes the second maturation division. As the head and middle piece of the sperm advance into the egg, these parts rotate through an angle of 180° so that the mitochondria and proximal centriole of the associated middle piece assume the leading position. Besides this rotation, the chromatin of sperm nucleus becomes finely granular. The nucleus itself starts swelling by absorbing fluid from the surrounding cytoplasm and becomes vesicular. It is now called male pronucleus.

As the male pronucleus and centriole move inward, they may be accompanied by some cortical and subcortical cytoplasm. If the latter is heavily pigmented, as in amphibian eggs, the path of the male pronucleus may be marked by pigment granules trailing along its path. This path is referred to as penetration path.

The centriole brought in by the spermatozoon subdivides into two and an achromatic spindle is established in the centre of the active cytoplasm.

With the production of the second polar body, the egg nucleus or female pronucleus is ready for union with the male pronucleus provided by the sperm head. It also migrates towards the site of union. Both pronuclei assume the general form of an interphase nucleus.

The male pronucleus which has been advancing along the penetration path, now moves directly toward the female pronucleus. This in many cases involves a slight change in the course of sperm. In such cases, the latter portion of its course is called the copulation path as distinguished from the first portion of entrance path.

Amphimixis: The fusion of male and female pronuclei is called amphimixis. The site of amphimixis lies in the centre of active cytoplasm at the animal pole in macro and telolecithal eggs, while in microlecithal eggs it lies near the centre of the egg.

In a few animal types, the two pronuclei actually fuse together. In mammals and other vertebrates the male and female pronuclei do not fuse as such. Instead, each pronucleus loses its membrane and its chromation resolves into the haploid set of chromosomes. The two sets of chromosomes then arrange themselves across the division spindle. This arrangement heralds the readiness for the first cleavage division.

Monospermy and Polyspermy

Monospermy: Fertilization performed by the penetration of one sperm only is called monospermic. This is the normal mode of fertilization in most classes of the animal kingdom *e.g.*, coelenterates, annelids, echinoderms, bony fishes, frogs and mammals.

Polyspermy: When more than one sperm establish contact and penetrate into the egg, fertilization is called polyspermic. It may be of two types :

(i) Pathological and (ii) Physiological.

(i) *Pathological Polyspermy:* It takes place under abnormal conditions when the egg is somehow adversely affected or if there happens to be an unusual high concentration of the spermatozoa around the egg. The development after such polyspermic fertilization is abnormal and the embryo is not capable of living.

(ii) *Physiological Polyspermy:* Several spermatozoa enter the large yolky eggs of molluscs, selachians, reptiles and birds as a rule, but of these only one takes part in the development of embryo. Rest of the spermatozoa degenerate sooner or later.

Significance of Fertilization

(1) Fertilization brings about reproduction, (a) by restoring the diploid number of chromosomes, and (b) by causing to develop a new kinetic division-centre.

(2) It brings about shuffling and recombination of the materna and paternal genes, producing genetic variations.

(3) Fusion of different strains of protoplasm which occurs during fertilization brings about revitalization in certain animals like *Paramecium.*

(4) The entrance of sperm activates the secondary oocyte to complete its second maturation division, hence it is of physiological importance.

(5) Fertilization causes separation of vitelline membrane which allows the rotation of the egg inside during gastrulation.

Explanation

Fertilization *is the penetration of a mature ovum by the spermatozoon and the fusion of the respective male and female pronuclei.* The penetration of a spermatozoon into ovum activates the egg to start the development, while the fusion of their pronuclei (amphimixis) results in restoring the diploid ($2n$) or parental chromosome number. The main idea of fertilization was enunciated by LEEUWENHOEK (1683), who emphasized that in order to make ovum fruitful (*i.e.* to develop into the embryo) its impregnation with seminal animalcule (the sperm) is essential.

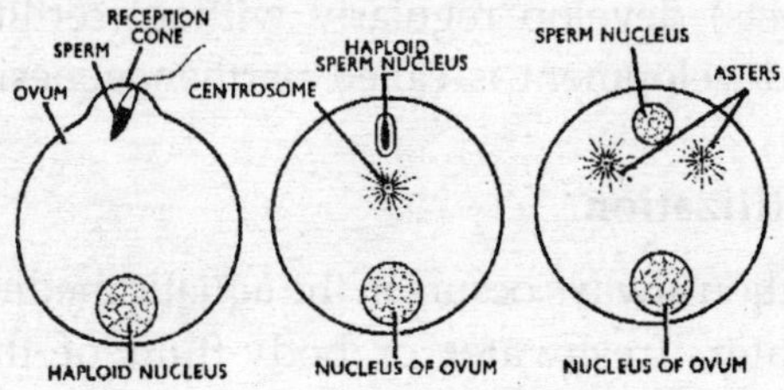

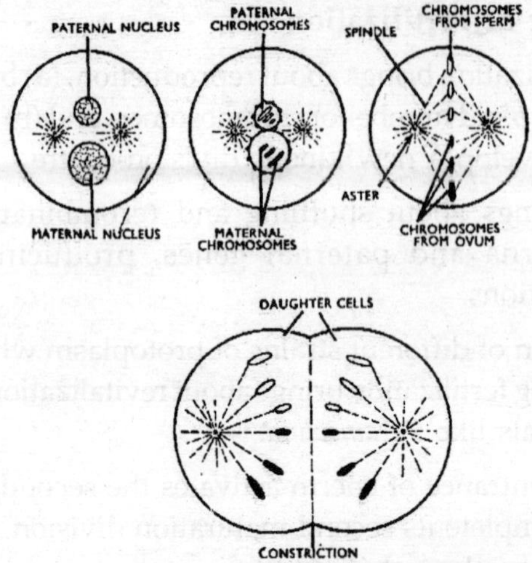

Diagrammatic representation of process of fertilization.

Dual Aspect of Fertilization

There are two Essentially Independent Aspects of Fertilization

Activation: Penetration of the sperm initiates a series of changes in the egg cortex and activates the egg cytoplasm by enhancing its metabolic activities.

Amphimixis: The fusion of the male and female pronuclei is known as amphimixis. It is not that essential for the development because even the single set of chromosomes of female pronucleus may control the development of a haploid embryo. Fertilization restores the original diploid chromosome number of the parents. Moreover, this brings about the intermingling of paternal and maternal hereditary material. The eggs of certain invertebrates (rotifers, crustaceans and certain insects) develop regularly without fertilization. The method of development is called parthenogenesis.

Site of Fertilization

Fertilization always occurs in the aquatic medium, whether it is sea-water, freshwater or body-fluid of the maternal organism. In many marine invertebrates and lower chordates, the sperm and ova are shed in water, where fertilization occurs. The type of fertilization where *gametes fuse outside the body of parent is known as* external fertilization. In a large number of terrestrial forms special organs are developed in male for depositing sperm in the genital tract of female. These organs are called copulatory organs. This facilitates the fusion of male and female gametes. *The fertilization completed inside the body of the female is termed as* internal fertilization. In still advanced forms, the fertilization of ovum and the subsequent embryonic and foetal development occurs inside the uterus of the female. The individuals that give birth to young ones are called viviparous, while those that lay eggs are called oviparous.

Mechanism of Fertilization

The process of fertilization can be separated into the following five steps:

1. Approach of spermatozoa to ova.
2. Capacitation and contact.
3. Acrosomal reaction and penetration.
4. Activation of ovum.
5. Amphimixis.

Approach of Spermatozoa to Ova : The male and female gametes are produced either in separate parents or in separate organs. The female gamete (ovum) is immobile, while the male gamete (sperm) is motile. The fertilizability and viability of gametes are often limited varying from a few minutes to a few hours. Eggs of aquatic animals with external fertilization survive only for a few minutes and in case of animals with internal fertilization for few hours and in case of man human egg survives for 24 hours. Lifespan of human sperm is 24 hours, cod's sperm 2 weeks, bat's sperm 3 to 4 months and honeybee's sperm many months. Moreover, the energy in the sperm is limited. Consequently, the major problem in sexual reproduction is bringing together of the ripe ova and the sperm.

Chemical Attraction or Trapping of Sperm by Chemotaxis: A chemical substance, the fertilizin secreted from the cortical region of egg cytoplasm of sea urchin egg was presumed to attract the sperm towards the egg. But an actual evidence for chemical attraction is lacking. The encounter between sperm and ova of sea urchin is brought about by swimming movements of spermatozoa. Their movements are at random and spermatozoa collide with the egg as a matter of pure chance. This applies for most animals. However, in certain cases the chemical secretion from eggs serves to trap spermatozoa, that accidentally enter their field of influence and are guided towards the eggs. For example, in two species of colonial hydroid, *Campanularia,* the cells of theca present near the gonangium produce sperm-attracting reagent. Similarly, a chemical sperm attractant is produced by fish eggs.

Mechanical Juxtaposition of Gametes : To facilitate an easy encounter of the sperm and ovum special devices are seen in animals with external as well as internal fertilization.

(a) *In Forms with External Fertilization :* In marine animals (like sea urchin) a large number of sexually mature males and females discharge their eggs and sperm in sea water in close vicinity and at the same time. Consequently, clouds of sperms and eggs are formed to ensure mass fertilization. Since the lifespan of gametes discharged in sea water is just a few minutes to a few hours, the discharge of ova and sperms at the same time is essential.

In fishes, amphibians and freshwater invertebrates, the lifespan of sperm is reduced to a few minutes only. Therefore, the sperms are discharged directly on the ova. These animals exhibit pseudo-copulation or amplexus.

(b) *In forms with Internal Fertilization* : The internal fertilization is found mostly in terrestrial forms. In them the spermatic fluid (semen) is delivered in the genital tract of female by the insertion of a specialized sexual appendage that acts as an intromittent organ. This organ is known as penis and the phenomenon of sperm deposition as insemination. The insemination occurs during sexual embrace, called copulation or coitus, which is exhibited in reptiles, birds, mammals and insects. In some amphibians, gastropods, turbellarians, trematods and cestodes, the sperms are received in a specialized receptacle after copulation.

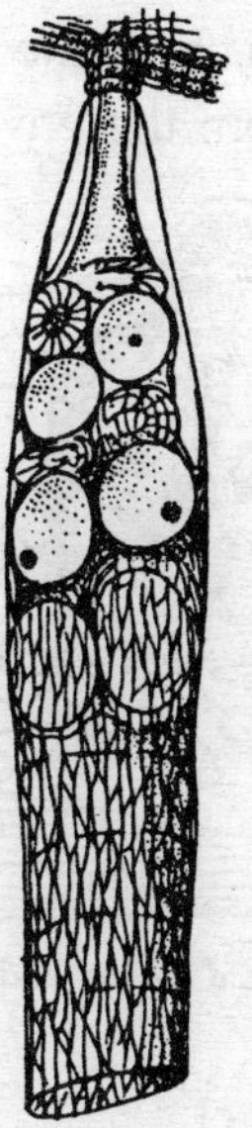

A theca of coelenterate campanularea

In majority of forms, the encounter of egg and sperm occurs in upper part of the oviduct. However, in some viviparous fishes *(Gambusia affinis* and *Heterandria formosa)* and certain eutherian mammals, it is accomplished inside the ovarian follicles. The sperms are deposited in the vagina and from here are transported to uterus by the contraction of uterine wall.

Special Devices: To bring together the eggs and spermatozoa, number of other devices have been encountered in animals. In spiders and crustaceans a forelimb or a pulp in male is modified for transferring semen into genital opening of female. In cephalopods, one of the arms is modified for holding spermatophores and transferring them to the female. Such a specialized arm is known is heterocotylized arm or heterocotylus. In *Peripatopsis,* the spermatophores are applied to any part of the body. The spermatozoa are released on contact, penetrate the body wall and make their way through the body tissue to reach the ovary.

In some animals spermatozoa are released in small packets, called spermatozeugmata. In it the sperms are held together by some mutual attraction, the enveloping sheath is absent.

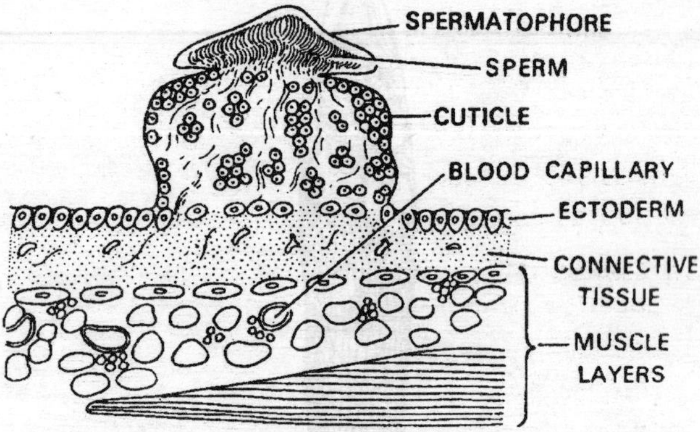

Spermatophore attached to the bodywall of Peripatopsis.

Capacitation and Contact

Capacitation : The egg of a particular species is fertilized only by the sperm of the same species. This is accomplished by a chemical mechanism. A species-specific chemical substance, called fertilizin is produced by the ripe egg, while another chemical substance antifertilizin is secreted by the sperm. Both fertilizin and antifertilizin are species-specific and form a sort of chemical lock like an antigen antibody reaction. The fertilizin acts as a receptor for antifertilizin and makes them capable of fertilizing the egg of the same species. This process is known as capacitation.

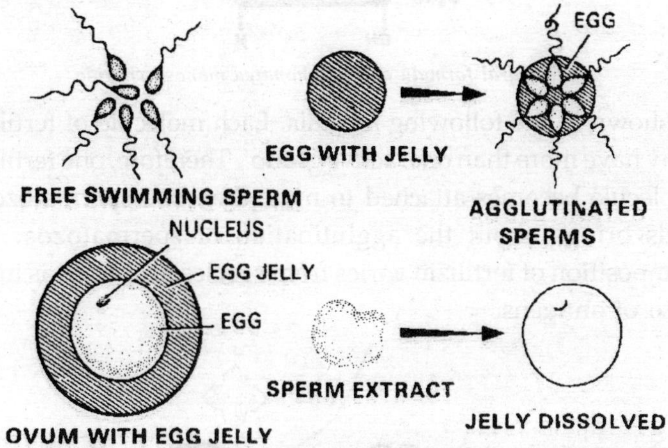

Fertilizin—antifertilizin reaction

Capacitation has been studied in sea urchin, where it occurs in sea water. In mammals the same is facilitated inside the genital tract of the female. Capacitation is essential for sperm penetration.

Adhesion: The adhesion of spermatozoan to the egg surface occurs due to the presence of fertilizin molecules in the surface layer of egg cytoplasm, which receive antifertilizin molecules present on the surface of spermatozoon.

Fertilizin and Antifertilizin Reaction : Structure and function of fertilizin was studied by F.R.LILLIE(1919). It is a glycoprotein or mucopolysaccharide. Its macromolecules have a molecular weight of about 82,000-300,000. Its proteinmoity is formed of a number of amino acids, while the polysaccharide component comprises of molecules of one or more monosaccharides like glucose, fructose, fucose or galactose. The monosaccharides are esterified by sulphuric acid as

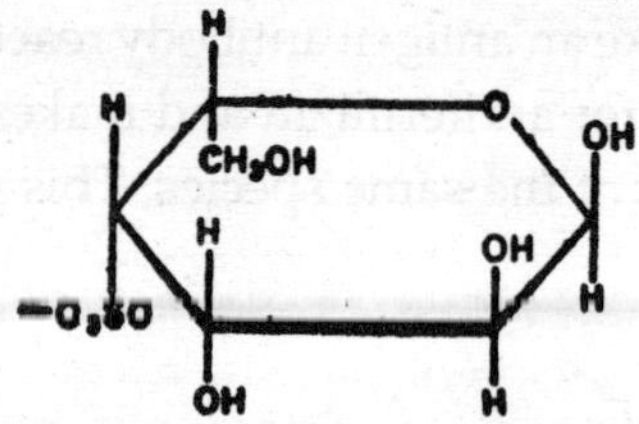

Structural formula of a sulphonated monosaccharide

is shown in the following formula. Each molecule of fertilizin may have more than one 'active group'. Therefore, one fertilizin molecule becomes attached to more than one spermatozoan. This brings about the agglutination of spermatozoa. The composition of fertilizin varies from species to species as in the case of antigens.

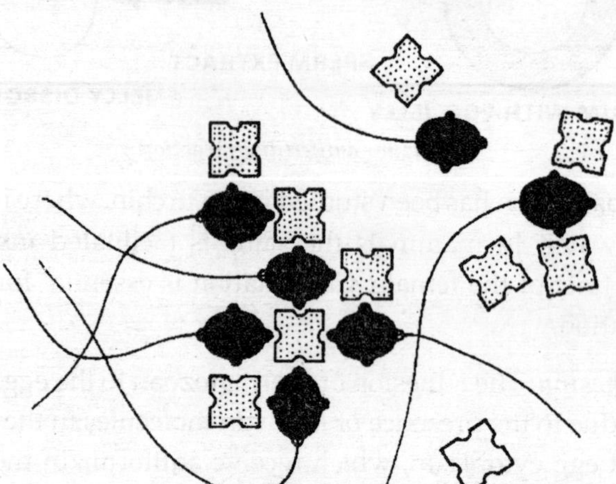

Clumping of spermatozoa due to their binding with fertilizin molecules (After Balinskey, 1976).

The fertilizin is produced by the ripe unfertilized eggs. It remains either in the plasma membrane or in the jelly, surrounding the egg. In sea urchin eggs, the jelly consists wholly of fertilizin and is produced by the follicle cells. In mammals, the cells of zona pellucida produce fertilizin. Functions: Fertilizin performs following functions :

(i) makes the sperm sticky so that they adhere to clumps.

(ii) makes sperm to adhere to the surface of egg and ensures fertilization.

(iii) clumping or agglutination of sperm thins out the number of spermatozoa around the egg to check the entry of any additional sperm into the egg.

(iv) leads to the capacitation of sperm, enabling it to penetrate the egg surface.

Antifertilizin is found on the surface membrane of the spermatozoa. It is also species-specific. Antifertilizin contains acid proteins with molecular weight of about 10,000. The antifertilizin molecules of sperm fit into the fertilizin molecules of egg in the same way as a key fits into the lock.

Sea water in which eggs have been allowed to stand for some time contains fertilizin and is termed as egg water. Sperms added to egg water are agglutinated, adhering by their head. These, later on, separate spontaneously, but their fertilizing power is greatly diminished. Eggs treated with antifertilizin also have reduced capacity for fertilization.

Acrosomal Reaction and Penetration : Almost all the animal eggs, except those of porifers and enidarians, are enveloped by one or more membranes or gelatinous layers external to the plasma membrane. A spermatozoon after attachment to the egg surface has to penetrate these membranes so as to reach the egg plasma membrane.

Sperm Entry by Way of Micropyles : In the eggs of nemertines, gastropods, pelecypods, echinoderms, insects, cephalopods and fish, the membranes surrounding the egg have pores, called micropyles. When micropyle is single, it represents the site at which the egg was originally attached to the ovary. In the eggs of insects, fish and cephalopods the sperm enters through the single micropyle. If pores are many, the spermatozoon may enter through any one of the pores on the egg surface. The sperm motility is increased when these approach the micropyle.

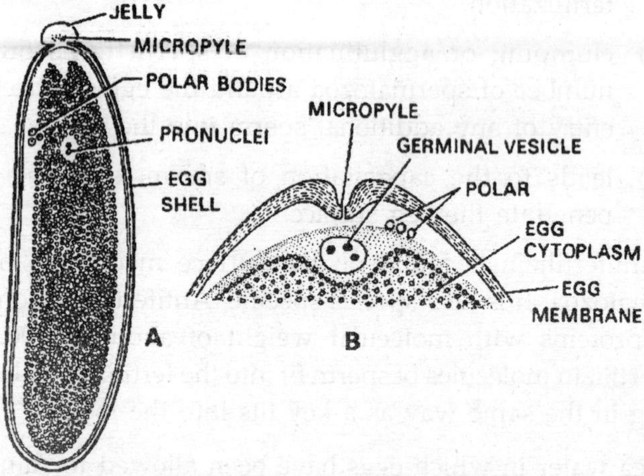

Few eggs with micropyle A- Egg of Musca B- Egg of a Cephalopod, (From Austin Fertilization)

Egg Membrane Lysins: The spermatozoa produce lytic substances which are enzymatic in nature. These sperm lysins are produced from the acrosome of the spermatozoa and are species- specific. The sperm lysins dissolve the membranes present around the egg in a local area and clear the path for sperm to reach the plasma membrane of the egg. Actual holes have been seen in the vitelline membrane of egg of *Mytilus* caused by the entry of sperm

Hyaluronidase: In mammals the covering around the egg is called corona radiata. It is formed of a single layer of follicular cells, cemented together by an adhesive substances the hyaluronic acid. The mammalian sperm produce enzyme hyaluronidase, which dissolves hyaluronic acid, separates the follicle cells of corona radiata and make way for the sperm.

In sea urchin, the egg jelly is dissolved by the acidification of sea water by carbondioxide that is produced by the spermatozoa.

In some mammals (horse, cow, sheep) the egg lose their corona radiata shortly after ovulation, enabling the spermatozoa to gain direct access to zona pellucida.

The acrosome is not able to release sperm lysin or hyluronidase till it has undergone capacitation or activation. This involves some specific change in the sperm acrosome.

Acrosome Reaction : The activated spermatozoon on reaching the egg plasma membrane, undergoes a number of changes in its acrosomal region. All these changes are collectively described under acrosome reaction. The details of the process are common to many animals with minor differences according to the structure of acrosome and egg membranes.

In *Saccoglossus* and also in other animals an acrosomal vesicle is present in the sperm head anterior to the nucleus. It is bounded by an acrosomal membrane. Inside the acrosomal vesicle is a large dense acrosomal granule which is surrounded by fine, granular material, except in the apical region where an apical space lies between the acrosomal granule and acrosome membrane.

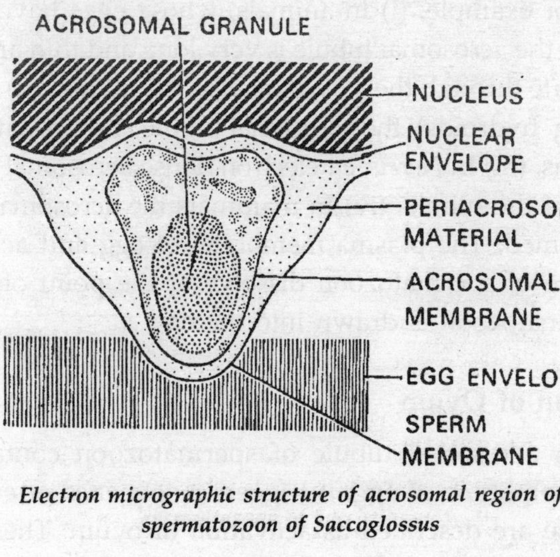

Electron micrographic structure of acrosomal region of spermatozoon of Saccoglossus

During the acrosomal reaction, the events occur in the following sequence: (i) The dissolution of plasma membrane and acrosomal membrane in the apical region forming an apical pore through which contents of acrosomal vesicle are passed on to the egg. (ii) The union of the plasma membrane and acrosomal membrane around the margin of the opening. (iii) Release of contents of the acrosomal vesicle *i.e.* the acrosomal granule that contains lytic enzymes, needed for sperm penetration. (iv) Deepening of the shallow depression of acrosomal membrane close to the nucleus and formation of an acrosomal tubule in the form of a projection from the inner surface of acrosomal membrane. (v) Lengthening of the acrosomal tubule by the eversion of the remaining acrosomal membrane and its addition to the tubule at its base. (vi) Liberation of the content of the acrosomal tubule. (vii) Penetration of acrosomal tubule gradually through the egg envelopes to reach the egg plasma membrane. (viii) Fusion of the membrane of acrosomal tubule with egg plasma membrane and activation of egg.

A number of modifications are seen in the pattern discussed above. For example, (i) In animals, whose eggs have a thick jelly coat, the acrosomal tubule is very long and thin and helps to penetrate through the jelly-coat as in sea urchin. (ii) In other forms (e.g. hydroids), the acrosomal tubule is short with many projections. (iii) In *Nereis, an* electron dense acrosomal rod fills the core of the tubule. (iv) In mammals the acrosomal tubule is not formed. The plasma membrane of egg and acrosomal membrane of spermatozoon dissolve at the point of contact and spermatozoon is drawn into the egg.

Activation of Ovum

When acrosomal tubule of spermatozoon contacts the plasma membrane of egg, it triggers a sequence of events in egg. These are described as activation of ovum. These are:

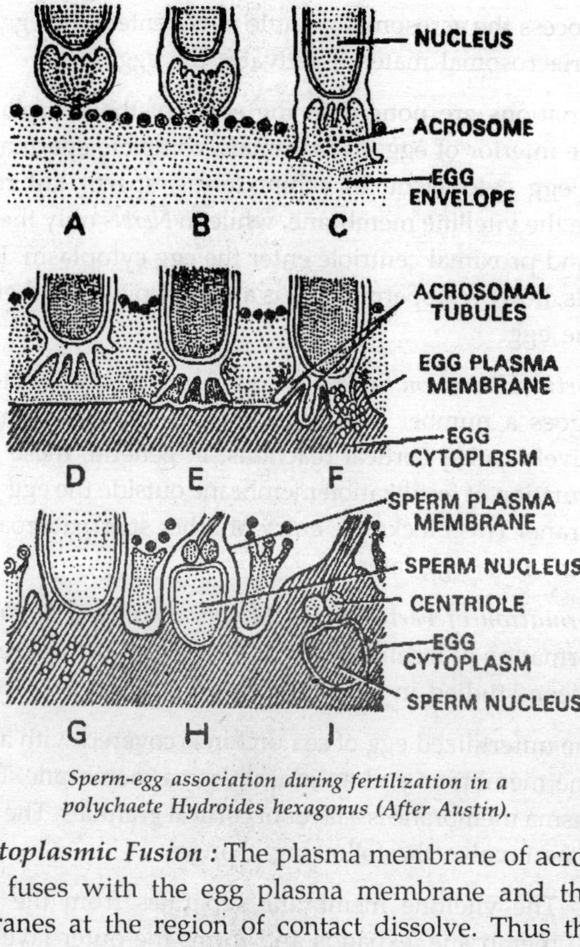

Sperm-egg association during fertilization in a polychaete Hydroides hexagonus (After Austin).

Cytoplasmic Fusion : The plasma membrane of acrosomal tubule fuses with the egg plasma membrane and the two membranes at the region of contact dissolve. Thus the egg cytoplasm becomes continuous with that of the sperm.

Formation of Fertilization Cone : The cytoplasm of the egg bulges forward in the region of cytoplasmic fusion and forms a projection of hyaline cytoplasm. This is known as fertilization cone. It may be in the form of a conical projection or a cytoplasmic cylinder or may consist of several pseudopodia-like processes.

The fertilization cone gradually engulfs the spermatozoon. It gradually subsides drawing the sperm within the egg. During this process the acrosomal granule never enters the egg, while the periacrosomal material activates the egg.

Variations are noticed in the entry of the spermatozoon into the interior of egg. In mammals, complete spermatozoon enters egg cytoplasm. In echinoderms, sperm tail remains outside the vitelline membrane, while in *Nereis* only the sperm head and proximal centriole enter the egg cytoplasm. In most animals, however, sperm nucleus and mid-piece get their entry into the egg.

Cortical Reaction: Soon, the cortical region of egg cytoplasm undergoes a number of physiochemical changes, which are collectively called cortical reactions. In general, these lead to the formation of fertilization membrane outside the egg plasma membrane. This blocks the entry of other spermatozoa which may strike the egg later.

Formation of Fertilization Membrane in sea Urchin Egg: The formation of fertilization membrane and cortical reactions have been studied in sea urchins and starfish.

The unfertilized egg of sea urchin is covered with an outer vitelline membrane and an inner plasma membrane. Beneath the plasma membrane is a layer of cortical granules. The cortical reactions involve the following changes:

(i) The vitelline membrane separates from the plasma membrane, expands and forms the outer layer of the fertilization membrane. The space formed between the two layers is the perivitelline space.

(ii) The contact of acrosome with egg surface is followed by the rupture of cortical granules. Their breakdown begins initially at the point of sperm entry and spreads through the cortex in all directions. The granules first swell up by imbibing water and the mucopolysaccharide contained in them liquifies. The breakdown of granules releases three components:

(a) The lamellar parts of the ruptured cortical granules appear as dark bodies or folded lamellae. These fuse with the vitelline membrane contributing to its thickening.

(b) The released globules fuse together and form a hyaline layer just outside the egg plasma membrane. It adheres to the egg surface and keeps the blastomeres together during cleavage.

(c) The liquid component of cortical granules forms the perivitelline fluid that fills the perivitelline space. It contains polymucosaccharides and water.

Formation of Fertilization Membrane in Nereis Egg : In unfertilized egg of Nereis, the vitelline membrane is traversed by microvilli. The cortical region has several layers of cortical alveoli. The rupture of cortical alveoli destroys the egg plasma membrane and releases jelly-like substance through the pores of vitelline membrane. The jelly forms a thick layer outside the vitelline membrane, that forms the fertilization membrane. The membrane fragments of cortical alveoli use to form a new membrane of the egg.

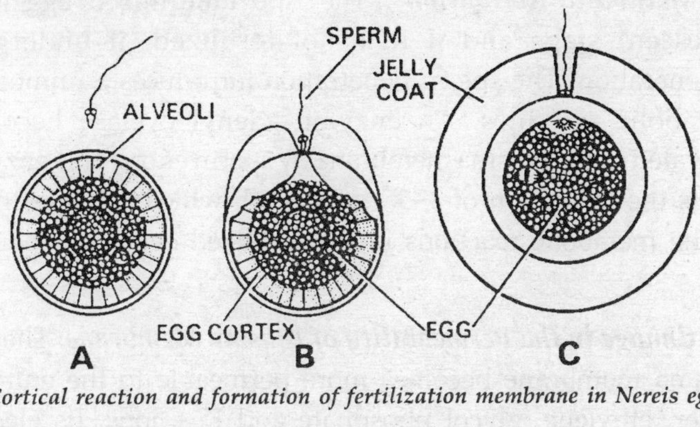

Cortical reaction and formation of fertilization membrane in Nereis egg

Bony Fish and Frogs : The unfertilized eggs of bony-fishes, and frogs have a narrow perivitelline space. The fertilization membrane is not formed but the rupture of cortical granules increases the amount of perivitelline fluid.

Mammalian Eggs : In mammalian eggs, the perivitelline space develops between zona pellucida and egg plasma membrane. The cortical granules that are present in some mammals only, release their content in the perivitelline space. Neither the fertilization membrane nor any other membrane is formed around the egg cytoplasm.

In the eggs of certain animals such as urodel amphibians and insects the cortical reaction does not occur at the time of fertilization.

In Pisces, the ectoplasm accumulates at the animal pole (the blastodisc) but at the vegetal pole in *Stylea* and annelids and at a point outside the poles in Amphibia. Normally, the ectoplasmic accumulation occurs at the point of sperm entry.

Significance of cortical reaction and formation of fertilization membrane: The formation of fertilization membrane and cortical reaction are defensive mechanisms against the penetration of additional spermatozoa after one has established contact with the egg plasma membrane.

Metabolic Activation : The ripe unfertilized egg is in quiescent stage and if it is not fertilized, it undergoes degeneration. The sperm penetration introduces a number of metabolic activities. An enzyme adenyl eyelase becomes activated in the plasma membrane by sperm entry. This enzyme starts the formation of 3'-5' cyclic AMP which activates most of the metabolic reactions in the fertilized egg. The changes are:

Change in the Permeability of Plasma Membrane: The egg plasma membrane becomes more permeable to the entry of water, ethylene, glycol phosphate and K + ions. Its electric potential changes first to positive and then negative.

Ionic change: The ionic concentration of sodium, potassium and calcium changes in fertilized egg.

Change in Coenzyme : In unfertilized egg, the enzyme NAD-kinase occurs in an inactive state. It is activated during fertilization. The activated NAD- kinase directs the interconversion of coenyzme NAD into NADP and NADPH.

$$\text{NAD} + \text{ATP NAD} \xrightarrow{\text{kinase NADP}} + \text{ADP}$$

NADP and NADPH are responsible for the oxidation-reduction reactions taking place during cell respiration and synthesis of energy. Thus increased NADP and NADPH contents initiate many synthetic pathways.

Respiration Rate : The oxygen consumption increases in the fertilized egg indicating an increase in the respiration rate. However, it does not change appreciably in starfish and amphibians, and it actually decreases after fertilization in eggs of mollusc *(Cumingia)* and annelid *(Chaetopterus).*

Increase in the Activity of Proteolytic Enzymes in the rate of Protein Synthesis: The cytoplasm of a ripe unfertilized egg contains complete machinery for protein synthesis but little or no protein synthesis takes place. Most probably, some inhibitor or repressor proteins are synthesized in later phase of orogenesis, which inactivate the chromosomal genes, mRNA molecules and ribosomes. During fertilization, some proteolytic enzymes remove these inhibitors and activate protein synthesis.

Initiation of Nuclear Divison : The eggs are ready for fertilization at different stages of meiosis in different animals. At one extreme, the eggs are laid with germinal vesicle intact and do not complete meiosis until fertilization. In them the germinal vesicle breaks down when sperm enters the egg and meiotic division is completed as in eggs *of Ascaris* and *Nereis.*

At the other extreme, the eggs ripen only after the completion of both meiotic divisions as in urchins and coelenterates. However, in majority of cases, the eggs are laid at metaphase of the first or second meiotic division. Nuclear division is delayed

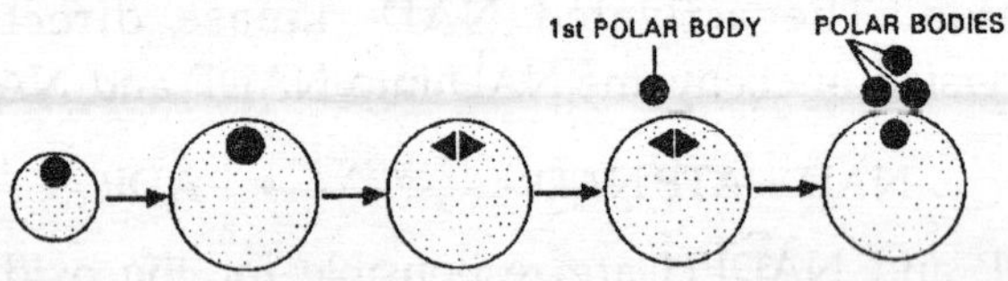

Young Primary Oocyte	Fully Grown Primary Oocyle	First Metaphase	Second Metaphase	Female Pronucleus
Branchiostoma	*Ascaris*	*Chaetopterus*	*Amphioxus*	*Coelenterates*
	Dog, Fox	*Dentalium*	*Most mammals*	*Echinoids*
Dinophyllus	*Grantia*	*Many insects*	*Siredon*	*(sea urchin)*
Hisriobdella	*Nereis*	*Cerebratulus*		
Periopatosis	*Thalassema*			
Saccocirrus				

Diagram to show the maturation stage of ovum at the time of egg laying until it is initiated by the sperm entry.

This is further proved by the following:

(a) DNA synthesis begins with sperm penetration. Its rate increases immediately after fertilization.

(b) Sperm entry initiates nuclear division by introducing its centriole. The unfertilized egg contains only one centriole and is unable to form mitotic spindle alone. With the entry of spermatozoon, the egg receives second centriole (the centriole of spermatozoon) and nuclear division is initiated.

Migration of Pronuclei and Amphimixis

Future of Spermatozoon in the Egg: Whether the whole spermatozoon or its head and middle piece enter the egg, only the sperm nucleus and centriole ultimately participate in future events of development.

Behaviour of Pronuclei: As the spermatozoon head moves inward from fertilization cone, it rotates through 180°, so that the mitochondria and centrioles of its middle piece assume the forward position. Both nucleus and centriole change in appearance.

(i) The nucleus swells up, becomes vesicular and its chromatin appears granular. This is known as male pronucleus.

(ii) The centriole gets surrounded by astral rays and forms the aster.

Simultaneously, the male pronucleus and centriole move through the egg cytoplasm to the site where union of male and female pronuclei is to take place. This site is near the centre in holoblastic microlecithal eggs and in the centre of active cytoplasm in telolecithal eggs. The movement of sperm in the egg cytoplasm is usually accompanied by the movement of cortical and subcortical cytoplasm. In frog egg the subcortical cytoplasm is heavily pigmented and the path taken by sperm nucleus is marked by pigment granules trailing along its path. This is known as penetration path.

Just after the second maturation division the egg nucleus lies in the peripheral cytoplasm in the form of several vesicles called karyomeres. These fuse to form female pronucleus, which swells up to become vesicular. Following the migration of male pronucleus, the female pronucleus from its peripheral position migrates towards the predetermined site of fusion.

What force governs the movement of male and female pronuclei to the site of fertilization has not been properly ascertained. It may be an attraction force between the two or the traction exerted by the astral rays. But both these explanations are inadequate as the experimental removal of either of the pronuclei does not prevent the other one from following the normal path.

Amphimixis (Union of Male and Female Gametes): The details of the fusion of male and female gametes differ in different animals:

(i) In sea urchin and vertebrates the two pronuclei actually fuse together. Their nuclear membranes break at the point of contact and their contents get surrounded by a common nuclear membrane forming the zygote nucleus. At the time of first cleavage the nuclear membrane dissolves, nuclear spindle is formed and the chromosomes of maternal and paternal origin get arranged on the equator of spindle.

(ii) In *Ascaris, some* molluscs and annelids the male and female pronuclei do not fuse. Their chromosomes get arranged on the equator of the spindle. In these animals the zygote nucleus is not formed. The paternal and maternal chromosomes get enclosed in the common nuclear membrane only after the completion of first cleavage in the nuclei of two blastomeres.

(iii) In few animals (e.g. Copepods *Cyclops*) the paternal and maternal nuclear contents remain separate even after cleavage. Therefore, each blastomere contains two nuclei lying side by side.

Changes in the Organization of Egg Cytoplasm after Fertilization : In addition to the activation of the egg cytoplasm and the restoration of diploid chromosome number, the fertilization causes reorganization of egg cytoplasm and also changes the symmetry of the egg. Due to the rupture of cortical granules, the outer egg surface is replaced by the inner cytoplasm lying below the cortical granules.

Site of Sperm Entry

The sperm may enter the egg at any point, usually the sperm avoids the yolk laden pole of the egg. In fish, mollusc and insect eggs the sperm entry is through a definite, funnel-shaped aperture, the micropyle.

Time of Fertilization

The eggs are fertilized at different stages of maturation in different species of animals as shown in the table given below:

Young Primary Oocyte	*Fully-grown Primary Oocyte*	*At Metaphase of first meiotic division*	*At Metaphase of Second meiotic division*	*Female Pronucleus*
Branchiostoma	*Ascaris*	*Chaetopterus*	*Amphioxus*	Coelenterates
Peripatopsis	*Grantia*	*Cerebratulus*	*Siredon*	Echinoids
Saccocrus	*Nereis*	*Petinaria*	Most mammals	
Octomesostoma	*Dicyema*	*Aphryotrocha*		
Histriobdella	*Myzostoma*	*Dentalium*		
	Spirula	*Many insects*		
	Thalessma			
	Dog and Frog			

Chemistry of Fertilization

Both egg as well as sperm contain certain chemicals that are necessary for fertilization. Since these chemicals are produced by the gametes and are of the nature of hormones, these are known as gamones. The hormones of the sperm are called androgamones and those found in the egg are termed as gynogamones. Two types of androgamones are found in the sperms. These are known as androgamone I and androgamone II. Similarly, the egg also contains two gynogamones namely, gynogamone I and gynogamone II.

The hormone androgamone I is responsible for conserving sperm's activity. The sperm contains limited amount of energy. If it were to swim as rapidly as it could from the very beginning its limited amount of energy would be utilized in too short a period and sperm may not be able to reach the ovum. By conserving the activity until the sperm approaches the egg, the probability of fertilization is increased. Androgamone II dissolves the gelatinous coating around the egg and is, therefore, indispensable for fertilization.

Both egg as well as sperm contain certain chemicals that are necessary for fertilization. Since these chemicals are produced by the gametes and are of the nature of hormones, these are known as gamones. The hormones of the sperm are called androgamones and those found in the egg are termed as gynogamones. Two types of androgamones are found in the sperms. These are known as androgamone I and androgamone II. Similarly, the egg also contains two gynogamones namely, gynogamone I and gynogamone II.

The hormone androgamone I is responsible for conserving sperm's activity. The sperm contains limited amount of energy. If it were to swim as rapidly as it could from the very beginning its limited amount of energy would be utilized in too short a period and sperm may not be able to reach the ovum. By conserving the activity until the sperm approaches the egg, the probability of fertilization is increased. Androgamone II dissolves the gelatinous coating around the egg and is, therefore, indispensable for fertilization.

Gynogamone I which is produced in the ovum neutralizes the androgamone I when sperm comes in contact with the egg and thereby increases the activity of the sperm. Gynogamone II makes the sperm head sticky and enables the sperm to stick to the egg surface and allows the androgamone II an opportunity to dissolve the gelatinous coating.

Summary of Chemistry of Fertilization

Gamone	*Gamete*	*Function*
1. Androgamone — I	Sperm	Conserves sperm activity.
2. Androgamone —II	Sperm	Dissolves vitelline membrane, allowing, sperm entrance into the egg.
3. Gynogamone — I	Ovum	Neutralizes androgamone-I thereby increasing sperm activity.

Contd...

Gamone	*Gamete*	*Function*
4. Gynogamone —II	Ovum	Makes sperm head sticky to facilitate attachment of sperm to egg surface.

Theories of Fertilization

Boveri's Theory: Boveri (1887 and 1895) suggested that the egg loses its power of mitotic division during maturation as its division centre degenerates. The sperm introduces the division centre into the egg during fertilization and makes the egg divide.

Loeb's Theory: Loeb (1913) suggested that sperm introduces two different types of substances in the egg cytoplasm. (i) The lytic substances bring about cortical cytolysis and (ii) the corrective factor regulates the oxidation.

LOVTRUP (1974) has supported LOEB'S view and has suggested that lytic substances act as activators by causing partial hydrolysis and perforation of plasma membrane, dissolution of cortical granules and subsequent swelling of perivitelline space.

Bimolecular Theory of Activation: R.S. LILLIE (1941) proposed that the entrance of sperm in egg leads to the formation of activating substance-A. It is formed by the union of two substances B and S. The substance-B is produced by the hydrolytic process taking place in the egg. Its production is stimulated by acid and heat. The substance-S is formed from the synthetic processes that are stimulated by hypertonicity. Entry of sperm increases production of these substances.

Bataillon's Theory : Bataillon (1910 & 1916) proposed that the unfertilized egg was inhibited from dividing due to the accumulation of metabolic products. The entry of sperm leads to the release of these substances from the cortex into the perivitelline space and thereby releasing the egg from the inhibition.

Sensitization to Calcium: The role of calcium in the activation of egg has been emphasized by two groups of embryologists. The theory `Sensitization to calcium' was proposed by DLACO, PASTEELS and BRACHET (1936) and the theory of 'calcium' release-protoplasmic clotting was put forward by HEIBRUNN (1930-40). The theories are based on the following observations:

(i) Isotonic calcium chloride solutions or solutions rich in calcium ions effectively activate the egg.

(ii) Activation of other chemical agents is dependent on the presence of calcium ions.

(iii) Eggs deprived of calcium become calcium-sensitive.

Heilbrunn's Theory: I.V. HEILBRUNN (1915,28 and 43) believed that an increase in viscosity of the egg cytoplasm is the cause for the initiation of division. This is almost similar to the coagulation of blood. Calcium brings about this effect and is, therefore, directly involved in egg activation. At the time of fertilization sperm liberates calcium that is bound to the egg cortex.

Runnstrom's Theory: J. RUNNSTROM (1949) pointed out that an inhibitor is present in the cortex and the vitelline membrane. This inhibitor is bound to a kinase. The kinase is released when the protein substances of sperm unite with the inhibitor. This enzyme initiates the development.

Repressor Theory of Activation: MONRAY and TYLER (1965) have suggested that during maturation of egg its energy-yielding system is blocked, which stops all the energy-requiring reactions. How such inhibitions occur and what is the mechanism of activation still remains to be discovered.

According to MONROY and TYLER (1963) in unfertilized egg either mRNA or ribosomes or both are inactivated in some way. Some proteins must be responsible for this inactivation because the ribosomes isolated from unfertilized sea urchin eggs and treated with trypsin for 30 minutes become active for protein synthesis. It means mRNA is attached to ribosomes even in the unfertilized egg but this mRNA is masked by a protein. During fertilization this protein is dissolved by proteolytic enzyme. There is an increase in the proteolytic activity in the egg immediately after the penetration of the sperm.

Significance of Fertilization

Fertilization Accomplishes following Significant Results

1. The gametes or the germ cells constitute the only physical bridge between the successive generations. The gametes posses haploid number (n) of chromosomes. As a result of fusion of a male and a female gamete, the diploid chromosomal configuration similar to parents is restored. This fertilization maintains the characteristic chromosome number.
2. Fertilization brings together the genes and chromosomes from two different lines of ancestry and results in new genetic recombinations, which ensure better adaptations to the changing environment.
3. The entry of sperm awakens the quiescent ovum and initiates the egg to divide the development to proceed.

The division may be initiated by artificial means either exposing the unfertilized egg to hypotonic, hypertonic or neutral salt solutions, acids, bases, alkaloids, heat, cold, etc., by radiation or by puncturing with a fine needle.

In addition to the above-cited aspects fertilization leads to: (i) Liberation of secondary oocyte to complete its second maturation division. (ii) Induces movement of cytoplasmic panicles and pigment granules to mark the fertilization track. (iii) Induces centriole which forms the nuclear spindle and initiates cleavage in the egg. (iv) Induces changes in the periphery of egg and this precludes the entry of other sperms. (v) Causes the separation of vitelline membrane which allows the rotation of egg inside. (vi) Enhances metabolic activities. (vii) Establishes a new plane of egg axis.

Monospermy

When fertilization is accomplished in nature or in the laboratory myriads of sperm surround each egg, yet only one enters and fertilizes the egg. This is known as monospermic fertilization. What prevents the entry of other sperms in the ovum? Can an egg be re-fertilized? It has been suggested that the formation of the fertilization membrane around the fertilized egg blocks the passage of other sperms. But the eggs of some species of sea-urchin can be re-fertilized as late as two-cell stage after the removal of fertilization membrane from *Saccoglossus* eggs permits re-fertilization even at eight or sixteen blastomere stage. The sperm receptor, fertilizin, present on the surface of egg is gradually covered by the hyaline layer after fertilization. This blocks the attachment of extra sperms to the egg.

Polyspermy

As a general rule, only one sperm enters an egg but in the large yolky eggs of birds, reptiles, some amphibians and insects many sperm enter the egg. However, only one fuses with the egg nucleus. This is known as polyspermic fertilization. Polyspermy can be of following two types :

Physiological Polyspermy : In physiological polyspermy more than one sperm nuclei and centrioles enter the egg cytoplasm, but only one sperm centriole and nucleus participate in the fertilization and initiation of cleavage.

Physiological polyspermy is found in moderately yolk-laden eggs (eggs of urodela amphibians and some insects) and very large yolky eggs of reptiles, birds and elasmobranch fishes.

Pathological Polyspermy : In this case more than one sperm centriole and nucleus enter the egg cytoplasm and become active. This leads to pathological development.

Over-ripe eggs permit entry of more than one sperm. Over ripeness is an abnormality and leads to pathological development. This is known as pathological polyspermy. It has been studied in the eggs of sea-urchin and certain mammals. Polyspermy can be induced by placing eggs in a dense suspension of spermatozoa, by treating eggs with toxic or narcotic substances (such as nicotine, alkaloids and chloral hydrate) or with heat and cold just before insemination. Polyspermy may lead to polyandry (fusion of more than one sperm nucleus with one female pronucleus). The polyandry is lethal.

Blocks to Polyspermy or Exclusion of Surplus Spermatozoa : Once a sperm has made its entry into the egg cytoplasm, the other sperm that contacts the egg surface later on, are not allowed to get in. Different mechanisms of exclusion of surface sperm have been noticed in different animals.

Elevation of Fertilization Membrane: In the eggs of annelids, sea-urchins, starfish, *Branchiostoma* and frogs, a fertilization membrane is formed around the egg. Formation or fertilization membrane begins from the point of sperm contact and is propagated over the entire egg surface. Finally it becomes about 800A° thick and impermeable to spermatozoa. In *Nereis,* the fertilization membrane is formed by the rupture of alveoli present in the cortex.

Property of Micropyle : In sturgeon and teleost eggs the micropylar canal is so narrow that only one spermatozoon at a time is able to pass through it. When one spermatozoon has entered the cytoplasm, a gelatinous substance blocks the canal blocking the entry of supplementary sperm. The egg membrane is tough and thick and unsurpassable by the sperm.

Change in Zona Pellucida: In mammals the zona pellucida becomes impermeable to spermatozoa after the contact with first spermatozoon. This is known as zona reaction. The cortical granules disappear after the penetration of sperm and occlude the entry of additional sperms in the ovum.

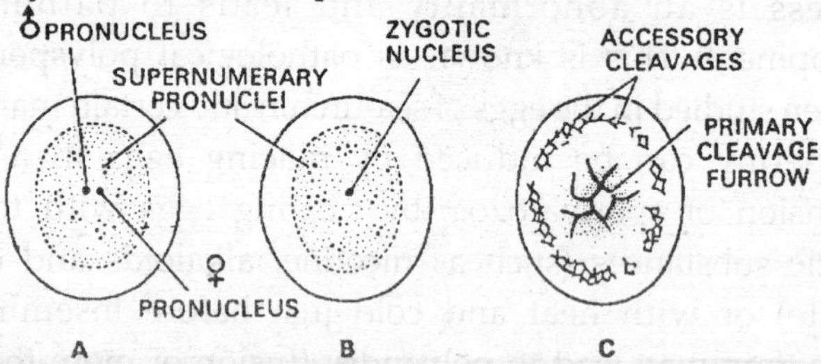

Diagram to show the mechanism that prevents entry of additional sperms, though lots of them may stick to egg surface.

It is now believed that cortical reaction of egg and formation of fertilization membrane is an imperfect protection because cortical reaction begins at one point and a wave travels around the egg. In sea urchin eggs it takes about 20 seconds and, therefore, cannot check the entry of additional sperms at different regions of the egg surface.

The two possible explanations believed to help in sperm exclusion are:-

1. Diaphasic changes in the egg cortex. The first reaction is fast and covers the entire egg surface within 1 or 2 seconds and confers partial protection.
2. Fertilization potential is established by sperm entry and avoids polyspermy. The role of fertilization potential is evidenced from those animal groups which have yolky eggs as in molluscs, selachians, urodels, reptiles and birds. In them extra spermatozoa degenerate after one fuses with the egg pronucleus.

Disposal of Supernumerary Male Pronuclei : In the eggs of elasmobranchs, urodels, reptiles, birds and a few insects, a number of additional spermatozoa enter the egg. These surplus spermatozoa form additional pronuclei in the egg. This phenomenon is known as physiological polyspermy. When one sperm pronucleus fuses with the female pronucleus, the supernumerary male pronuclei are either suppressed or rejected. In bird eggs, these rejected pronuclei are seen on the periphery of the blastodisc, where some of them induce cell division in the early cleavage stages of embryonic development.

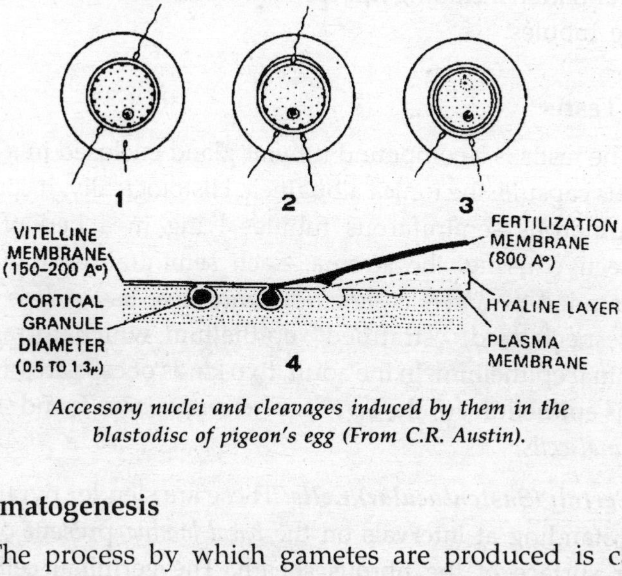

Accessory nuclei and cleavages induced by them in the blastodisc of pigeon's egg (From C.R. Austin).

Spermatogenesis

The process by which gametes are produced is called gametogenesis or, more particularly, spermatogenesis in the case of male and oogenesis in the case of the female. Gametogenesis is the first phase in the sexual reproduction of animals. *Spermatogenesis* begins at puberty and is a steady process throughout life until senility. *Oogenesis,* on the other hands, is a cyclic process, and the "raw material" is present from the start. At birth each ovary contains upto 5000,000 *immature* germ cells, but only few hundreds go on to become mature gametes.

Spermatogenesis (Gr. *Sperma* — sperm or seed ; *genesis*— origin) is the process of the development of spermatozoa in the male gonads, the testes. In the vertebrates and insects, the testes are composite organs consisting of numerous seminiferous tubules. Spermatogenesis is a continuous process, and various stages of development of the sperm may be observed in the seminiferous tubules at the same time. In vertebrates, early stages (the *spermatogonia)* are located at the inner surface of the tubule in an epithelium like arrangement next to the basement membrane, whereas the later stages of differentiation including ripe *spermatozoa* lie nearer to the lumen of the tubules.

The Testis

The testis is a compound tubular gland enclosed in a thick fibrous capsule, the tunica albuginea. Histologically, it consists of numerous seminiferous tubules lying in a bed of lose connective tissue, the stroma. Each seminiferous tubule is surrounded by a *fibrous sheath* of connective tissue. It is lined by a specialized, "stratified" epithelium which forms the germinal epithelium. In the adult, two kinds of cells are present in this epithelium: *(i)* the *Sertoli* or *sustentacular cells* and *(ii)* the *germinal cells.*

Sertoli (Sustentacular) Cells: These are slender pyramidal cells standing at intervals on the *basal lamina* present on the inner surface of the fibrous sheath. The germinal cells are crowded between the Sertoli cells. The function of Sertoli cells is to support and nourish the developing spermatozoa and the germinal cells.

Germinal Cells: The germ cells or sex cells make up a stratified layer of 4 to 8 cells deep. The cells differentiate progressively, from periphery to lumen, in the tubule. Germ cells nearest the lumen transform into spermatozoa which detach as motile cells. This sequence of events is known as spermatogenesis. Next to the basal lamina lie the *spermatogonia* : these have clear cytoplasm with their nuclear chromatin usually appearing as a network. Following the spermatogonia are *spermatocytes,* their nuclei frequently showing active division. The outer layer of *primary spermatocytes,* formed from the spermatogonia, are large and spherical with big nuclei; the inner layer, formed from these by meiosis are the much smaller *secondary spermatocytes.* Next to these and formed by their division, are the *spermatids,* appearing as several layers of small round cells with round nuclei. In some places these spermatids may be seen developing into the *spermatozoa,* a process known as *spermiogenesis.* During this differentiation, the spermatids first develop short tails and then elongate, the nucleus being situated at the head end, remote from the tail.

The somatic number of chromosomes in the human is 46. When the spermatogonia divide there are 22 ordinary pairs and one XY pair, all of which split longitudinally. At the reduction division of primary spermatocytes the XY chromosomes separates so that the secondary spermatocytes are of 2 kinds, each having 22 ordinary chromosomes (or *autosomes)* and either an X or a Y chromosome *(Sex chromosomes).*

The interstitial tissue or stroma fills the spaces between the seminiferous tubules. It consists of lose connective tissue with blood vessels, a lymphatic network and various kinds of cells. Fibroblasts and macrophages are always present. In addition, there are groups of specialized epithelial-like cells, the interstitial cells or "Cells of Ley dig". These cells form the endocrine tissue of the testis. They secrete male hormones, the androgens under the influence of pituitary *leuteinizing hormone (LH).*

(a) *Multiplication Phase:* The undifferentiated primordial germ cells are larger in size and their chromatin-rich nuclei are distinct. They undergo repeated mitotic cell divisions to produce *sperm mother cells* or *spermatogonia* (Gr., sperma—sperm or seed ; gone — offspring). These cells contain a diploid (2*n*) number of chromosomes and enter the next phase of spermatogenesis : the phase of growth.

(b) *Growth Phase:* During this phase, a limited growth of spermatogonia takes place. They increase in volume roughly by a factor of 2. The cells in this stage are called *primary spermatocytes* which are still diploid (2n) in nature.

Events in Spermatogenesis : The entire process of spermatogenesis can be divided into two stages namely, (I) Formation of spermatids and (II) Spermiogenesis.

Formation of Spermatids

Spermatogenesis begins in the germinal epithelial cells of the seminiferous tubules. The germinal cells which develop into spermatids are called primordial germ cells. There are three phases in the conversion of primordial germ cells into spermatids. They are (A) *Multiplication phase* (B) *Growth phase* and (C) *Maturation phase.*

(a) *Multiplication Phase :* The undifferentiated primordial germ cells are larger in size and their chromatin-rich nuclei are distinct. They undergo repeated mitotic cell division to produces *sperm mother cells* or *spermatogonia* (Gr., sperma-sperm or seed; gone offspring). These cells contain a diploid (2n) number of chromosomes and enter the next phase of spermatogenesis : the phase of growth.

(b) *Growth Phase:* During this phase, a limited growth of spermatogonia takes place. They increase in volume roughly by a factor of 2. The cells in this stage are called *primary spermatocytes* which are still diploid (2n) in nature.

(c) *Maturation Phase:* In this phase, a *diploid primary*

spermatocyte produces four *haploid spermatids.* The reduction is accomplished by *Meiosis* which consists of 2 consecutive cell divisions:

(i) *First Meiotic* or *Maturation Division* : It is reductional in nature and reduces the number of chromosomes from *diploid to haploid*. The nuclear DNA is duplicated in the beginning of division. In the first division homologous chromosomes pair up at *prophase* in a process called synopsis, each such pair being referred to as a bivalent. Nevertheless, a bivalent consists really of four chromatids closely joined together in one complex unit. While the chromatids are in close proximity, breakage occurs along the length of the chromatids and their parts join up in new combinations. .This phenomenon is called crossing over which enables an exchange of parts of the chromosomes to take place. At the site where a crossing over has occurred the chromosomes are connected by a chiasma.

The centromere become attached to the spindle fibres during *metaphase* and the bivalents are placed in the equatorial plate of the achromatic figures. At the start of *anaphase,* the two chromosomes forming a bivalent separate from one another and are drawn to the opposite poles. Thus at the end *oftelophase* two haploid (re) daughter cells emerge from a primary spermatocyte. These are known as the secondary spermatocytes. A secondary spermatocyte contains a member of each homologous pair of chromosomes originally present in the parent cell.

(ii) *Second Meiosis* or *Maturation Division* : It is equational or mitotic in nature and produces two haploid (n) spermatids from each secondary spermatocyte. At *metaphase* the centromeres align themselves along the equatorial plate and duplicate ; at *anaphase* the daughter centromeres, with the assistance of the spindle fibres, move to the respective poles, dragging along the two chromatids (now called chromosomes).

As a result of two meiotic divisions, four cells are formed from each primary spermatocyte. These are called spermatids. Each spermatid gets one chromatid from a bivalent, therefore, it possesses one chromosomes for each pair of chromosomes present in somatic cells. In other words we can say that the spermatids have a haploid set of chromosomes.

The spermatids are still not capable of functioning as male gametes. They have to undergo a process of differentiation to become the spermatozoa.

Spermiogenesis

The transformation or differentiation of the spermatid into spermatozoon is called spermiogenesis. The haploid spermatid is a typical cell containing nucleus and cytoplasm with mitochondria, centrioles and Golgi bodies. Since the sperm is a very active and mobile cell, therefore, to provide greater mobility to the sperm, the superfluous material of the spermatid is discarded and a high degree of specialization is attained by the sperm cell during spermiogenesis. Following changes occur:

Changes in the Nucleus

(a) The nucleus gradually diminishes in size by losing water from the nuclear sap, and the chromosomes become closely packed into a small volume. The weight is reduced to enhance the motility of the spermatozoon.

(b) Whole of the ribonucleic acid (RNA), especially in the nucleolus, is eliminated, leaving only the genetic material, the deoxyribonucleoproteins.

(c) The shape of the nucleus changes from the usual spherical to an elongated and narrow form—an adaptation for the propulsion in any fluid medium. The head of the spermatozoon assumes different shapes in different animals.

(i) *Ovoid and flattened from the sides* : man and bull.

(ii) *As a short curved sword with pointed tip* : rodents and amphibia.

(iii) *Spirally twisted like a corkscrew* : birds and some molluscs.

(iv) *Round,* bivalve molluscs.

Acrosome Formation : The acrosome of the spermatozoon is derived from the *Golgi bodies.* In an early spermatid, the Golgi body is concentrated near the anterior end of the nucleus. It consists of a series of membranes arranged concentrically around a cluster of small vacuoles. One of the vacuoles starts enlarging and a small dense body, the proacrosomal granula (mucopolysaccharide) appears in it. The vacuole with its granule becomes closely applied to the tip of the nucleus. The pro-acrosomal granule increases further and becomes the acrosomal granule. The latter forms the core of the acrosome. In the next stage the vacuole loses its liquid content and its wall spreads over the acrosomal granule and the front half of the nucleus, covering them with a double membranous sheath called the cap of the spermatozoon. The remaining part of the Golgi body is gradually reduced and ultimately discarded from the spermatid as *"Golgi rest"*, along with some cytoplasm. According to L.H. Colwin and A.L. Colwin (1961), the acrosomal granule contains a supply of enzymes which are used to dissolve the egg membranes during fertilization.

Changes in the Centrosome : The centrosome of a spermatid after the second meiotic division consists of two *centrioles.* The centrioles are in the form of two cylindrical bodies, lying at right angles to each other. During early stages of sperm differentiation, the two centrioles move to a position just behind the sperm nucleus in the neck region. A depression is formed in the posterior surface of the nucleus and one of the two centrioles becomes placed in this depression with its axis at right angles to the main axis of the sperm. This is the proximal centriole of the spermatozoon. The other centriole called the distal centriole get positioned behind the proximal centriole with its axis parallel to the longitudinal axis of the sperm. The distal centriole gives rise to the *axial filament* of the flagellum of the spermatozoon for which it serves as a *basal granule.*

Changes in the Mitochondria : In many animals, particularly mammals, the mitochondria of the spermatid join in one continuous body which becomes twisted spirally around the axial filament and the distal centriole. In other animals, the mitochondria fuse together to form one or more massive clumps called *mitochondrial bodies.*

Changes in the Cytoplasm : The abundant cytoplasm of the spermatid is reduced to a condensed layer known as the manchette in sperm. The manchette is confined to the periphery of the middle piece. It is also present at the posterior part of the head of the spermatozoon.

Ring Centriole : In some species the posterior end of the middle piece is marked by dark ring called the *"ring centriole".* It is different from the centriole in its structures. The ring centriole forms the boundary between the middle piece and the tail. The function of the ring is not known.

Axial Filament : It starts from the distal centriole of the spermatid. The axial filament of the sperm has the same organization as the axial filaments of the flagella and kinocilia present in other animal and plant cells. It has a pair of longitudinal fibres in the centre and a ring of nine pairs of longitudinal fibres surrounding it. In mammals, the nine pairs of longitudinal fibres are accompanied on the outside by 9 much thicker fibres in the middle piece. Besides, there is a set of semicircular ribs articulating with each other on the opposite sides of the sperm tail.

The spermatozoon is totally devoid of stored food and protective envelopes, which characterise female gametes.

Factors Controlling Spermatogenesis : The production and liberation of spermatozoa in animals are governed by environmental or physiological factors. Spermatogenesis is controlled mainly by the anterior pituitary gonadotropin, *follicle stimulating hormone* (FSH). Temperature, light, and psychological state of the animal exert some influence upon spermatogenesis in different animals like birds, rodents and many other vertebrates. In some instances, pituitary itself is subject to external influences.

Morphology of a Mature Spermatozoon : A spermatozoon is a highly specialized type of cell. The greater part of its total volume is represented by nuclear material. The sperm is characterized by the presence of a propulsive system in the form of an axial filament powered by energy obtained from the mitochondria. Unlike female gametes, the sperm cell is totally devoid of stored food and protective envelopes. Thus a spermatozoon may be looked upon as hardly more than a motile nucleus whose fate is to carry the paternal chromosomal elements to the ovum and to activate ovum.

A typical mammalian spermatozoon consists of the following main parts:

the head

the middle piece,

the tail or flagellum.

Head : The head is spoon-shaped in man and many other mammals. The anterior tip of the head is differentiated as the *acrosome* which plays an important role in the penetration of the spermatozoon through the egg membranes and the activation of the egg during fertilization. The *nucleus* occupies the major part of the head. It contains genes and is thus responsible for the transmission of the hereditary characters from the male parent. A depression is formed on the posterior surface of the nucleus which contains two centrioles, lying at right angles to each other. During fertilization, *the proximal centriole* of the sperm gives rise to a spindle system inside the egg and is necessary for the initiation of the cell division in the fertilized egg. The *distal centriole* lies behind the proximal centriole. Its axis coincides with the longitudinal axis of the sperm. The distal centriole gives rise to the axial filament of the flagellum of the spermatozoon for which it serves as a basal granule or a starting point.

The cytoplasm forms a condensed layer known as the *manchette* around the posterior part of the nucleus.

Middle Piece

Electron microscopy reveals a highly complex architecture in the middle piece. The most internal structure is the *axial filament* which consists of two *central fibres* surrounded by ring of nine double *inner fibres.* In mammals the nine pairs of longitudinal fibres are surrounded by nine thick *outer fibres.* Still more external are *mitochondria,* arranged spirally around the rings of filaments. The mitochondria, being carriers of oxidative enzymes, are the "power plants" furnishing the work energy for the fibre system of the spermatozoon.

A dark ring known as the *ring centriole* is sometimes seen at the posterior end of the middle piece forming the boundary between the middle piece and the tail. However, it does not in any way resemble an centriole in its structure. The function of the ring is not known.

The *manchette* is present around the inner periphery of the middle piece. All these structures, as well as those in other regions of the sperms cell, are encased by the *sperm plasma membrane.*

Tail of Flagellum

The tail is subdivided into two regions —*principal piece* and *end-piece.* In these region's the fibre system is reduced to the axial complex of two *central fibres* surrounded by the ring of nine *inner fibres.* Throughout the principal piece there is also present *a fibrous helix* surrounding the longitudinal fibres. The helix is composed of semicircular ribs articulating with each other on the opposite sides of the sperm tail. The tip of the end-piece consists only of the axial filament covered with cytoplasm and plasmalemma. It lacks any other type of filaments.

Types of Sperms

The sperms are classified into two types namely: (a) flagellate spermatozoa and (b) non-flagellate spermatozoa.

***Flagellate Spermatozoa*:** Flagellate sperms contain one or two flagella. All vertebrates produce flagellate sperms. Many vertebrates produce monoflagellate spermatozoa but the sperm of some animals *e.g.*, toad-fish *(Opsanus)* is provided with two tails. Such sperms are called *biflagellate* sperms.

In some animals two or more sperm heads adhere closely to form conjugate sperms *e.g., Oppossum,* a beetle *Dytiscus* and a gastropod *Turritella.* In the grasshopper *Poecilocercus* many sperm-heads aggregates together to from a *sperm-boat.* After ejaculation by the male, all conjugate sperms normally dissociate from each other in the female genital tract.

***Non-flagellate Spermatozoa*:** Flagella are absent in non-flagellate spermatozoa. Such spermatozoa resemble with common body cells. This type of sperms occur in some invertebrates such as *Procambarus* (cray fish) and *Ascaris* (round worm). In the latter, spermatozoa are unique in being amoeboid in nature.

regions of the sperms cell are encased by the *sperm plasma membrane*.

Tail of Flagellum

The tail is subdivided into two regions—principal piece and end piece. In these regions the fibre system is reduced to the axial complex of two central *fibres* surrounded by the ring of nine outer *fibres*. Throughout the principal piece there is also present a *fibrous helix* surrounding the longitudinal fibres. The helix is composed of semicircular ribs articulating with each other on the opposite sides of the sperm tail. The tip of the end-piece consists only of the axial filament covered with cytoplasm and plasmalemma. It lacks any other type of filaments.

Types of Sperms

The sperms are classified into two types namely (a) flagellate spermatozoa and (b) non-flagellate spermatozoa.

Flagellate Spermatozoa: Flagellate sperms contain one or two flagella. All vertebrates produce flagellate sperms. Many vertebrates produce monoflagellate spermatozoa but the sperm of some animals e.g., toad fish (*Opsanus*) is provided with two tails. Such sperms are called *biflagellate sperms*.

In some animals two or more sperm heads adhere closely to form conjugate sperms e.g., *Opisthorchis*, a beetle *Dytiscus* and a gastropod *Turritella*. In the grasshopper *Parthenogenesis* many sperm heads aggregates together to from a spermatozeugma. After ejaculation by the male, all conjugate sperms normally dissociate from each other in the female genital tract.

Non-flagellate Spermatozoa: Flagella are absent in non-flagellate spermatozoa. Such spermatozoa resemble with common body cells. This type of sperms occur in some invertebrates such as *Cambaridae* (crayfish) and *Ascaris* (round worm). In the latter, spermatozoa are unique in being amoeboid in nature.

2

The Gradients

Polarity

All animal eggs and some plant eggs are strongly polar structures. The two opposite poles are differentiated as animal pole and vegetal pole. The imaginary axis passing through these two poles is called polar axis or animal-vegetal axis. It is the main axis of the egg.

Polarity in Animal Eggs

Polarity in animal eggs may be evident in the primary oocyte. But it is distinctly established either in secondary oocyte or in the fertilized egg. In telolecithal eggs it is evident even before fertilization. Polarity is basically displayed in three forms:

(i) Eccentric position of nucleus, which lies in the animal hemisphere or towards the animal pole.

(ii) Release of polar bodies at the animal pole.

(iii) Accumulation of yolk granules towards the vegetal pole.

Polarity is usually expressed as a gradient in the ratio of cytoplasm and yolk from animal to vegetal pole. Whatever may be the amount of yolk, it is never uniformly distributed in the egg cytoplasm. Its density gradually increases from animal towards the vegetal pole. Polarity is responsible for the differentiation of egg as a bipolar structure.

Bipolar Differentiation

In Telolecithal Eggs : During growth phase, the oocytes establish bipolar differentiation because of unequal distribution of various substances and cellular constituents. In telolecithal eggs the yolk or deutoplasm is not distributed evenly throughout the ooplasm. Usually at one end of the oocyte, an area is relatively free of yolk and contains the egg nucleus. When the nucleus of oocyte undergoes meiosis, the meiotic spindle is formed in this region and the polar bodies are discharged here. The end of oocyte which contains nucleus and yolk free cytoplasm is called animal pole. The end opposite to the animal pole is referred to as vegetal pole, where the concentration of yolk is greatest. The establishment of animal and vegetal poles is called bipolar differentiation. It is caused by the unequal distribution of deutoplasm. The imaginary axis that passes through animal and vegetal poles is called the polar axis or animal-vegetal axis.

In Oligolecithal and Centrolecithal Eggs : In oligolecithal eggs that have very little yolk distributed uniformly and also in centrolecithal eggs the animal pole and vegetal poles are not distinct. In them, the animal pole is distinguished by the discharge of polar bodies. In these types of eggs, there is little or no gradient in yolk distribution along the animal-vegetal axis. However, in telolecithal eggs, that have greater concentration of yolk, the animal-vegetal axis is characterised by a gradient in yolk concentration which increases from animal to vegetal pole. It affects changes in the distribution of other cytoplasmic contents and imposes changes in the structural organization of egg or establishes some type of differentiation.

In some cases, the animal and vegetal halves are made more distinct by unequal distribution of pigment granules. For example, in frog the animal half or animal hemisphere contains black or brown pigment while the vegetal half is clear white with no pigment. Similarly, in *Nereis dumerilii* a violet pigment is concentrated in the vegetal half.

An Example of Bipolar Differentiation : Bipolar differentiation has been studied by JOSEPH SPEK (1934) in *Nereis dumerilli.* In *Nereis,* during bipolar differentiation, the ooplasmic substances become distributed in such a way that the alkaline substances with high *p*H accumulate in the animal pole, while substances with low *p*H migrate towards the opposite or vegetal pole. In an undifferentiated oocyte, a yellow pigment is uniformly distributed in the ooplasm. This pigment remains yellow in alkaline medium but turns violet at *pH.* During bipolar differentiation, the pigment migrates and accumulates in the vegetal half. As a result, the animal pole becomes colourless. With the accumulation of substances in the vegetal half, the yellow pigment turns violet indicating an increase of acidity in this part.

Origin of Polarity

In the beginning of growth phase the primary oocyte is an undifferentiated cell. Polarity develops during growth and differentiation of primary oocyte within the ovary. There is definite relationship between the position of oocyte within the ovary and the direction of future animal-vegetal axis.

Various factors are attributed for differentiation and polarity in the egg. These are:

Direction of How of Nutrients: In molluscs and echinoderms, the end of the oocyte which is attached to the wall of the ovary and receives nutrients from it, grows into the vegetal pole. It was, therefore, concluded that the greater amount of yolk is deposited in the part of the oocyte nearest to the proximal surface of the ovary, which then differentiates as vegetal pole. However, this concept does not apply to those ova which receive their nourishment from the follicle cells that surround the ovum from all the sides as in mammals and amphibians.

Direction of Oxygen Supply: CHILD (1941) believed that the end of oocyte which is near the blood vessel would get more oxygen than its opposite end. Therefore, this end develops into the animal pole.

Electric Field Concept: According to SPEK (1934) an electric field is established inside the egg cell. This causes the migration and orientation of the microscopical and ultramicroscopical particles entering egg cell at polar region according to their electric charge.

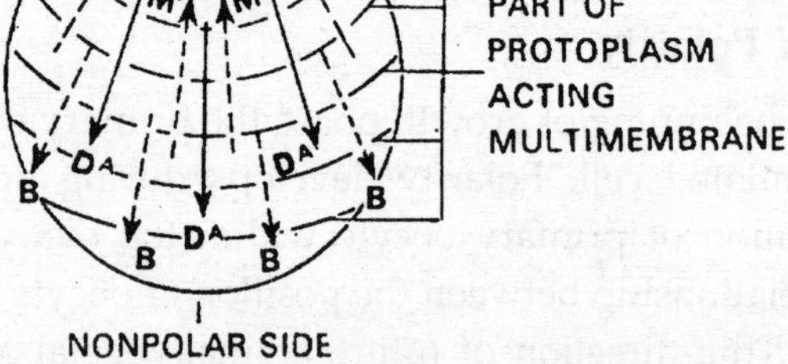

Hypothetical scheme of diffusion of electrically charged particles entering egg cell at polar region (After Berrill).

Polarity as a Characteristic of Every Cell: BALINSKY (1970) suggested that polarity is a phenomenon found not only in egg cells but in all other cells of the organisms. The position of centrosome with respect to the nucleus establishes a general form of polarity with the main axis or polar axis passing through the centrosome and nucleus. This polarity influences the distribution of cytoplasmic inclusions and even the structure of nucleus.

Factors Determining Polarity in Eggs

Though deposition of yolk is responsible for polarization, a number of environmental agents were found to influence egg polarity- (LUND (1923), WHITAKER (1931-44).

These factors may be :

(i) Direct electric current (ii) Unilateral exposure to light (iii) Presence of neighbouring eggs (iv) p*H* gradient (v) Temperature gradient (vi) Position of sperm entry.

The eggs of *Fucus* and *Pelvetia* (both algae) provide considerable insight into the factors determining polarity in eggs. There is no sign of polarity in *Fucus* egg when it is laid in sea water. The first indication of visible differentiation appears about 12 hours after fertilization as a protuberance at one pole. The egg becomes pear-shaped and the end with protuberance forms the rhizoidal cell.

Study of various factors responsible for polarization in *Fucus* egg reveals that it is determined by the direction of incident light, *p*H differential or CO_2 differential. The chemical gradient also induces polarity in eggs.

According to L.F. JAFFE localized changes in plasma membrane potential are the cause of polar differentiation. The non-homogeneity in the membrane potential of plasma membrane causes local currents in the egg cytoplasm. JAFFE suggested that in *Fucus* egg there is a flow of positive ions into the egg at rhizoidal end and out at the opposite end. This is established by self cataphoresis.

Inversion of Polar Axis

TADANO in Japan has worked on the inversion of animal-vegetal axis. The egg is deeply centrifuged before first cleavage. Its material stratifies into five layers. When egg is strongly centrifuged, the first of the five layers separates into mitochondrial layer and a heavy hyaloplasmic layer. After centrifugation these layers become indistinct because the stratified material regains its original distribution. If the eggs are not fixed in place, these rotate bringing animal pole towards the centrifugal end of the tube. But if the eggs are first held in such a way that the heavier vegetal pole is towards centrifugal end, the centrifugation inverts the vegetal pole and also the gradient polarity of the egg.

Significance of Polarity

1. The regional differentiation of egg serves as guideline for the development of major axes of an organism. Primary polarity leads to the visible polarity of differentiation of oocyte.
2. Polarity affects the direction of cleavage. The first and second cleavage furrows coincide with the animal-vegetal axis.
3. In sea urchin the polar axis becomes the axis of radial symmetry during cleavage.
4. The animal pole generally forms the anterior end and differentiates into external covering (ectoderm) of the embryo. The elements of vegetal pole differentiate into endodermal structures.

Gradients

Organisms, whether unicellular or multicellular are highly polarised. These have antero-posterior or apico-basal axis. All animal eggs are also distinctly polarized. The gradual differentiation of egg cytoplasm along the animal-vegetal axis indicates an axial gradient. The axial gradient is a manifestation of metabolic gradients or physiological gradients.

History of Gradient Concept

During development, one cell (zygote) gives rise to many cells. Each of these cells (blastomeres) has a specific composition and gives rise to cells of differentiated properties.

Experiment 1: Wilhelm Roux (1888) Killed One Of The Blastomeres Of Two-celled Frog Egg. The Result Was Half Embryo That Developed From The Living Blastomere. It Was Concluded That Each Cell Produces A Specific Part Of The Developing Embryo.

Experiment 2 : Hans Driech (1892) Separated Blastomeres Of Sea Urchin Embryo At Two And Four Cell Stages By Vigorous Shaking. Each Blastomere Developed Into A Complete And Normal Embryo When Developed In Isolation. Driech Concluded That Egg Is A Harmonious Equipotential System. Each Part Of The Egg Has A Potency To Form The Whole Embryo. The Fate Of A Cell Is The Function Of Its Position In The Entire Embryo.

Experiment 3 : A sea urchin embryo at eight cell stage was separated into two halves lengthwise. Each group of four blastomeres developed into one complete larva.

Next the eight-celled sea urchin embryo was separated into two halves horizontally. The animal half differentiated into a hollow ball of cells with very long cilia. It was Next

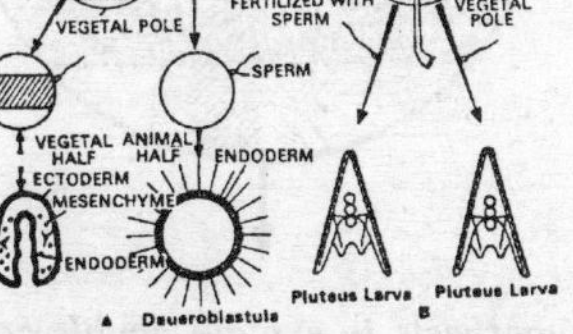

HORSTADIUS experiment on sea urchin egg showing effect of animalizing and Vegetalizing factors

the eight-celled sea urchin embryo was separated into two halves horizontally. The animal half differentiated into a hollow ball of cells with very long cilia. It was called a dauerblastula. It was devoid of endodermal and mesodermal components. The vegetal half developed into an ovoid body without arms. It had an enlarged and often evaginated outward gut. It was named exogastrula.

From the above experiment it was concluded that animal and vegetal halves of an egg have different future. The animal half contains ectodermal contents, while vegetal half has mesodermal and endodermal components.

Gradient Theory

HORSTADIUS (1955) and RUNNSTROM (1967) proposed the existence of a double-gradient system to control the morphogenesis and differentiation during early development of sea urchin embryo. An animal gradient is maximum at the animal pole and is responsible for the formation of structures characteristic of that region. Similarly, the vegetal gradient, which is most intense at the vegetal pole, controls processes like invagination, formation of archenteron and mesenchyme.

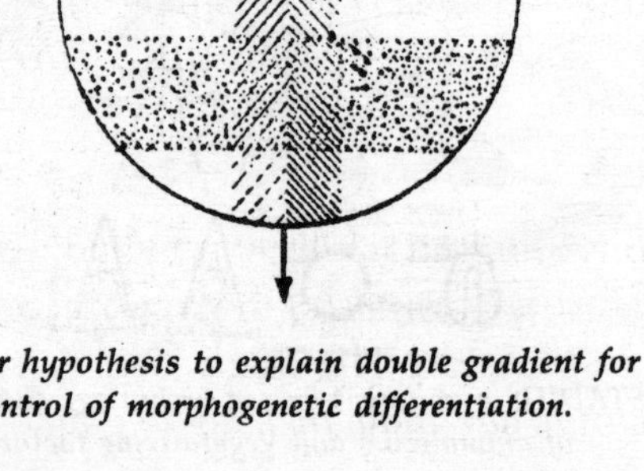

Two-factor hypothesis to explain double gradient for the control of morphogenetic differentiation.

If the animal gradient is weakened or suppressed, the vegetal gradient becomes preponderant and the embryo is vegetalised; and if the vegetal gradient is weakened, the animal gradient becomes preponderant and embryo becomes animalized. A normal development results only when two gradients are in correct equilibrium. HORSTADIUS and JOSEFSSON (1969) have shown the existence of specific animalizing and vegetalizing substances (such as tryptophan and nucleotide) in the matured fertilized eggs. The animalizing agents are presumed to promote synthesis of ribonucleic acid and proteins, while the vegetalizing agents inhibit the onset of these processes.

Conclusion : The regional differentiation of the cytoplasm early in the development appears to coincide with the animal-vegetal axis of the egg. An interpretation of the organization is based upon qualitative differences in the cytoplasm. According to this concept, an animal gradient, with its centre in the animal hemisphere, and a vegetal gradient, with its centre in the vegetal hemisphere, are requisites to normal development.

Those gradients appear to be based on physico-chemical differences. It is thought that contrasting metabolic systems have centres of greatest intensity at the opposite poles of the egg and exert their effect in decreasing quantity along the animal-vegetal axis.

The graded interaction of the antagonistic systems underlies normal development. The removal of the animal or vegetal hemisphere results in a deficient larva. But the separation of the egg along the meridional axis which preserves the balanced system of gradients, gives rise to two embryos.

Furthermore, according to the gradient concept, the animalizing or vegetalizing influence of various chemical agents result from the depression of the metabolic system representing the opposite gradient with the result of an inordinate development of one gradient.

It is now clear that the concept of qualitative and quantitative differences in the cytoplasm of the egg are not enough for the fundamental organization of the egg. But a stimulus is necessary to convert the organization into the adult structure. This stimulation is the process of activation, which is normally introduced by the sperm.

3

The Gametogenesis

The process by which gametes are produced in the gonads is known as gametogenesis. In all animals, heterogametes (dissimilar) are produced which is of great adaptive value. To carry out their function most efficiently, gametes should be motile (so that they can come together and unite) and be supplied with food reserve to furnish energy and material for developing embryo. The two requirements are rather incompatible. The solution is: one (male gamete) the sperm is motile and small and the other one, the egg or ovum is filled with food reserve. The process of formation of male gametes or sperm is known as spermatogenesis and that of female gametes or ova as orogenesis.

The process of gametogenesis is of great significance because the gametes are the only link between the generations. Their nuclear DNA is the depository of all those genetic informations that are needed in the development of new organism. In monoecious or hermaphroditic animals both male and female gametes are produced in the same individual, but in dioecious animals, the sperm and ova are formed in different individuals of the same species. This separation of sexes is called gonochorism.

Spermatogenesis

The process of maturation of primordial germ cells in the testes of male to form spermatozoa (sperm) is known as spermatogenesis. The testes are formed of numerous tubular seminiferous tubules, held together in connective tissue. Each seminiferous tubule shows an orderly arrangement of cells undergoing different phases of maturation. The peripheral layer of cells next to the basement membrane is formed of spermatogonia or the sperm mother cells and is often described as germinal epithelium. The spermatogonia undergo spermatogenesis to produce sperm.

In between the groups of spermatogonia are tall columnar cells, the sertoli cells, attached proximally to the basement membrane and projecting distally into the lumen of the tubule. The spermatids undergoing differentiation into spermatozoa remain partially embedded in the cytoplasm of Sertoli cells which provide nourishment to the developing sperm.

Interspersed in the connective tissue in between the seminiferous tubules are present groups of interstitial cells or Leydig cells which secrete maie hormone.

The process of spermatogenesis is a continuous process and is much complicated.

(A) From the cell of germinal epithelium produced are as a result of meiotic division.

(B) Metamorphosis of spermatids into spermatozoa, the spermateliosis.

Formation of Spermatids : The formation of spermatids starts from the primordial germ cells of testis or the primary germ cells. The entire process can be separated into three phases :

1. Mitotic Multiplication phase
2. Growth phase
3. Maturation phase or Meiotic phase.

Multiplication Phase : The spermatogonia or sperm mother cells lie next to the basement membrane. These divide repeatedly by mitosis producing new sex cells throughout life. Some of these cells move towards the lumen of the seminiferous tubule and enter the growth phase. These are called primary spermatocytes or proleptotene spermatocytes while others produced by the mitotic division of spermatogonia remain in the original condition and continue to produce new spermatogonia throughout the reproductive life of the animal. These cells are known as 'stem cells'.

Thus, there are two types of spermatogonia : (i) *Type-A spermatogonia* represent stem cells. These are dark non-cyclic cells (Ad). (ii) *Type-B spermatogonia* (AP) develop by the differentiation of some of Type-A and undergo spermatogenesis.

There is no fixed number of spermatogonia, unlike the female, where number of germ cells destined to differentiate as ova *i.e.* oogonia is limited and is fixed during embryogenesis.

Growth Phase: The spermatogonia, formed as a result of repeated divisions of the primordial germ cells, stop dividing and prepare themselves for maturation division. They increase in size by accumulating nourishing material obtained from germinal cells. The enlarged cells are known as primary spermatocytes. Initially, the nucleus of each primary spermatocyte is of ordinary size, but soon it imbibes material and enlarges considerably. At the end of growth phase, when the primary spermatocyte is ready to undergo first maturation division (*i.e.* the reduction division) its nucleus is much larger than that of spermatogonial cell.

Maturation Phase: Each diploid primary spermatocyte

undergoes the first maturation division which is a reduction division, with its long drawn-out and complicated prophase. The pairing and splitting of homologous chromosomes take place during zygotene and pachytene and this leads to the formation of tetrads. Due to crossing over, the exchange of homologous chromosomes also takes place. According to some, all these chromosomal events are completed in the growth phase only, so that during first maturation division the chromosomes are equally distributed to the two daughter cells. As a result of reduction division, (1st maturation division) the two cells formed are haploid, having *n*-number of chromosomes. These haploid cells are called secondary spermatocytes.

The secondary spermatocytes undergo second maturation division which is a simple mitotic division. As a result, each secondary spermatocyte divides into two equal cells, the spermatids. Each spermatid consists of only one set of homologous chromosome pairs and is, therefore, haploid. It undergoes metamorphosis to form the mature motile sperm. At the end of maturation phase four haploid spermatids are formed from each diploid primary spermatocyte.

Spermiogenesis or Spermatolysis : It is the gradual differentiation of a stationary rounded and undifferentiated spermatid into an active and motile sperm. The spermatids formed as a result of maturation divisions are typical undifferentiated animal cells containing mitochondria, Golgi body and centriole but with a haploid set of chromosomes. In this from it is incapable of functioning as a male gamete, which has to reach the ovum. The changes which transform spermatid into a spermatozoon are briefed as under and the account pertains to that found in cat:

Nuclear Changes : During spermiogenesis, the nucleus undergoes following changes:

(i) The nucleus shrinks by losing water from the nuclear sap and the chromosomes are closely packed. The step is essential, since it reduces the weight of spermatozoon and enhances its motility. Even RNA and other accessory materials are also removed leaving only the hereditary material.

(ii) The nucleus changes from its usual spherical form and becomes elongated and narrow. This is an adaptation for propulsion in liquid medium. In different animals the nucleus assumes different shapes which determine the shapes of the sperm.

Formation of Acrosome : The acrosome of spermatozoon is derived from Golgi complex of the spermatid.

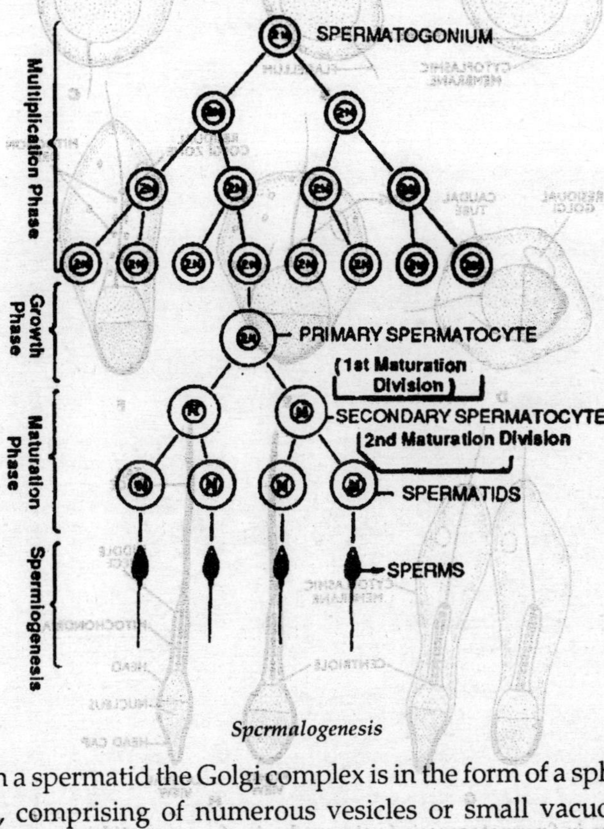

Spcrmalogenesis

In a spermatid the Golgi complex is in the form of a spherical body, comprising of numerous vesicles or small vacuoles in the centre surrounded by several rows of concentrically-arranged cisternae. As the differentiation proceeds, the arrangement of cisternae becomes irregular and one or two vacuoles enlarge to replace the vesicles. Inside each large vacuole appears a small dense body, the proacrosomal granule. The proacrosomal granule and vacuole are formed of polymucosaccharides. If more than one vacuoles and proacrosomal granules are formed, these fuse together so that only one is left in the end.

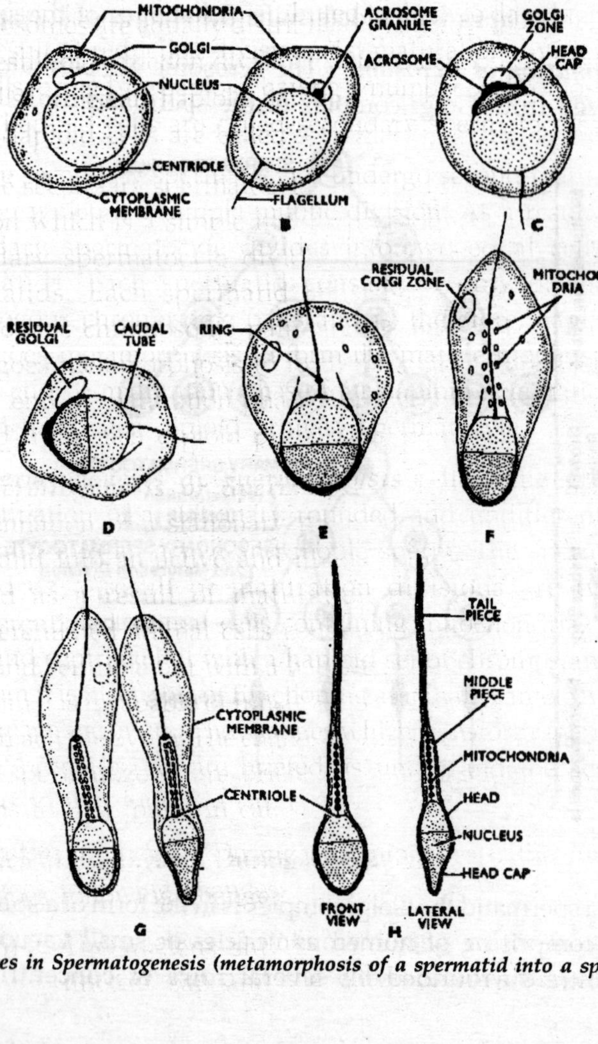

Stages in Spermatogenesis (metamorphosis of a spermatid into a sperm)

The vacuole with its acrosomal granule enlarges in size, migrates towards the anterior pole and gets attached to the tip of elongated nucleus forming a sort of cap (cap stage). The proacrosomal granule enlarges further and forms the acrosomal granule. It forms core of the acrosome, (acrosomal stage). The vacuole loses its liquid content, spreads over the acrosomal granule and half of the nucleus forming a double sheath at the terminal end of the head of spermatozoon. It is known as the acrosome cap. The remainder of Golgi body undergoes a gradual regression and is discarded as 'Golgi rest' together with the cytoplasm of spermatid.

The above description is based on cat. In other animals the development may be complicated by the formation of a second component, the axial body or acrosomal cone between the acrosomal granule and the nucleus. This is regarded to be the rudiment of acrosomal filament that develops when spermatozoon approaches the egg.

The acrosomal granule contains lytic (tissue dissolving) enzymes which are used to dissolve the egg membranes during fertilization (L.H. COLWIN and A.L. COLWIN, 1961). The acrosome, therefore, helps in penetration of sperm into ovum.

Formation of Axial Filament of Spermatozoon : The axial filament of the tail of spermatozoon is formed from the centriole of spermatid. The spermatid consists of two centrioles. During spermiogenesis these move and come to lie behind the nucleus. One of them enters in the depression developed in the posterior part of nucleus and is known as the proximal centriole. It lies at right angles to the main axis of sperm. The second or the distal centriole lies next to the proximal centriole with its axis coinciding with the longitudinal axis of the spermatozoon. The distal centriole gives rise to the axial filament of the flagellum and acts as a basal granule. The proximal centriole enters the ovum alongwith sperm nucleus and initiates spindle formation for the first division of the zygote nucleus.

Formation of Mitochondrial Spiral or Mitochondrial Helix : All the mitochondria from different parts of the spermatid accumulate in the middle piece of spermatozoon around the proximal part of axial filament and distal centriole. These partly fuse forming two densely-packed bodies one on either side of axial filament. Finally, these get twisted spirally forming a sheath around the axial filament and proximal centriole. This sheath is known as nebenkern. The spiral arrangement of sheath is seen in mammals only. In other animals, the mitochondria are joined into one or more massive clumps or mitochondrial bodies.

The mitochondrial spiral provides energy to the vibratile flagellum of sperm when it swims or moves towards the ovum.

Formation of Manchette : Much of the cytoplasm of the spermatid is lost. Due to acrosome formation, the cytoplasm of the anterior end moves into the middle piece and forms a condensed layer around its periphery. This is known as manchette or cytoplasmic droplet. An extremely thin layer is also left with the plasmalemma over the acrosome and nucleus, but there is no cytoplasm in sperm tail.

Protein Synthesis during Spermiogenesis : According to BRINK (1968) protein synthesis occurs during spermiogenesis but to a limited extent. Since no RNA is synthesized during this period, it is presumed that spermatid contained some stable form of *m*RNA.

Factors Controlling Spermatogenesis : The formation of sperm and their liberation is precisely controlled by the environment in primitive animals and by environment and hormones in chordates. The environmental factors include temperature, light and season, etc. The proper functioning of testes and the maturation of spermatozoa in vertebrates is controlled by gonadotropic hormones secreted by the adenohypophysis of the anterior lobe of pituitary gland. The functioning of pituitary is influenced by day length and intensity of light. The specific hormones have not been isolated in invertebrates for proper functioning of testes, certain chemical factors are presumed to control the process.

Structure of Spermatozoon

The spermatozoon is a single specialized cell, modified for swimming and delivering itself into the ovum to complete the act of fertilization. It is very small, only a few microns in size but has a long tail or flagellum. It is enclosed in a plasma membrane. Some form of extraneous coat is also present, which is responsible for some of the antigenic properties of the spermatozoon and for the specificity of sperm-egg interaction.

The shape, size, and structure of male gamete varies greatly in different animals.

However, it can be differentiated into following three parts: The head, middle piece and tail or flagellum.

Head

It is the anterior-most part of the spermatozoon. It is often conical but its shape varies considerably. It may be long and slender *(Rhomalium)*, spheroidal (teleosts), rod-shaped or lens-shaped (amphibians), spoon-shaped or short and flat (man), thin and crescentric (nemertine *worm-Cerebratulus)*, cork-screw shaped (in certain toads and elasmobrach fish) or hooked (mouse and rat). The head is formed of acrosome and nucleus.

Acrosome : The anterior tip of the sperm head is differentiated as acrosome. The acrosome is a cap-like structure varying greatly in size and appearance. It is formed from the Golgi complex and helps the spermatozoon to penetrate through the egg membranes and to establish connection with the egg cytoplasm. Some investigators have named it perforatorium, a term to indicate its function.

The acrosome is bounded by an acrosomal membrane. It contains proteases enzymes and some acrosomal polysaccharides. The enzymes proteases are tissue-lytic enzymes which help in the penetration of nucleus and centriole of the sperm in the egg.

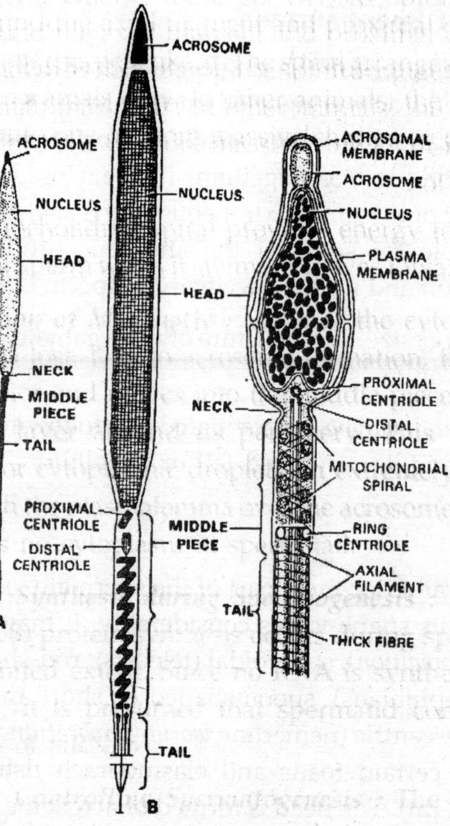

Structure of a mammalian sperm A-Under light microscope; B-Under electron microscope. (After Burgos & Fawcett, 1955)

In the sperm of certain animals like *Nereis*, cricket, oyster and fowl, etc., a cone-shaped structure is present in between the acrosome and nucleus. This is called axial body or acrosomal cone. It lies in the indentation at the anterior end of the nucleus. It develops into an acrosomal filament at the time of fertilization.

A very thin layer of cytoplasm is present in between the nucleus and acrosome and also in between the membrane of acrosomal vesicle and sperm plasma membrane. This is known as periacrosomal cytoplasm.

Nucleus : The sperm nucleus consists almost entirely of DNA and protein. The DNA is present in quiescent state and is so densely packed that the clear structure pattern cannot be distinguished. The protein present is primarily of basic or histone type. The shape of the nucleus also differs in various groups. The nucleus is a truncated cone in sea urchin sperm, oval and disc-shaped in rabbit sperm and bilobed in oyster *(Crassostrea)* sperm. The posterior margin of nucleus is depressed to accomodate the proximal centriole.

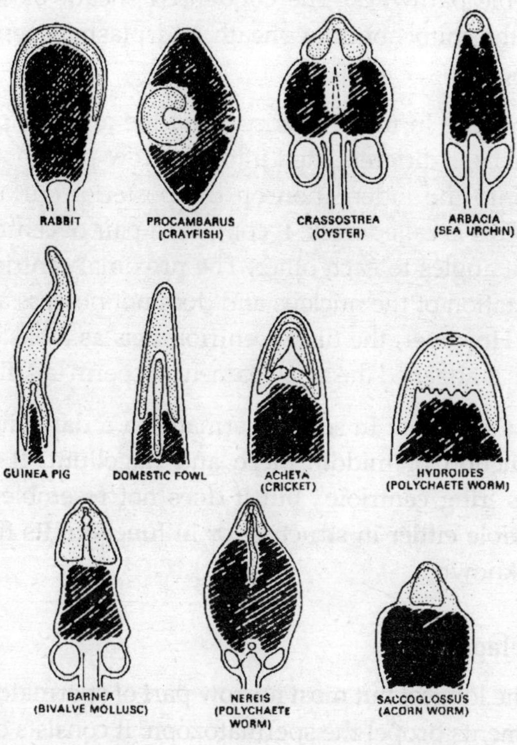

Structure of acrosome in various spermatozoon as seen under electron microscope.

Middle Piece

Lying immediately behind the head is the middle piece. It varies greatly in form. It may be so short as to contain only the centrioles as in *Sturgeon* (fish). In sea urchin, it is represented by a single mitochondrion arranged around the posterior aspect of the nucleus. In rabbit's spermatozoon the middle piece is very prominent and consists of the distal centriole and the apical part of the tail filament in the middle line, surrounded by a tightly coiled spiral of elongated mitochondria. The mitochondrial spiral lies between the proximal and ring centriole. It contains oxidative enzymes and provides energy for sperm motility. The energy can be derived from exogenous as well as endogenous substrates and through aerobic as well as anaerobic pathways. The condensed sheath of cytoplasm between the mitochondrial sheath and plasma membrane is called machete.

Centrioles : In many spermatozoa the anterior portion of middle piece is differentiated into a narrow part that remains inserted into the indentation on the posterior surface of the nucleus. This is called neck. It contains a pair of centrioles that lie at right angles to each other. The proximal centriole lies in the indentation of the nucleus and does not possess any active function. However, the distal centriole acts as a basal granule and to this is attached the axial filament of sperm tail (flagellum).

Ring Centriole : In some spermatozoa a dark ring is seen at the junction of middle piece. and flagellum. It has been known as 'ring centriole', but it does not resemble with the true centriole either in structure or in function. Its function is also not known.

Tail or Flagellum

It is the longest but most narrow part of spermatozoon and its movements propel the spermatozoon. It consists of an axial filament, a thin layer of cytoplasm and an outer sheath of plasmalemma. The structure of axial filament is very much similar to that of cilium or flagellum. It consists of 9 peripheral and 2 central longitudinal fibres. In mammals these 9 + 2 pairs of longitudinal fibres extend upto the tip of the flagellum and are accompanied by another set of nine much thicker fibres present on the outer-side. These are called coarse fibres.

They appear wedge-shaped in cross-section. These fibres do not reach the tip of the flagellum (YASUZUMI 1956, TELKKA, FAWCETT and CMRISTENSEN 1961). Another set of threads or flattened bands are present around the longitudinal fibres of the spermatozoon tail. Each fibre is composed of semicircular ribs articulating with each other on the opposite sides of sperm tail.

The free end of sperm tail lacks the additional covering filaments. It is called the end piece. It contains the axial filament surrounded by cytoplasm and plasmalemma.

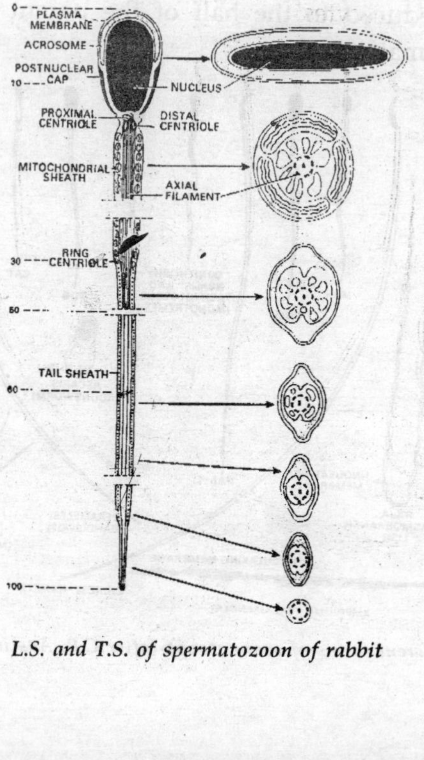

L.S. and T.S. of spermatozoon of rabbit

Variations in Sperm Structure

In some fishes and amphibians, the spermatozoa possess an undulating membrane almost all along the length of the tail. It assists the spermatozoa in locomotion. In *Opsonus* (toad fish) the sperm is biflagellate. In some animal groups such as nematodes, decapod crustaceans, myriapods and arachnids sperm are without flagella and therefore, unable to swim. These lack centrioles and mitochondria as well. In *Ascaris* (nematode) and *Polyphemus* (crustacean) sperms are amoeboid.

Significance of Spermatogenesis

1. As a result of spermatogenesis haploid male gametes or spermatozoa are formed. The first maturation division during maturation phase is a reduction division which produces haploid cells, the secondary spermatocytes. In them the number of chromosomes is reduced to the half of the parent cell (primary spermatocytes).

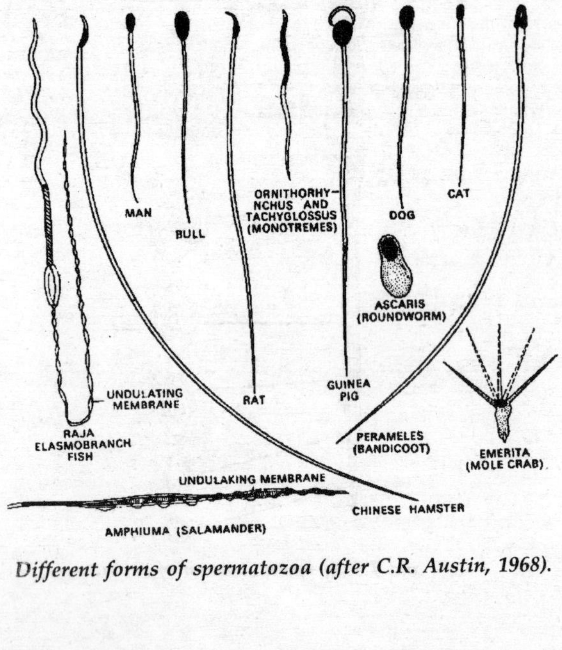

Different forms of spermatozoa (after C.R. Austin, 1968).

2. At the end of spermatogenesis four haploid spermatids are formed from each primary spermatocyte.
3. As a result of spermiogenesis, the non-motile spermatid changes into a motile sperm which can approach the non-motile ovum to fulfil the act of fertilization and formation of zygote which develops into the adult.
4. Spermatogenesis is a means of maintaining species-specific chromosome number constant.

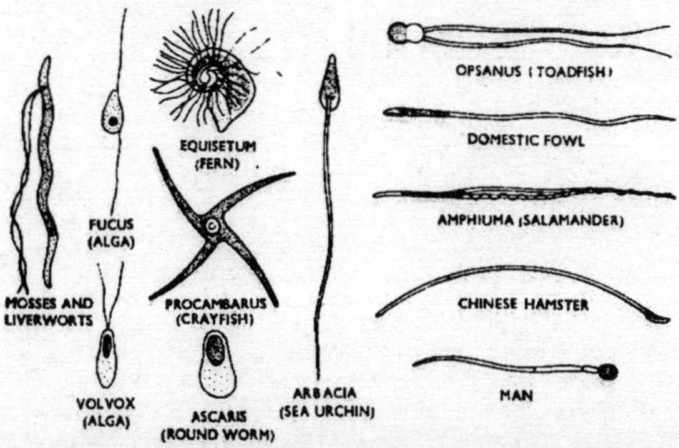

Male gamete of some plants and animals

Non-seasonal and Seasonal Breeders

In non-seasonal breeders the act of reproduction continues uninterrupted. In them spermatogenesis is a continuous process. The process of differentiation of stem cells, spermatogonia and spermatozoa continues throughout reproductive span of the male. As a result the sperm are produced uninterrupted and male is always fertile. There is no synchronization with the cyclic ovulation in female, as for example, man.

In seasonal breeders there is a testicular cycle similar to ovarian cycle. The sperm are produced only when female is ready to receive them. The testicular cycle is differentiated into (i) breeding phase (ii) regressive phase, (iii) refractory phase and (iv) the progressive phase.

4

The Oogenesis

The process of formation and maturation of ova is called *oogenesis* (Gr. *Oon-egg;* genesis-origin). It is fundamentally similar in all animals except for minor difference related to the amount of yolk in the ova produced. The process of oogenesis is somewhat more complicated and different than spermatogenesis. It involves not only the production of the haploid nucleus but also the acquisition of food reserves and preliminary organization of the cytoplasm from which the embryo will be formed.

The ova are derived from the germinal epithelium lining, the ovary. These germinal cells are diploid. Some cells in the germinal epithelium are larger than others and have bigger nuclei. These are called primordial germ cells which eventually give rise to the eggs.

The Ovary

The ovary is a solid organ attached by its antero-lateral border to the *broad ligament*. In the region of attachment, known as the hilus are found smooth muscle fibres, numerous large blood vessels and lymphatics. The tissue of the broad ligament is continued into the ovary, where it spreads out as the stroma. The free surface of the ovary is covered with surface epithelium, the modified mesothelium of the visceral peritoneum. In young women this is a cuboidal epithelium; it usually becomes flattened in later life. Immediately beneath the epithelium the stroma is condensed to form a tunica albuginea.

The stroma consists of cortex and medulla, which are not sharply delimited from each other. The cortex occupies the greater part of the ovary. It is a primitive type of connective tissue, in which large, spindle-shaped fibroblasts predominate. Coursing in all directions between them are compactly arranged fine collagenous and reticular fibres. Scattered throughout the cortex are vesicles of different sizes : these are the developing Graafian (or ovarian) follicles. It also contains transformed discharged follicles—the corpora lutea (singular, corpus luteum) and degenerating atretic follicles.

If the ovum has perished on its way to the exterior the corpus luteum survives for about 14 days and then degenerates : this is the corpus luteum of menstruation or *corpus luteum spurium.* If the ovum has been fertilized the corpus luteum enlarges and persists during pregnancy as the corpus luteum of pregnancy or *corpus luteum verum.*

If fertilization of the ovum has not taken place, slight haemorrhage into the corpus luteum occurs at the next menstruation and this is the beginning of its involution. The wide structure shrinks, and after about three months is represented by fibrous hyaline scar, the corpus albicans. A corpus luteum may sometimes give rise to a cyst.

The interior of the ovary, or medulla *is* a vascular and fibrous core. Abundant blood vessels enter at the hilus and then take spiral course inwards. The medulla reaches the "surface" only at hilus where it merges with the mesovarium.

Events in Oogenesis

Oogenesis is a complication operation. It can be divided into three phases. They are (A) Multiplication phase, (B) Growth phase, and (G) Maturation phase.

Multiplication (Proliferation) Phase: The primordial germ cells undergo proliferation by mitotic divisions and the resulting cells are called oogonia or egg mother cells. The oogonia multiply by repeated mitotic divisions. When the division stops, the cells are termed primary oocytes which enter a period of growth. The nucleus of a primary oocytes is diploid.

Growth Phase: Egg contributes the greater part of the substances used in development, therefore, growth plays a much greater role in oogenesis than in spermatogenesis. During oogenesis, first meiotic division starts and then goes into a suspended state, while the nucleus and cytoplasm carry out major synthetic activities. As a result of these activities, the oocyte increases greatly in size and volume. Besides, important qualitative changes also occur.

The period of growth in the female gametes is very prolonged and the increase in size is appreciably high. In frog, a young oocyte may be about 50 microns in diameter while the fully developed egg is upto 2000 microns in diameter. The diameter of ovum is about 40,000 microns in birds but in mammals it is only 200 microns.

The rate of growth of oocytes varies in different animals. In *Rana pipiens,* the growth takes place over a period of three years. In the hen the last rapid growth of oocytes takes place in the 6 to 14 days proceeding ovulation. During this time the volume of the oocyte increases 200 fold. In mammals the proliferation of the oogonia is restricted to the intra-uterine period of life. The growth period of oocytes may be divided into two stages *(i) Previtello genesis* and *(ii) Vitellogenesis* (Raven, 1961).

Pre-vutelliogenesis

During this period of growth, the nucleus and cytoplasm of primary oocyte increases tremendously in volume.

Growth of Nuclear Substances: The nucleus of the oocyte becomes enlarged mainly because of the production of a large amount of nuclear sap. Due to this the nuclei of advanced oocytes appear to be bloated with fluid and are often referred to as *germinal vesicles.*

The chromosomes increase in length. In oocytes of animals having large eggs (notably in the amphibian oocyte), the chromosomes acquire a very characteristic appearance. Numerous paired threads or loops project transversely from the main chromosomal axes. The shaggy appearance given to the chromosomes by these loops has led to their being called lamp brush chromosomes. The loops of lamp brush chromosomes represent loci of gene activity *i.e.,* at these sections *messenger RNA* is synthesized which subsequently controls the synthesis of proteins in the cell. However, the amount of DNA in the chromosomes does not increase in proportion to the enlargement of the nucleus.

The nucleolus in the germinal vesicle is concerned with the synthesis of *ribosomal RNA.* The nucleolus of a growing oocyte increases greatly in size, in many animals, for example in amphibians, instead of one large nucleolus, many smaller nucleoli are formed in the germinal vesicle. It is believed that RNA passes out of the nucleus into the cytoplasm during the growth of the oocyte.

Growth of Cytoplasmic Substances: The amount of cytoplasm increases quantitatively during the growth of the oocyte. Besides, it also changes in quality by the elaboration and regular distribution of various cell inclusions like mitochondria, Golgi bodies, endoplasmic reticulum, cortical granules etc.

Mitochondria: The mitochondria are fewer in young oocytes but increase in numbers quite appreciably during the growth of oocytes. In some animals, *e.g.*, amphibia, birds, they are aggregated in the form of large *mitochondrial clouds* (Romanoff, 1960; Wartenberg, 1962; Balinsky and Devis, 1963). Mitochondria are carriers of oxidative enzymes, therefore, the overall oxygen consumption increases during the growth of the oocyte.

Golgi Bodies: In younger oocytes, Golgi bodies are found around the centrosome. In mature oocytes they sometimes disappear completely (Odor, 1960). This indicates that Golgi bodies are transformed into some other structures like *cortical granules.*

Endoplasmic reticulum. The cytoplasm of the young oocytes contains numerous vesicles surrounded by a simple membrane. Ribosomes are often attached to the surface of the vesicles. These vesicles are often supposed to be equivalent to or to be a modification of the endoplasmic recticulum. Oocytes often have a different kind of membranous structure. It takes the form of stacks of double membranes, either in parallel or in spiral arrangement. The membranes usually do not have ribosomes attached to them but instead are perforated by pores. These pores closely resemble the pores of the nuclear membrane.

Cortical Granules: In mature oocytes, formation of special structures known as the *cortical granules* takes place on the inner side of the plasma lemma. These are spherical bodies, surrounded, by a simple membrane and containing acid mucopolysaccharides. They vary in diameter from 0.8 μ (in sea urchins) to 2 μ (in frogs). The acid mucopolysaccharides of the cortical granules synthesize fertilization membrane during fertilization. The cortical granules are present in sea urchins, frogs, fishes, bivalve molluscs, some annelids, and some mammals (*e.g.*, hamster, rabbit and man), but they are absent in rat, guinea pig, gastropod molluscs, urodele amphibians, insects and birds.

Vitellogenesis

Yolk appears in the oocytes in the second period of their growth called the vitellogenesis period. Yolk is the most usual form of food storage in the egg. In *amphibians* (Ward 1962 ; Balinsky and Davis, 1963) and fishes Yamamoto and Oota, 1967) the vitellogenesis or synthesis of different yolk components takes place inside modified mitochondria. In other vertebrates, the yolk is not synthesized in the oocytes at all but is produced in the liver of the body of the female. It is then transported in a soluble form via the blood stream and the follicle cells to the oocytes when it is finally deposited in the form of yolk platelets or yolk granules.

Physio-Chemical Nature of Yolk : Yolk is a complex of variably assembled components, rather than a definite chemical substance. The principal components are *proteins, phospholipids and fats* in different combinations. Depending on which of these components predominate, the yolk is distinguished as *"protein yolk"* or *"fatty yolk."* These two kinds of yolk are present side by side in the eggs of many animals. The avian yolk as a whole contains 48.7% water, 16.6% proteins, 32.6% phospholipids and fats and 1% carbohydrates. The fatty portion of avian yolk is mainly neutral fat (50% of the dry weight), the remaining being phosphatides and cholesterol. In animals, yolk is found in three forms as given hereunder :

Granular Yolk: Protein yolk of many invertebrates like echinoderms and of lower chordates (*Amphioxus,* Tunicates) consists of fine yolk granules which are fairly evenly distributed in the cytoplasm of the eggs.

Yolk Platelets: In *amphibians* eggs, the yolk is found in the form of large granules called *yolk platelets.* The yolk platelets are oval and flattened in one plane. They contain two main proteinaceous substances : phosvitin and lipovitellin. Phosvitin is a highly phosphorylated protein (phosphorus 8.4%), whereas lipovitellin contains a considerable amount of bound lipid

(17.5%). In the yolk platelets 2 molecules of phosvitin are associated with 1 molecule of lipovitellin in a structural unit. Electron micrographs of amphibian yolk reveal that these units are arranged in the platelet in a crystalline lattice work with regular hexagonal packing (Wallace, 1963).

In addition to the yolk platelets the amphibian egg contains lipid and glycogen. Lipid is found in the cytoplasm in the form of *lipochondria,* which consists of an internal core of lipid surrounded by a thin protein layer.

Cyclostomes, elasmobranchs, gonads and the *lungfishes* have eggs with a distribution of food reserves much the same as in amphibians.

Yolk Spheres: The yolk of birds, reptiles and bony fishes lies in a compact mass in the interior of the egg. The cytoplasm is restricted to a thin layer on the surface, with a thickened cap on the upper side. Most of the yolk is liquid, but about 23% is in the form of solid *"yolk spheres."*

Function of Yolk:

(1) Yolk is the most usual form of food storage in the egg.

(2) It influences the differentiation of ooplasm and the patterns of cleavage.

(3) The size of the egg is determined by the amount of yolk present in it.

(4) Yolk exercises an important influence on the morphogenetic movements of blastomeres during gastrulation.

(5) The nature of development whether *indirect* with larval forms or *direct* with juvenile stages is governed by the amount of yolk present in the egg.

Role of Follicle/Nurse Cells in Oogenesis : The growing oocytes are surrounded by special nutritive cells which immersely help their growth in various ways. Their are two main types of nutritive cells, viz., *follicle cells* and *nurse cells.*

Follicle Cells: In mammals particularly and some other vertebrates, the oocytes are surrounded during growth and maturation phases by special cells of the ovary, the *follicle cells.* These are derived from the germinal epithelium of the ovary. Initially, the young oocyte is surrounded by a single layer of follicle cells but later, the number of follicle cells increases greatly, the cells becoming arranged in several rows. In a mammal, the follicle cells and the developing oocyte together constitute a Graafian follicle. As the egg approaches maturity, an eccentric cavity called *ant rum* appears in the mass of the follicle cells. This cavity is filled with a fluid known as *liquor folliculi* which is secreted presumably by the cells of the follicle.

In the beginning, there is a simple apposition of the follicle cells and the oocyte. The cytoplasmic membranes of the adjoining cells remain separated by a narrow gap of about 80 A. The plasma membrane of oocyte and that of follicle cells show close connections at some points in the form of desmosomes. At a later stage a wider space appears between the follicle cells and the oocyte. However, the follicle cells maintain their contact with the oocytes at the points where the desmosomes were observed in the earlier stage. The surface of a young oocyte is drawn out into numerous finger-like microvilli which project into the space between the oocyte and follicle cells. These microvilli interdigitate with cytoplasmic processes of the follicle cells. (Fig.). The presence of the microvilli greatly increases the surface area of the oocyte. This increase in area facilitates metabolic turnover between the oocyte and the surrounding cells. *He believed that the follicle cells actively help in the growth of the oocyte by secreting substances which are taken up by the oocyte.*

The individual microvilli cannot be seen with the optical microscope and the zone of microvilli appears as a radially striated layer known as the *zona radiata.* The presence of small pocketings of the oocyte cytoplasm at the base of the microvilli points out that the oocyte takes in fluid and dissolved substances from the space between itself and the follicle cells by way of "cell drinking" or pinocytosis.

Nurse Cells: In some invertebrates like annelids, insects and molluscs the oocyte is surrounded, in addition to follicle cells, by special nurse cells. Derived from the egg cell, the nurse cells supplement the function of follicle cells in providing nutrition to the growing oocyte. In *Drosophila* an oogonial cell divides by four successive mitotic divisions into 16 cells. One of these cells becomes an oocyte whereas the other 15 becomes nurse cells an nourish the oocyte. Nutrients from the cytoplasm of the nurse cells pass into the oocyte through gaps developed in the cell membranes of two cell types. This type of relationship is different from that found between oocyte and follicle cells because in this case no microvilli or cytoplasmic processes are developed at the interface between the oocyte and the nurse cell. In some insects and annelids the nurse cells are gradually consumed during the growth of the oocyte. In molluscs *e.g.,* the snail *Helix,* the entire nurse cells are engulfed in the cytoplasm of the oocyte.

Maturation Phase

The primary oocyte contains diploid number of chromosomes. After the oocyte completes its growth, it is ready for meiosis or reduction division during which the diploid chromosome number is reduced to haploid number. In this process, the primary oocyte is changed into haploid ovum or egg. This is called maturation. The maturation process of oogenesis is somewhat different from that of spermatogenesis. In spermatogenesis, the primary spermatocyte divides into four cells of equal size which eventually give rise to four sperms. In oogenesis only one ovum is produced out of the four unequal cells derived from the primary oocyte.

At the beginning of the maturation phase, the nuclear membrane breaks up and the contents of the nucleus get mixed up with the surrounding cytoplasm. The chromosomes which have become greatly contracted and concentrated towards the centre of the germinal vesicle, are carried to the periphery of the oocyte. An achromatic spindle is formed at the periphery, which takes up a position perpendicular to the surface of the oocyte. The bivalents are stationed on the equatorial plate and subsequently separate into the two component chromosomes. Next, a bulge appears at the surface of the oocyte.

The outer pole of the spindle with half of the chromosomes enters into this cytoplasmic bulge during anaphase of *first meiotic division.* The bulge is then pinched off from the rest of the oocyte as a small cell called the first polar body or polocyte. It receives only a very small quantity of cytoplasm, while all the rest goes to the oocyte which is now distinguished as the secondary oocyte. The secondary oocyte is of the same size as that of primary oocyte. Thus, as a consequence of the first meiotic division the primary oocyte divides into a large and a very small cell, each with a *haploid* number of chromosomes.

In the *second meiotic division* an achromatic spindle is again formed at the surface. When division takes place, half of the chromatids are given off, along with a small quantity of cytoplasm to form a secondary polar body or polocyte. The larger cell, which receives the major part of the cytoplasm together with one half of the chromatids, represents the fully mature ovum.

As the secondary oocyte is dividing, the first polar body divides into two cells. Therefore, in the maturation of egg, four cells are produced from one oocyte: one cell, the egg, is a functional gamete, the second and third cells are produced by the division of the first polar body, and the fourth cell is the second polar body. All the polar bodies disintegrate later because they have very little cytoplasm with no food reserves.

The unequal cytokinesis (cytoplasmic division) during oogenesis has the great significance for the egg. These unequal divisions allow one cell out of the 4 daughter cells to inherit most of the cytoplasm and reserve food material which is essential for the developing embryo.

Nuclear Transplantation

During the process of development the nucleus performs varied tasks from the time of cleavage of the egg to that of organogeny. Does it mean that the nucleus of blastula cell possesses properties different from that of the nucleus of gastrula cell or that a differentiated cell of the intestinal wall? WEISMANN had proposed that the diversification among the cells during development arises through differential or quantitative division of nuclei during cleavage. His conclusion was based on the observations that during early development in *Ascaris,* the nuclei of prospective somatic cells undergo chromosomal diminution, whereas those of prospective reproductive cells do not.

However, the cytological observations soon established that during cleavage, nuclei of all the daughter cells descending from a zygote are equivalent in every way. DRIESCH demonstrated the equivalence of nuclei in sea urchin.

The present approach to test the equivalence and totipotency of nuclei includes nuclear transplant experiment. The transplant of the nuclei from different cells are made to the enucleated egg and the course of development is followed carefully.

Nuclear Transplantation Experiments in Amphibians : BRIGGS and KING (1953) transplanted the nuclei of the embryonic cells of frog *Rana pipens.* Their first experiment involved the transplantation of blastula cell nuclei into enucleated egg. This involves three steps :

Enucleation of Recepient Egg

The fully ripe eggs of frog are pricked with a fine glass needle to activate them. The nucleus now moves towards the surface in preparation of the second maturation division. At this time with the help of a sterile fine glass needle the nucleus is slowly removed. The egg may also be enucleated by irradiating it with ultraviolet rays which kill the nucleus. The egg must be kept in Niu and Twitty solution.

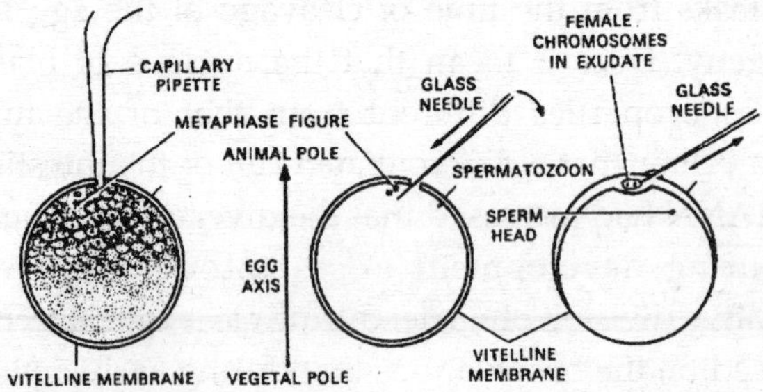

Enucleation of frog egg with a capillary pipette or glass needle.

Removal of Donor Nucleus

The egg membrane is slowly removed from the blastula. With the help of a fine glass needle the centre of the animal hemisphere is prodded to remove the sub-surface cell. This is placed over the intact surface of the adjoining cells. A sterile micropipette is selected which has a slightly smaller diameter than that cell. When cell is sucked with the help of the micropipette, the cell membrane breaks and nucleus alongwith a very small portion of the cytoplasm enters the pipette. The whole process requires careful manipulation and care must be taken not to damage the nucleus.

Transplantation of the Donor Nucleus : The donor nucleus that has been sucked from the blastula cell is slowly introduced into the enucleated egg. At the time of introduction the nucleus must be nearer to the tip of the micropipette but not at the tip. Once the nucleus has entered the enucleated egg the pipette is slowly withdrawn. When the pipette comes out it draws the surface coat of the egg against the vitelline membrane and a small quantity of the egg cytoplasm flows out as the exovath.

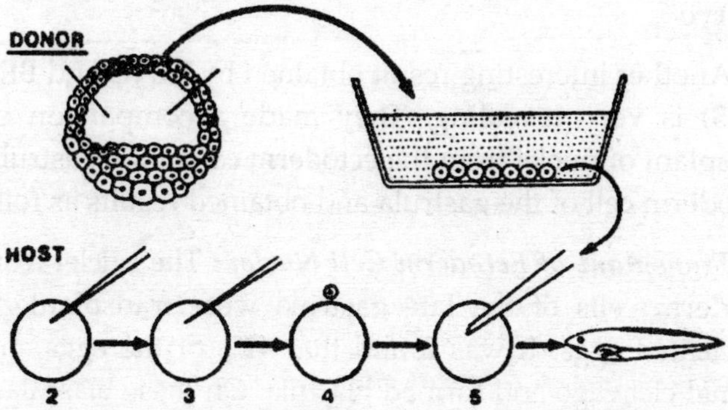

Diagram representing transplantation of donor nucleus from blastula into the enucleated egg and its development into a tadpole.

Effects of Transplantation

BRIGGS and KING studied the effect of transplantation of the nuclei taken from different stages of growth.

Transplantation of Cleavage and Blastula Cell Nuclei : Nuclei taken from cleavage cells as well as those from blastula cells were transplanted to enucleated egg of *Rana pipens*. About 80% of the eggs show segmentation, but all the eggs which start cleaving do not develop normally. In actual experiments out of a total of 204 injected eggs, 116 showed normal cleavage and out of this only 69 produced complete embryos. This showed a success rate of 34%. In further experiments it was noticed that the nuclei of cells of earlier stages of development showed better success rate than those taken from later stages of development.

Transplantation of Gastrula Cell Nuclei : Nuclei taken from the blastocoels roof of the early gastrula produce all types of differentiation necessary for formation of a complete embryo. However, success rate was low. Out of a total of 135 eggs injected, 52 showed normal cleavage and only 8 became complete embryos, thereby giving a success rate of 15% only. According to BRIGGS and KING there is "decreasing success in nuclear transplantation with increasing age of the donor embryo".

Another interesting result obtained by KING and BRIGGS (1955) is very revealing. They made a comparison of the transplant of nuclei from the ectoderm cell of the gastrula and endoderm cell of the gastrula and obtained results as follows :

Transplant of Ectoderm Cell Nuclei : The nuclei from the ectoderm cells of the late gastrula were transplanted into enucleated eggs. It was found that 41% of the eggs showed normal cleavage and formed blastula. On these blastulae 80% developed into normal tadpoles.

Transplant of Endoderm Cell Nuclei : A similar transplant was made with the endoderm cell nuclei of the late gastrula. About 40% of the eggs showed normal cleavage and formed blastulae. Of these blastulae only 20% developed into normal tadpoles while 30% were blocked at the gastrula stage and 50% formed embryos with ectodermal deficiencies, reduced sense organs and small nervous system and became inviable.

These experiments show that the endoderm nuclei have already undergone some "genetic restriction", when compared to the ectoderm nuclei.

Serial Transplantation of Blastula Nuclei : In serial transplantation, the experiments are conducted successively to give continuity so that the cumulative effect can be studied for generations. A nucleus from the micromere of the blastula is transplanted to the enucleated egg, which is activated to parthenogenetic development. When this egg reaches the blastula stage, nuclei from the micromeres are taken and transplanted to a series of enucleated eggs. The eggs developed into tadpoles. This is called the first blastula generation. If from one of the blastulae the nuclei of the micromeres are again removed and transplanted to a series of the enucleated eggs. The eggs show development leading to the tadpole stage. This is the second blastula generation like this and get an idea of the effects of development on the nucleus and the changes it may undergo during development. The experiments with blastula nuclei clearly prove their totipotency as may be seen in the diagrams.

Serial Transplantation of Gastrula Nuclei : The endoderm nuclei are taken from the late gastrula and transplanted to a series of enucleate eggs. The nuclei thus taken from adjacent cells, produce different varieties of development like blocked blastulae, irregular gastrulae, abnormal embryos and one or two tadpoles. If the nuclei from one of the arrested blastulae are transferred to a series of enucleated eggs, they show uniform development in the second blastula generation. Here the variation is less and none develops into tadpoles. This test clearly reveals that a certain amount of differentiation takes place in the nuclei at the late gastrula stage. The generation of cells produced from the blocked blastula nucleus that was transplanted is called a clone, as all of them were derived from a single endoderm nucleus.

Transplantation of Nuclei from Cells of the Postgastrular Stages : DIBERARDINO and KING (1967) transplanted the nuclei from the neural plate of a frog embryo to enucleated eggs and these developed into normal tadpoles. Another interesting observation was made by KING and DIBERARDINO (1965) when they transplanted the nuclei taken from the adrenocarcinoma cells of frog and obtained almost normal embryos. GURDON (1968) transplanted nuclei taken from the alimentary tract of the tadpole of *Xenopus laevis* to enucleated egg and obtained normal embryos.

A comparison of the studies made of *Rana pipiens* and *Xenopurs laevis* show an interesting contrast. In *Rana* the differentiation starts at an early stage and the nucleus looses its totipotency soon, while in *Xenopus* it appears to be taking place very late and the nuclei retain their totipotency for a long time.

Nuclear Transplunt between Species : HENNEN, SALLY (1965) tried nuclear transplant between two species of frog viz *Rana pipens* and *R. palustris* and were successful. The nucleus of *R. palustris* if transplanted into enucleated egg of *R. pipens* develops into normal adult showing the character of both its parents. On the other hand the nucleus of *R. pipiens* when transplanted to the enucleated egg of *R. palustris* the development stops at the early larval stage.

Nuclear Transplantation in Insects : ILLMESEE (1955) made nuclear transplantation work in *Drosophila*. He transplanted nuclei from the late cleavage stage into enucleated eggs. Development proceeded normally and larvae hatched out.

Nuclear Transplantation in Amoeba : DANIELLI (1955) made some very interesting transplantation experiments between two species of *Amoeba*. *Amoeba proteus* differs from *Amoeba discoides* in three important characteristics: (i) shape, (ii) nuclear diameter, (iii) division rate.

The nucleus taken (form *proteus* was transplanted into the cytoplasm *of discoides* resulting in a hybrid $p_n d_c$ (proteus nucleus and discoides cytoplasm). This hybrid had a shape intermediate between proteus and discoides while in nuclear diameter and the division rate it resembled more like the discoides. After this hybrid form with proteus nucleus has undergone many divisions a reverse transplant was done *(i.e.)* the nucleus from the hybrid form was transplanted back to enucleated proteus. The amoeba that is formed as a result of this transplant shows division rate characteristic of discoides and not that of proteus. It is possible that the nucleus has acquired some of the characters of discoides due to its continued stay for many generations in the discoides cytoplasm.

Nuclear Transplantation in Acetabularia : *Acetabularia* is a marine alga, formed of single cell and is differentiated into *rhizoids, stalk and cap*. Early experiments on *Acetabularia*, mostly by HAMMERLING, showed that-

(i) Its stalk can regenerate the imputed cap even when the rhizoidal part containing nucleus is also amputate.

(ii) When a non-nucleated piece of *A. mediterranea* stalk (*i.e.* without cap and rhizoid) is grafted on the nucleus containing rhizoid of *A. crenulata*, the first cap developed was similar to mediterranea, showing character of the species represented by stalk; but in the second regeneration the cap was intermediate. If this cap is also removed, the successive caps resembled *A. crenulata*, the nucleus containing part.

The above experiments show that nucleus produces some substance which moves through the stalk and produces caps according to the genes present in the nucleus.

(iii) When one rhizoid each of *A. mediterranea* and *A. crenulata* were grafted the resulting plant had a cap intermediate between both.

(iv) In another experiment two rhizoids of *A. mediterranea* were grafted to one rhizoid of *A. crenulate* and the hybrid plant produced cap which resembled more that of *A. mediterranea*.

(v) In the third experiment two rhizoids of *A. crenulata* were grafted to one rhizoid of *A. mediterranea* and the hybrid plant produced a cap which resembled more that of *A.crennlata*. It is clear from these experiments that the shape and size of the cap depends on the nucleus present.

The Ovum

The ovum or female gamete is much larger than the sperm. It is nonmotile and laden with different types of energy-rich materials, like yolk, glycogen and proteins, accumulated during its growth period in its cytoplasm. The size and yolk contents vary considerably in the eggs. The small eggs can be 10 to 100 μ in diameter while the larger ones may be several centimetres in size. For example, eggs of many polychaete worms are about 50 μ and those of ascidians about 150 μ. The yolky eggs of birds, reptiles and some fish, particularly sharks and rays are very large.

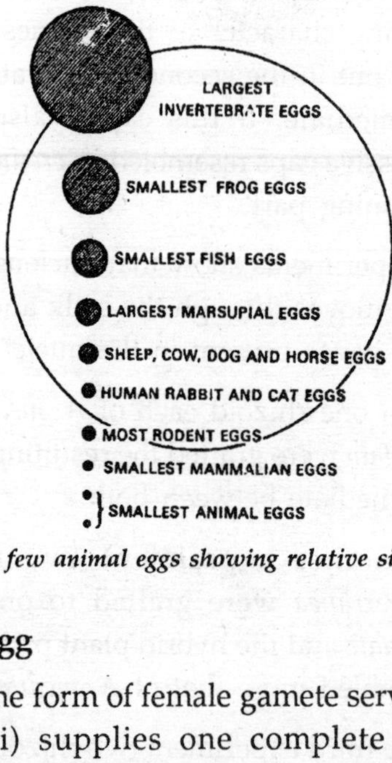

A few animal eggs showing relative size

Functions of Egg

The egg in the form of female gamete serves the following purposes: — (i) supplies one complete haploid set of chromosomes from female parent to the future embryo. (ii) supplies all the cytoplasm to the future embryo upon union with the spermatozoon which contains practically very little cytoplasm. (iii) supplies reserve food material for the developing embryo in oviparous animals.

To perform the above-mentioned functions, the egg cell is enlarged, is packaged with reserve food stuff and is programmed during its maturation. Moreover, it is covered with membranes of various kinds, that protect the embryo during its development. Thus, the formation of ovum is more complex than the formation of sperm. It usually requires a long period for maturation.

Maturation of Ovum

The maturation of ovum takes place from the primary oocyte, produced by the division of cells of germinal epithelium in the ovary of female organism. The process of development and maturation of ovum is known as oogenesis. It includes essentially the same steps as in spermatogenesis, but the steps are greatly modified and the end products of the process are different from those of spermatogenesis. The process of oogenesis is broadly separated into three phases:

1. Multiplication phase 2. Growth phase 3. Maturation phase.

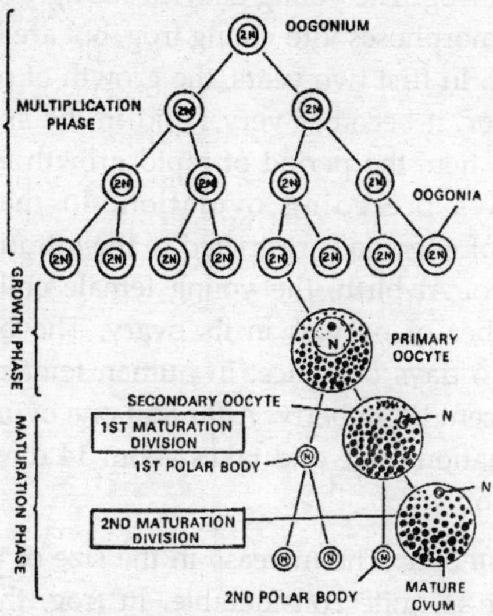

Diagrammatic representation of stages during oogenesis.

Multiplication Phase

During multiplication phase, the cells of germinal epithelium divide and detach to produce oogonia. These undergo repeated mitotic divisions and the final products are known as primary oocytes. These are diploid cells containing the same number of chromosomes as in the parent somatic cells. The primary oocytes cease to divide and enter the growth phase.

Growth Phase

Owing to the fact that the egg cytoplasm is stuffed with food substances needed during development, the growth phase or accumulation phase is very long and elaborate. The differentiation of egg takes place simultaneously with the growth rather than after the maturation as is seen in spermatogenesis.

Period of Growth : The growth phase of a female gamete is very long, varying from few days to many years. It lasts for three years in frog. The young oocytes start growing after the tadpole metamorphoses into young frog, but are laid down by the third year. In first two years, the growth of oocyte is very slow. However, it becomes very rapid in the summer of the third year. In hen, the period of rapid growth is confined to last 6-14 days preceding ovulation. In mammals, the proliferation of oogonia is restricted to the intrauterine period of the embryo. At birth, the young female child contains a definite number of oocytes in its ovary. The oocytes attain maturity in 16 days old mice. In human female the oocytes remain quiescent till puberty. After that one ovum matures in each menstruation cycle and takes about 14 days for growth and maturation.

Increase in Size: The increase in the size of ovum during growth phase is quite considerable. In frog, the increase is about 27,000 times. Its young oocyte is about 15 μ in diameter whereas the fully developed egg in most species ranges between 1000 μ to 2000 μ.

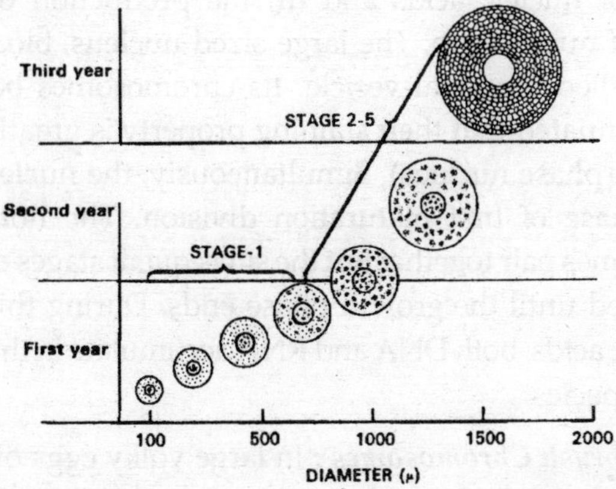

Growth of frog's oocyte showing increase in its diameter in three successive generations (Ater Berries, 1976),

In mice, the oocyte is about 20 μ in diameter and a fully mature ripe ovum is about 70 μ showing an increase of about 43 times. In man the oocytes increase from 0.02 mm to 0.14 mm *i.e.* about 7 times. In birds the increase in size is tremendous reaching upto 40,000 μ. This tremendous increase in size is largely due to the deposition of food reserve in the form of yolk.

Substages of Growth Phase : The growth of oocyte involves: (i) increase of nuclear and cytoplasmic substances and (ii) accumulation of food reserve. The events occurring during growth phase are separated into two periods:

(A) Previtellogenesis, the period of synthesis of nuclear material and cytoplasm.

(B) Vitellogenesis, the period of synthesis of yolk.

Previtellogenesis : The period of previtellogenesis is characterised by the tremendous increase of the nuclear and cytoplasmic contents with no addition of yolk. The major events that occur during this period are:

Increase of the Nuclear Material : During growth phase, the nucleus of the oocyte increases considerably by (i) the increase of nucleic acids and (ii) the production of a large amount of nuclear sap. The large sized nucleus, bloated with fluid is called germinal vesicle. Its chromosomes become so much attenuated that their staining property is greatly diluted (as in interphase nucleus). Simultaneously, the nucleus enters the prophase of first maturation division. The homologous chromosomes pair together but the subsequent stages of meiosis are arrested until the growth phase ends. During this period, the nucleic acids, both DNA and RNA accumulate in the nucleus of most species.

Lampbrush Chromosomes : In large yolky eggs of reptiles, birds and bony fishes and even in the amphibian eggs, the chromosomes of the oocyte increase greatly in length and develop long-side loops, which correspond to the two chromatids and extend transversely to the axis of the chromosome. The loops resemble to the bristles of a lampbrush. Therefore, chromosomes in this stage are described as lampbrush chromosomes. Altogether in a nucleus their can be as many as 5000 loops and these represent only 2-3 per cent DNA of the oocyte in extended condition.

Each loop of lampbrush chromosome represents a completely despiralized section of chromosome in which histone and non-histone proteins become displaced, exposing the DNA strand. The exposed DNA loop synthesizes *m*RNA which contains the genetic information copied from DNA. *m*RNA governs the protein synthesis taking place in the oocyte cytoplasm. A large number of mRNA molecules are synthesized during growth phase because of extraordinary increase in the oocyte volume.

Alongwith the synthesis of *m*RNA other types of RNAs i.e. transfer RNA (*t*RNA) and ribosomal RNA (*r*RNA) are also synthesized in the primary oocyte to facilitate protein synthesis.

Informosomes : Some of these *m*RNA molecules become inactive and are ensheathed by protein. These form informosomes (SPIRIN, 1965). The informosomes bring about protein synthesis during early cleavage, when chromosomal DNA remains condensed and involved in nuclear division and as such is not able to synthesize *m*RNA.

Nucleolus : Normally a cell has one nucleolus per haploid set of chromosomes. As such an ovum is supposed to have only one nucleolus, but it increases greatly in size. In amphibian oocytes, instead of one, a large number of nucleoli are seen on the periphery of germinal vesicle immediately below the nuclear membrane. There may be as many as 600 nucleoli in *Triturus,* 1000 in *Siredon* and 1200 in *Xenopus laevis* (toad). The enlargement of the nucleolus or increase in the number of nucleoli is because of the increase in the number of genes coding for ribosomal RNA (*r*RNA). This increase in the number of genes without mitosis is referred to as amplification of genes (EPEL, 1973) or redundancy (DE ROBERTBS, 1975). The increase in the number of nucleoli is associated with the need to produce large amounts of ribosomal RNA required for the formation of large number of ribosomes, necessary for future protein synthesis during cleavage and the accumulation of yolk reserve in the growing oocyte.

Gene Amplification : During growth period of oocyte, the nucleolar genes located in the nucleolar organizer region for 28S and 18S RNA multiply several times so as to produce large number of these loci. All of them are associated with the rapid synthesis of ribosomal RNA. The increase in the number of genes without mitosis has been described as gene amplification or redundancy. The gene amplification is evident from the following observations. (i) appearance of lampbrush chromosome having transcriptionally active loops of DNA for the active synthesis of *m*RNA (ii) movement of nuclear material through the nuclear pores into the cytoplasm. (iii) movement of large masses of nucleolar material through nuclear pores (pores in the nuclear membrane.) (iv) RNA can be elected in the oocyte cytoplasm in the form of large number of ribosomes.

Growth of Cytoplasmic Substances : During growth phase both quality and quantity of cytoplasm increases. The young oocyte possesses a finely granular cytoplasm. It is poor in inclusions and possesses practically none of those specialized structures found in the mature oocyte. It contains a few mitochondria, Golgi complex saccules and a few cisternae of endoplasmic reticulum. During growth phase all of them undergo following changes:

Mitochondria : These are very few in the younger primary oocyte, but increase in number considerably during growth phase. In some oocytes (amphibian and avian) these aggregate to form large 'mitochondrial clouds'.

Ribosomes : These become very numerous in the growing oocyte. All of them participating actively in the synthesis of protein, require in the formation of yolk.

Endoplasmic Reticulum: The vesicles and annulate lamellae of ER act as storage site of RNA in the cytoplasm. These break down and disappear during late oogenesis.

Golgi Complex : It takes active part in the formation of vesicles and cortical granules. Its saccules are found to contain acid mucopolysaccharides. These vesicles form cortical granules.

Cortical Granules : These are membrane-bound spherical bodies filled with mucopolysaccharides. These are formed from the small vesicles of Golgi complex and get arranged in the cortical region of ooplasm underneath the egg plasma membrane. The cortical granules play an important role during fertilization. These are found in the oocytes of molluscs, anurans and sea urchins.

Vitellogenesis : Vitellogenesis is the second period in the growth of oocyte characterised by the synthesis and accumulation of large amount of yolk. Growth is very much accelerated during vitellogenesis and oocyte attains giant proportion in some animals. For example, a hen's egg contains about 55 gms of yolk. Egg even larger than this and with more yolk are found in a few birds and certain fishes. The yolk is not a definite chemical substance, rather it is a morphological term used to describe the reserve food in the oocyte. Chemically, it consists of proteins, neutral fats, phospholipids, certain carbohydrates and glycogen.

Nature of Yolk : The main components of yolk are proteins, phospholipids and neutral fats. Their proportion varies in the oocytes of different animals. When yolk contains proportionately more protein, it is called 'protein yolk', and yolk with proportionately more lipids is 'lipoid yolk'. Both the varieties of yolk are present side by side in the eggs of many animals. Mainly protein yolk is present in the eggs of many invertebrates and lower chordates *(Amphioxus)*. It occurs in the form of yolk granules. In mature amphibian oocyte protein yolk constitutes roughly 45 per cent of the dry weight and lipids 25%.

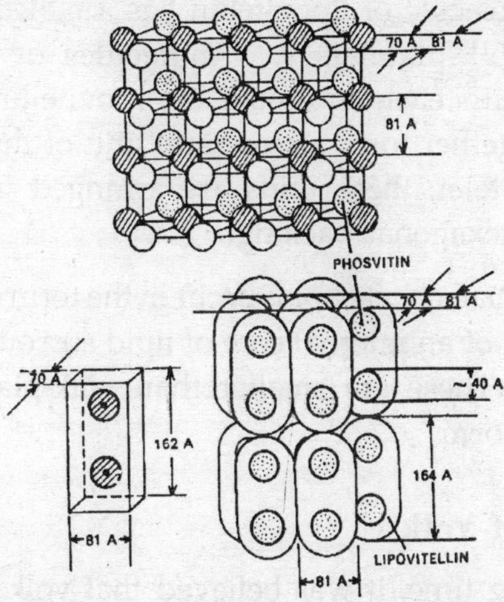

Diagrammatic representation of the crystalline structure in the yolk platelets of an amphibian oocyte, (After Balinskey).

Fatty yolk is more abundant in oligolecithal types of eggs of bony fishes, reptiles and birds. The phospholipids and fats are about 32.6 per cent whereas proteins are 16.6 per cent. (ROMANOFF and ROMANOFF, 1949).

Granular Yolk : The yolk occurs in the oocyte cytoplasm in the form of fine granules. In the eggs of invertebrates and lower chordates (*Amphioxus* and tunicates), the yolk granules are uniformly distributed. In them the yolk is less in amount and uniform in distribution (isolecithal eggs).

Yolk Platelets : In the oocytes of most of the vertebrates like cyclostomes, cartilaginous fishes, bony fishes, lung fishes, amphibians, reptiles and birds, the yolk is found in the form of large granules, called yolk-platelets. The cytoplasm is densely packed with yolk-platelets. In amphibian oocytes the yolk-platelets are denser in the lower part. The yolk-platelets are formed of two different types of proteinaceous substances—phosvitin and lipovitellin.

The phosvitin is highly phosphorylated protein with 8.4% phosphorus with a molecular weight 35,000. The lipovitellin is a combination of protein and lipids. The lipids are 17.5 per cent. Each molecule of lipovitellin has a molecular weight of 40,000. In yolk-platelets two molecules of phosvitin are associated with each molecule of lipovitellin. These three molecules together form a structural unit of the yolk-platelet. In a yolk-platelet, these units are arranged in a crystalline lattice with hexagonal packing.

In amphibian oocyte lipids occur in the form of lipochondria which consist of an internal core of lipid surrounded by a thin protein coat. These are smaller than yolk-platelets and are spherical in form.

Formation of Yolk

For a long time, it was believed that yolk is synthesized inside the oocyte by a special body, the 'yolk nucleus'. The yolk nucleus has been observed in the young oocytes of many animals lying next to the nucleus, but in later stages, it breaks up. The yolk nucleus in amphibian and avian oocyte is formed of a cloud of mitochondria and it actually converts the soluble phosvitin yolk into insoluble form that is deposited in the form of yolk platelets.

Apart from yolk nucleus, the Golgi complex, the endoplasmic reticulum and even mitochondria are presumed to be associated with the synthesis of yolk in the oocyte.
(i) Vitellogenesis in solitary type of oocytes : In Spirorbis, the growing oocyte develops numerous elongated mitochondria, free ribosomes and dense annuli, indicating the movement of material from nucleus into the cytoplasm. In the second phase, the outer egg membrane is produced into numerous microvilli. The pinocytosis begins in the pits at the bases of microvilli. The pinocytic vesicles detach and move inward to fuse with the rough endoplasmic reticulum and thus transport metabolites necessary for yolk formation.

Vitellogenesis in Vertebrates and Insects : Both in insects and in vertebrates, the yolk is found to be synthesized elsewhere in the body of female. In some insects yolk proteins are synthesized in the midgut region of the intestine and are carried by blood to the ovaries. In other insects yolk proteins are synthesized in follicle cells. In vertebrates protein-yolk is synthesised in the liver. It is transported through blood in soluble form to some special ovarian cells, such as follicle cells or nurse cells.

The growing oocyte collects yolk from these follicle cells by the process of micropinocytosis. The pinocytic vesicles with extracellular yolk pinch off into the cytoplasm, lose their coat, and fuse to form crystalline yolk droplets, which coalesce to form yolk platelets. The platelets are first deposited in the centre of the ooplasm and then progressively outward towards the periphery. In amphibian oocyte the yolk deposition begins near the cell surface and fills the peripheral cytoplasm. Progressively the entire cytoplasm gets studded with yolk from the peripheral zone inward except the perinuclear cytoplasm. The yolk protein phosvitin is insoluble in water when it is fully phosphorylated, but if a part of phosphate is removed by the action of phosphatase, the remaining phosvitin becomes water soluble. Therefore, partially phosphorylated phosvitin is transported by the blood. On reaching the oocyte, it is phosphorylaled by an enzyme protein-kinase.

The phosphate molecule is collected from ATP inside the mitochondria.

$$\text{Portially phosphorlated} \xrightleftharpoons{\text{Protein kinase}} \text{Fully phosphorylated protein}$$

$$\text{protein} + \text{ATP Mg+} + +\text{ADP}$$

The presence of enzyme protein-kinase in the mitochondria supports the view that synthesis of phosvitin takes place inside mitochondria.

Amount and Distribution of Yolk and Types of Eggs : The amount of yolk in a fully-grown oocyte varies greatly in different animal groups and so also its distribution. Based on the amount and distribution of yolk the animal eggs have been classified into following categories:—

Egg Types Based on Amount of Yolk

Microlecithal: These are small sized eggs with only a small amount of yolk or reserved food. The microlecithal eggs are found in *Amphioxus,* other cephalochordates, tunicates and eutherian mammals. KENT (1969) has described such eggs as alecithal. But this term is not appropriate as no egg is without yolk.

Mesolecithal : The eggs with moderate amount of yolk are described as mesolecithal eggs. Such eggs are found in *Petromyzon,* Dipnoi and Amphibia.

Macrolecithal or Polylecithal: These eggs contain enormous amount of yolk or reserve food and just a little yolk free cytoplasm. These are found in Myxinoidea, cartilaginous and bony fishes, reptiles, birds and Prototherian mammals and in insects.

Egg Types Based on the Distribution of Yolk

Homolecithal or Isolecithal: In microlecithal eggs, the amount of yolk is so little that it is found scattered almost uniformly throughout the egg cytoplasm. Such microlecithal eggs are described to be homolecithal or isolecithal.

Telolecithal : In telolecithal eggs the yolk is not evenly distributed. The mesolecithal and macrolecithal eggs are telolecithal. Because of its gravity, the yolk tends to concentrate in the lower part of the egg, leaving a somewhat yolk-free cytoplasm in the anterior or upper part of the egg. This unequal distribution of yolk leads to the differentiation of animal and vegetal poles. The animal pole contains the nucleus and the active cytoplasm with a little or no yolk. The vegetal pole is concentrated with yolk. The telolecithal eggs can be of two types :

(i) Mesolecithal eggs with moderate amount of yolk distributed unevenly in the ooplasm as discussed above, are moderately telolecithal eggs. For example, eggs of Amphibia, Petromyzontia and Dipnoi.

(ii) Macrolecithal eggs with enormous amount of yolk that occupies most of space of egg; so that the active cytoplasm and germinal vesicle (nucleus) form a small cap in the region of animal pole are strongly telolecithal. For example eggs of cartilaginous and bony fishes, reptiles and birds.

Centrolecithal Eggs: In insects the eggs are of macrolecithal type with massive yolk that occupies the centre of the egg and the cytoplasm forms a thin peripheral layer around the yolk. Such eggs are called centrolecithal eggs.

Functions of Yolk

The Yolk Serves the Following Purposes:

1. Yolk supplies energy to the developing embryo.
2. Yolk provides material for the synthesis of those substances that are required for the elaboration of embryonic body.
3. Yolk excercises important influence on
   (i) the size of egg
   (ii) the differentiation of ooplasm
   (iii) the pattern of cleavage
   (iv) the early morphogenetic movements of blastomeres during gastrulation
   (v) on the type of development (direct or indirect).

Cleidoic and Non-cleidoic Eggs : Cleidoic eggs like those of reptiles, birds and Prototherian mammals contain sufficient amount of nutritive material and water for the developing embryo. The embryo hatches out into a fully formed young animal or juvenile. In the developing embryo, the foetal membranes (allantois, chorion, amnion and yolk sac.) are formed. Only oxygen gets in and carbon dioxide diffuses out of these membranes.

Noncleidoic eggs do not contain sufficient amount of nutritive material for the complete development of the embryo and embryo does not have extra-embryonic membranes or foetal membranes. These eggs hatch into larvae. Non-cleidoic eggs are present in fishes, and amphibians.

Based on the presence of cleidoic or non-cleidoic types of eggs sub-phylum vertebrate is divided into two groups :

1. Amniota— with amnion and with cleidoic eggs.
2. Anamniota — without amnion or with noncleidoic eggs.

Role of Follicle Cells or Nurse cells in Vitellogenesis : The nutritive materials that accumulate in the ooplasm of developing oocyte are not synthesized completely by the oocyte itself. A

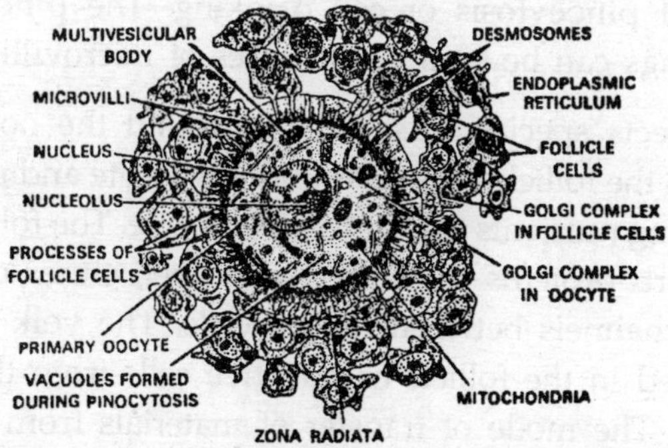

Young mammalian oocyte surrounded by follicle cells. (After Balinskey, 1976)

major portion of these substances is synthesized in some extroversion tissue of the female body (in the liver in vertebrates and in the fat bodies in insects). These are brought to the gonads by the blood stream and are deposited in the follicle cells or nurse cells that surround the developing oocyte. The oocyte collects these substances from the follicle or nurse cells either by pinocytosis or by engulfing them.

The developing egg cell is surrounded by follicle cells in majority of animals. These are derived from the germinal epithelium. In the beginning, these lie in simple apposition with the surface of egg cell having few close connections in the form of desmosomes. At a later stage a wider space appears between the follicle cells and the oocyte except in the regions of desmosomes. The whole surface of the oocyte is produced into fine finger-like processes, the microvilli which increase the surface area. At the same time the basal follicle-cell membrane extends downward as fine branching processes, the macrovilli. The region occupied by interpenetrating macrovilli and microvilli presents striated appearance under light microscope and is called zona radiata or zona pellucida.

In mammals, the yolk is synthesized in the liver cells. It is transported by the blood to the follicle cells. The oocyte collects yolk and other nutrients from the follicle cells by the process of pinocytosis or cell drinking. The pinosomes or inpocketings can be seen at the bases of microvilli.

In insects special nurse cells surround the oocyte. This alongwith the follicle cells surround the oocyte and participate in providing nutrients to the growing oocyte. The follicle nurse cells absorb proteins from the haemocoel, either directly or through channels between follicle cells. The yolk protein is synthesized in the follicle or nutritive cells from the protein absorbed. The mode of transfer of materials from the nurse cells to the oocyte is different from those of follicle cells.

The microvilli and cytoplasmic processes are not produced. Rather, special apertures appear between the oocyte and nurse cells and through such gaps the nutrients, cytoplasm and even mitochondria of the nurse cells are drawn into the oocyte. As a result the nurse cells are used up during growth of oocyte.

What causes the Oocyte to Grow so Large : A normal body cell cannot grow unlimited. After attaining a specific size, it must divide or it should stop growing. Question arises how can the oocyte grow beyond certain limits without dividing? To answer this question one is expected to know the cause for the onset of normal cell division.

One of the factors that affects cell division may be the ratio of surface area to cell volume. The gaseous exchange necessary for cell metabolism takes place through the cell membrane, whereas the cell metabolism takes place unit volume or per unit of cytoplasm becomes smaller. This directly affects the rate of basal metabolism and the cell is pressed to divide, so that with the formation of new cell wall the surface per unit volume of cytoplasm is increased. In oocytes the division fails either because of some inhibition or from lack of stimulation.

The growing oocyte usually bogs down before completing the maturation. The oocytes grow rapidly for a while, then progressively more slowly until a characteristic terminal size is reached. The maturation division follows but it is arrested in the metaphase stage of first or second meiotic division. Hence, self increase in the size of oocyte. Any further increase is actually assisted either by the follicle cells or nurse cells which deposit nutrients in the ooplasm. Another way of increase in the size of oocytes into a large mass of cytoplasm is by its fusion with the nurse cells or fusion of a number of growing oocytes with a single nucleus which survives, while others disintegrate.

Differentiation of Oocyte

In the beginning of growth phase the primary oocyte is a simple undifferentiated cell. During growth phase, when nutrient materials and nucleic acid, etc. start accumulating in the ooplasm, a pattern of organization gradually sets in. The differentiation involves the following phenomena :

Establishment of Polar Axis

All animal eggs have the polar structure. The two opposite poles that can be distinguished are referred to as the animal and vegetal poles of the egg. The imaginary line connecting the poles defines the main axis of the egg and is known as the animal-vegetal axis.

The polarity of the egg is often apparent in the arrangement of its cytoplasmic inclusions. In many eggs, the yolk is not evenly distributed; often its density increases from the animal pole towards the vegetal pole with corresponding structural changes. In some cases, there are substantial differences in the degree of pigmentation. In many amphibians, the animal region of the egg surface is heavily pigmented, whereas the vegetal region is essentially unpigmented.

Establishment of Symmetry

In addition to the establishment of polarity along the main axis, the dorsal and ventral sides also become differentiated, resulting in the establishment of bilateral symmetry in the primary oocyte or the unfertilized eggs. The bilateral symmetry is seen in the eggs of tunicates, cephalochordates and amphibians and even in mammals.

In mammalian oocyte, the 'yolk nucleus' containing RNA and mitochondria lie next to the nucleus somewhat to one side of the main axis nearer to the vegetal axis. Later on in the middle-sized oocyte, the mitochondria and RNA spread out in about half the surface of oocyte, on one side of the animal-vegetal axis. This RNA-rich side represents the dorsal side of the embryo, while the opposite half with vacuolated cytoplasm represents the ventral side of the embryo (JONSES SEATION 1950 & DALEQ 1954).

During growth phase, the oocytes establish bipolar differentiation because of an unequal distribution of various substances and cellular constituents. In telolecithal eggs, especially the yolk or deutoplasm is not distributed evenly throughout the ooplasm. Usually at one end of the oocyte, an area is relatively free of yolk and contains the egg nucleus. When the nucleus of oocyte undergoes meiosis, the mitotic spindle is formed in this region and the polar bodies are discharged here. This end of oocyte which contains nucleus and yolk-free cytoplasm is called animal pole.

The end opposite to the animal pole is referred to as vegetal pole, where the concentration of yolk is greatest. The establishment of animal and vegetal poles is called bipolar differentiation. It is caused by the unequal distribution of deutoplasm. The imaginary axis that passes through animal and vegetal poles is called the polar axis or animal-vegetal axis.

However, in oligolecithal eggs that have very little yolk

distributed uniformly and also in centrolecithal eggs the animal and vegetal poles cannot be easily differentiated. The animal pole is then, is distinguished by the discharge of polar bodies. In these types of eggs, there is little or no gradient in yolk distribution along the animal-vegetal axis. However, in the telolecithal eggs, that have greater concentration of yolk, the animal-vegetal axis is characterised by a gradient in yolk concentration which increases from animal to vegetal pole. It affects changes in the distribution of other cytoplasmic contents and imposes changes in the structural organization of egg or establishes some type of differentiation.

In some cases, the animal and vegetal halves are further differentiated by unequal distribution of pigment granules. For example, in frog the animal half contains black or brown pigment while the vegetal half is clear white with no pigment. Similarly, in *Nereis dumerilli* a violet pigment is concentrated in the vegetal half.

An Example of Bipolar Differentiation : Bipolar differentiation has been studied by JOSEPH SPLK (1934) in *Nereis dumerilli.* In *Nereis,* during bipolar differentiation, the ooplasmic substances become distributed in such a way that the alkaline substances with high *p*H accumulate in the animal pole, while substances with low *p*H migrate towards the opposite or vegetal pole. In an undifferentiated oocyte, a yellow pigment is uniformly distributed in the ooplasm. This pigment remains yellow in alkaline medium but turns violet at *p*H 5.4. During bipolar differentiation, the pigment migrates and accumulates in vegetal half. As a result, the animal pole becomes colourless. With the accumulation of substances in the vegetal half, the yellow pigment turns violet indicating an increase of acidity in this part.

Factors Imposing Polarity in Oocytes : Several attempts have been made by the embryologist to explain the origin of polarity of the eggs.

Cortical Differentiation

The homogeneous cytoplasm or ooplasm of the young primary oocyte, in cephinoderms, molluscs, annelids and amphibians, during the course of differentiation, gets separated into two distinct regions:

(i) The outer peripheral layer of hyaline cytoplasm just underneath the plasma membrane is differentiated into cortex or the cortical layer.

(ii) The inner mass of cytoplasm is the endoplasm.

Egg Cortex : The cortical layer of egg is formed of gelatinous cytoplasm which is more viscous than the endoplasm. It does not exhibit streaming movement. It is 2-3 μ in thickness. It is traversed with microfilaments which are linear polymers of tensible protein (TP). These resemble the muscle protein-actin found in the muscles. These are described under the name of 'tectins' by MAZIA and RUBY (1958) and 'tensilines' by LOVTRUP (1974). The TP polymers may occur as microfilaments, microtubules (the one-dimensional or linear structures) or as membranes (the two- dimensional structures). These are either embedded in the cortex or remain attached to it, thereby occupying a fixed position.

The egg cortex provides fixed form to the egg. It fixes the position of parts of the oocyte cytoplasm. It is the bearer of some differentiations which are highly characteristic of the late oocyte and mature egg.

Cortical Granules : These are spherical bodies of varying size, ranging from 0.8 μ – 2 μ. These contain acid mucopolysaccharides, enclosed in a simple membrane. In a mature oocyte, these are arranged in a layer close to the plasma membrane of oocyte. The cortical granules are formed in the endoplasm of the oocyte, most probably from the Golgi bodies (as in sea urchins, frogs and man), and migrate towards the periphery to the egg cortex.

The cortical granules are found in the oocytes of sea urchin, frogs, fishes, bivalve molluscs, some annelids and some mammals including rabbit and man. However, these are absent in rat, guinea pig, gastropod molluscs, insects, birds and urodel amphibians. In general, these may present homogeneous, finely granular or floccular appearance. But in sea urchin, these are formed of concentric or spirally arranged dense lamellae, separated by less dense material. The cortical granules play an important role at the time of fertilization. When sperm comes in contact with the egg surface, the cortical granules rupture liberating their contents which accumulate around the fertilized egg between the egg surface and fertilization membrane.

Ooplasmic Pigment

In the growing oocyte of certain animals, pigment granules are deposited in addition to the yolk. The pigment is yellow in case of ascidian, *Stylea (Cynthia)* and its granules are distributed in the cortical layer of cytoplasm all over the egg surface. In sea urchin, *Paracentrurus lividus,* the pigment is red, though the distribution is the same. During the course of development, it concentrates in specific parts of the embryo, like muscles and mesenchyme in *Stylea* and in the gut wall in *Paracentrurus.*

In the eggs of most amphibians' dark brown or black pigment is present in the cortical layer of cytoplasm. The pigment is more concentrated in the animal hemisphere, so that it appears black or dark brown. The vegetal hemisphere which is densely packed with yolk contains very little or practically no pigment, so that it appears clear white. The formation of pigment granules starts somewhat later than the yolk platelets.

The pigment granules do not have any significant role in the process of development. However, its distribution acts as an indicator of qualitatively different areas in the ooplasm. For example, in *Nereis dumerilli,* the yellow pigment indicates the alkaline medium of the ooplasm and its change into violet colour shows that the medium has become acidic.

Polarplasm and Ooplasmic Segregation : In the mollusc, *Dentalium,* the ooplasm of the oocyte is differentiated into three distinct regions:

(i) A pigment-free colourless area in the region of animal pole, the animal polarplasm.

(ii) A pigment-free colourless area in the region of vegetal pole, the vegetal polarplasm, with no yolk granules.

(iii) The remaining cytoplasm is filled with densely-packed yolk granules and contains a pigment which varies in different individuals from olive green to brick red.

The vegetal polarplasm extends inward and surrounds the nucleus. It is also connected with the cortical layer of the ectoplasm. Both animal and vegetal polarplasm are necessary for the normal development of the larva, the vegetal polarplasm is seen to give rise to the mesoderm of the larva.

In gastropod eggs, it has been observed that the various components of the ooplasm during growth period organise in such a fashion that the egg cytoplasm is regionated and these regions differ in their chemical composition. This phenomenon of ooplasmic differentiation is known as ooplasmic segregation. In these eggs, glycogen gets concentrated in the animal polarplasm, RNA in both the polarplasms and vitamin-C presumably bound to the Golgi complex, tends to concentrate near the equator into an annular band. Such differentiated eggs are called mosaic eggs because their blastomeres get different substances and have a predetermined fate.

Maturation

With the commencement of growth in the oocyte, its nucleus enters the prophase of meiosis. The homologous pairs of chromosomes synapse, but further steps are postponed until the end of growth period. By the time the growth phase is completed, the chromosomes reach the diakinesis stage. Further events can be evoked only by some stimulus. The stimulus may be the contact of the egg with the sperm or with some external medium. In mammals it is accomplished by the pituitary hormones.

On entering the maturation phase, the nuclear membrane of the germinal vesicle breaks up liberating the chromosomes and the nuclear sap. The nuclear sap or nucleoplasm contains substances like *m*RNA, *t*RNA, *r*RNA, riboproteins, informosomes and certain stimulating agents. The RNAs are vitally important for the normal development of the embryo. The stimulating agent enables the egg cytoplasm to respond to the entry of spermatozoon and initiate the formation of microtubules.

The liberated chromosomes are by now greatly concentrated and contracted. From the periphery of the germinal vesicle, these move towards the centre and get arranged on the equator of the achromatic figure, which is formed perpendicular to the surface of oocyte. The chromosomes of the tetrad finally separate into two chromosomes which reach the poles of the meiotic spindle. A bulge appears at the surface of oocyte in the region of animal pole.

The outer pole of the meiotic spindle with half of the chromosomes in anaphase stage enters into this cytoplasmic protuberance. The protuberance with one set of chromosomes and very little cytoplasm is pinched off from the oocyte. The resulting small cell is called first polar body or first polocyte. The oocyte now contains haploid set of already duplicated chromosomes. It is known as secondary oocyte.

A- Nucleus of ovum in growth phase (i.e. before entering the maturation phase) B- Nucleus of ovum after entering the maturation phase. C- and D- First maturation division E- First maturation division completed. A polar body is formed. F, G and H stages of 2nd maturation division.

The haploid polar body receives complete one haploid set of chromosomes, but very little amount of cytoplasm. Usually this remains attached to the animal pole of the oocyte. It may undergo the second meiotic division or the homoeotypic division dividing into two polocytes or it may remain undivided.

The secondary oocyte undergoes second maturation division, which is a mitotic division. Here again the cytoplasm divides unequally producing one small cell, the second polocyte and a large- sized cell, the ovum.

Significance of Unequal Cytokinesis during Maturation Divisions in Oocyte : The process of equal karyokinesis but unequal cytokinesis is a unique feature of the orogenesis and is of great significance. After the maturation of oocyte four cells are formed, three of them are small-sized polocytes or polar bodies each of which receives the same number of chromosomes as by the ovum or the fourth cell. However, these contain very little cytoplasm with no reserve food. The ovum is very large and contains practically all the yolk and cytoplasm. If the cytoplasmic division of the primary and secondary oocyte has been equal, the reserved food accumulated with great efforts during growth phase, would have been equally distributed to the four daughter cells. That amount of yolk might have proved quite insufficient for the developing embryo. Therefore, unequal cytokinesis helps in conserving nutrient material in one cell only. The polocytes with so little cytoplasm and no food reserves are unable to start development and die off in course of time.

Egg Membranes

Formation of Egg Membranes : Like all other animal cells, the egg or ovum is covered by a plasma membrane or cell membrane. In most animals, except sponges and coelenterates, the special protective membranes are deposited outside the plasma membrane. These membranes are described as accessory membranes. Depending on their origin these may be divided into following types.

Primary Egg Membranes: The primary egg membranes are formed outside the plasma membrane of the oocyte between it and the follicle cells in the space occupied by the interdigitating microvilli. These membranes are believed to be secreted by the follicle cells, but the oocyte may also contribute to it. In the initial stages of their formation, these appear to be formed of mucopolysaccharides. However, in later stages of development the fibrous proteins are deposited. In insects, the primary membrane becomes sclerotized. In different animals, eggs, the primary egg membranes have different structure and are known by different names. These are:

Vitelline Membrane: The primary membrane of the oocyte in insects, molluscs, amphibians and birds is called vitelline membrane. It is formed of mucopolysaccharides and certain fibrous proteins. It is closely applied to the plasma membrane.

Zona Radiata : In the oocytes of shark, some bony fishes, some amphibians and reptiles, the primary membrane is striated in appearance. It owes its striations from the degraded microvilli of the growing oocyte. In fishes, the zona radiata is perforated by minute pores, caused by the withdrawal of microvilli in the mature egg. These pores are called micropyles.

Zona Pellucida: It is found in the eggs of mammals and is formed of secretions both from the ovum and the follicle cells. It has unstriated appearance.

Jelly Envelope : In the eggs of echinoderms and many marine invertebrates, the primary egg membrane is formed of jelly and is much thicker. This is known as jelly coat.

The primary membranes closely adhere to the plasma

membrane of the oocyte, but at a later stage a fluid-filled space appears between the two. This space is known as perivitelline space and fluid is called vitelline fluid.

Secondary Egg Membranes: The secondary envelope is secreted outside primary egg membrane by a layer of follicle cells that surround the oocyte. It occurs in the form of a chitinous shell surrounding the egg in insects ascidians and cyclostomes and is known as chorion. However, in amphibians it forms a thin membrane outside the vitelline membrane.

Corona Radiata : No secondary membranes are found in the eggs of urodeles, reptiles and birds and even in mammalian eggs. In mammalian eggs a layer of follicle cell lies outside the zone pellucida and is known as corona radiata. The corona radiata is not a true membrane, because its cells are peeled off as the egg descends the oviduct.

Tertiary Membranes: The tertiary egg membranes are formed either by the oviduct or some other maternal tissue other than ovary, when the egg passes down through the oviduct to the exterior. The examples of tertiary membranes are:

(i) Albumen around the eggs of oviparous elasmobranchs and the horny egg capsule outside are tertiary membranes in the eggs of sharks and rays. The horny egg capsule is secreted by the egg-shell glands of the oviduct.

(ii) Jelly-coat around the amphibian oocyte is secreted by the oviduct.

(iii) Albumen or egg white, the shell membranes and the shell around the eggs of reptiles and apes are secreted by different parts of the oviduct.

Function of Egg Membranes or Extraneous Membranes : The egg membranes serve the following purposes:

(i) Main function of egg membranes is protection of the egg contents or the developing embryo from different ecological hazards i.e. *pH*, temperature variations and radiations etc., from the mechanical injuries and from the enemies.

(ii) Provide buoyancy to the eggs as in amphibian eggs.

(iii) Prevent self-fertilization as in ascidians.

(iv) Prevent entry of more than one sperm (avoid polyspermy).

(v) Egg white in the eggs of birds and reptiles acts as an extra source of nourishment.

(vi) The tertiary membranes, if stick, fastens the egg mass (spawn) to a twig or water plant.

(vii) Zone pellucid of mammalian eggs serves following purposes:

(a) It maintains normal cleavage of the egg serves following purposes.

(b) Prevents egg fusion.

(c) Prevents polyspermy.

5

Development of the Mammal

Oviparity, Ovoviviparity and Viviparity

Oviparity: It is a form of reproduction in which all or most of the development of the embryo in the egg takes place after the egg has been laid. Most *fishes, amphibians, reptiles* and all *birds* are oviparous. The eggs are shed to the outside, either in an unfertilized or in a fertilized state. Among vertebrates, many fishes are oviparous and externally fertilizing, whereas all birds are oviparous and internally fertilizing. In oviparity, the eggs develops on their own, independent of the parents. The food is obtained by yolk within each egg. The developing eggs ultimately *hatch* as larvae or as small, immature adults. If development proceeds in water, the zygotes are often surrounded by layers of jelly *(e.g., frog).* Zygotes that develop on land are usually protected against dessication by cocoons *(e.g., earthworm, spider* and *insects* like *cockroaches* or shells *(e.g., reptiles* and *birds).*

Ovoviviparity: The bearing of youngones developed from the eggs which have been retained the female reproductive system, but without the maternal organism providing additional nourishment of the embryo, is known as ovoviviparity. The fertilization is internal. The young are *born* rather than hatched, and the females released fully formed animals instead of eggs. The examples are *some* of the fishes *(e.g., Mustelus vulgaris)* amphibia, reptiles and mammals *(e.g., Echidna).*

Viviparous: In this reproductive pattern, fertilization is internal, zygotes are retained inside the female and the embryo establishes a direct connection with the maternal body, so that nutrition can pass from the mother to the embryo. The female in this case is said to be *pregnant* and the young are *born* as developed animals.

Notable examples of viviparity among the anamniotes (lacking the other membranes including amnion) are found in the Chondrichthyes. In some sharks, the highly vascular yolk sac like in close contact with the inner surface of the uterus, with a resultant transfer of metabolic products. In some amphibia, *e.g., Pipa americana,* the Suriname toad, the females have small pits on their back in which eggs are carried till hatching. In others, connection between the mother and the embryo is established through a special organ, the placenta. It is an outgrowth of the embryo joined to uterus of the maternal body. Placentae are found in the protracheates *(e.g. Peripatus),* in the tunicates *(e.g., Salpa)* in several elasmobranchs *(i.e., Mustelus laevis)* and in eutherian mammals. However, the mode of origin and the structure of placenta is different in each group. In reptiles, although egglaying is the common practice, *some snakes* and *lizards* are viviparous. Certain of them utilize the yolk sac in association with the lining of the uterus, while others utilize the chorion.

Evolution Of Viviparity In Mammals : Palaentological evidences indicate that the mammals are derived from ancestors which were closely related to the early reptiles. It is expected, therefore, that they must have had large yolky eggs and their developmental history must have resembled with that of the reptiles. At some stage of their evolution some of the mammals switched from oviparity to viviparity. In such cases embryo received sufficient supply of nourishment from the mother while it was retained in the uterus, and the yolk supply of the egg became unnecessary. As a result, there was a progressive decline in the yolk supply and eventually it disappeared altogether. In this respect, there is a distinct graduation in the three subclasses of the class Mammalia.

Subclass Prototheria: Mammals of this subclass are mostly *oviparous* as they lay eggs that develop outside the maternal body, *e.g., Ornithorhynchus.* However, some of them are ovoviviparous, *i.e.,* though developing in the maternal body, they are not supplied with nourishment, *e.g., Echidna.* The eggs, therefore, have a large amount of yolk. They meroblastic and develop in a reptilian pattern (Flynn and Hill, 1939).

Subclass Metatheria (the Massupials): The quantity of yolk in the egg is insignificant and it becomes unnecessary for the development of the embryo. Nevertheless, it is ejected at the beginning of cleavage. Although the developing embryos receive nourishment from the mother in the uterus, but the adaptations for this procedure are not much advanced and the young are born poorly developed.

Subclass Eutheria (Placental mammals): The microlecithal egg is devoid of yolk right from the very beginning. Therefore, the embryos of these mammals develops inside the uterus and draw their nutrition from the maternal body through a 'physiological bridge', the placenta.

Maturation and Fertilization

In mammals the first maturation division generally occurs before ovulation and fertilization. With the exception of a few mammals e.g., the Mole, Rabbit and Man, the second maturation division is completed after sperm penetration. After coitus, sperm are introduced into the vagina of the mammal. Soon after, they ascend into the uterus and up the oviducts. Within a period of a few hours or even less, they reach the upper ends of these ducts where the actual process of fertilization is consummated.

Cleavage

With the disappearance of the yolk, cleavage of the eggs of eutherian mammals is complete or holoblastic, but despite a microlecithal condition the blastomeres tend to show size differences from the start. Although total, the cleavage is irregular as the synchronization of mitosis in the blastomeres is lost very early. Even the first two blastomeres divided at different rates. Therefore, the numbers of blastomeres do not increase by a regular doubling sequence but tend to show arithmetical progression. Consequently, a 3-cell stage is found and, subsequently stages with 5, 6, 7 blastomeres, and so forth.

In the majority of mammals, cleavage results in the formation of a solid mass of cells known as the morula, in which some cells are superficial and others lie inside. The cells lying in the interior are known as the inner cell mass. They are the main source of material for the body of the embryo proper. The cells of the enveloping layer give rise mainly to the extra-embryonic membranes.

Blastocyst

At about 70 to 75 hours after mating a cavity appears inside the compact mass of tells of the morula. The cavity is formed of crevices which appear between the inner cell mass and the cells of the enveloping layer. Fluid passes from the uterine cavity through the zona pellucida and begins to accumulate between the cells. The enveloping layer of cells gets lifted off the inner cell mass on most of its inner surface and remains attached on one side only. This side later on gives rise to the dorsal side of the embryo. Gradually, the fluid-filled intercellular spaces become confluent forming a single cavity. The morula has now become a blastocyst, which corresponds in a general way to the blastula of lower forms. The cavity of the blastocyst may be compared to the blastocoel. As subsequent development exhibits, the inner cell mass lying above the fluid virtually plays the role of a blastoderm. However, the blastocyst as a whole differs essentially from a blastula because its cells are already differentiated into two types : (*i*) the inner cell mass, and (*ii*) the cells of the enveloping layer.

Gastrulation

The term gastrulation in a mammal is used to denote the formation of an archenteric cavity and the differentiation of epiblast and hypoblast (McEwan, 1923). During the progressive differentiation of the mammalian blastocyst, a layer of flat cells appears on the interior surface of the inner cell mass *i.e.,* on the surface facing the cavity. This layer of cells, representing the presumptive endoderm is called the hypoblast.

There are two views regarding the origin of the hypoblast (endoderm) cells : (*i*) the more generally accepted view is that the endoderm cells arise by a splitting off (elimination) of cells from the ventral side of the inner cell mass, (*ii*) the endodermal cells in some mammals such as elephant shrew (Van der Horst, 1942) or even in all mammals (Dalcq, 1954) are derived by an infiltration from the enveloping layer of cells. Some of the enveloping cells, near the edge of the inner cell mass, move inward along the internal surface of the inner cell mass and arrange themselves in a continuous layer, the hypoblast.

With the origin of the hypoblast the remainder of the inner cell mass may now be termed, the epiblast. It consists of a thick plate of columnar cells, clearly distinguished from the more flat cells of the enveloping layer. The hypoblast cells on the underside of the epiblast may become cuboidal or even columnar. The epiblast may become cuboidal or even columnar. The epiblast and hypoblast together constitute the blastodisc which becomes quite sharply delimited from the remainder of the embryo. The cells of the blastodisc are often referred to as the formative cells because the embryo proper will be developed at the expense of these cells. As regards the enveloping layer, it does not directly contribute any longer to the formation of the embryo proper. The function of the cells of this layer is to establish a connection of the embryo with the maternal body so that the nutrition can pass from the mother to the embryo. This layer of cells, therefore, from now onwards is known as the trophoblast (Greek *trophe,* nourishment; blast, layer). The layer of trophoblast corresponds in position to the chorion of the later embryos of the reptiles and birds. The hypoblast becomes specially thick near one edge of the blastodisc. This thickening is called prechordal plate. It is destined to become the anterior end of the embryo.

The hypoblast cells are at first found in the region of the inner cell mass only but later they multiply and spread along the inner surface of the trophoblast and surround the internal cavity of the blastocyst. This extension of the hypoblast and later mesoderm around the inside of the blastocyst converts a part of this cavity into archenteron, while part of it becomes the yolk sac (McEwen, 1923). The yolk sac, in this case, however, instead of being filled with yolk, is filled with fluid.

It becomes apparent from the account given above that the mode of gastrulation in the mammal is entirely one of elimination or infiltration, and proliferation. It does not involve any involution, invagination, epiboly or concrescence. However, a well-marked blastopore is lacking in connection with the actual process of hypoblast formation.

In the next phase of gastrulation, a primitive streak is formed as a thickening in the epiblast. A Hensen's node is seen as its anterior end. The primitive streak is, however, much shorter than in birds and, is confined to the posterior part of the blastodisc. The cells of the primitive streak migrate downward and on the sides between the epiblast and the hypoblast. Some of the migrating cells join the hypoblast and thus contribute to the formation of the endoderm (Heuser and Streeter, 1941). The loose cells migrating sideways eventually give rise to the layer of mesoderm.

The cells that migrate forward from Hensen's node are aggregated more closely and give rise to the head process, which is the rudiment of notochord. The primitive streak in mammals is a structure of short duration. It starts shrinking after giving rise to the mesodermal layer and the notochord rudiment. On the other hand, the germinal layers begin to form the primary organ rudiments in the anterior parts of the blastodisc. The first of these become visible is the neurafplate followed by mesodermal segments.

Neurulation

The neurulation proceeds in an anteroposterior direction. As the primitive streak starts shrinking and Hensen's node recedes farther and farther back, parts of the neural plate become differentiated. The anterior parts of the neural plate proceed to close into a tube, the neural tube. The notochord becomes separated from the adjoining mesoderm. The dorsal mesoderm becomes subdivided in somites.

Extraembryonic Membranes of Mammals : The embryos of rabbit and other mammals develop four types of foetal membranes as in Chick. They are amnion, chorion, yolk sac and allantois. However, they are characteristically different from that of the Chick in the mode of their formation, structure and function. The modifications are mainly due to the intrauterine development and the absence of yolk in eutherian mammals. All the foetal membranes are discarded at parturition or birth.

Amnion and Chorion Development : The amnion and chorion develop simultaneously. There are two chief methods by which the amnion is formed in the mammal.

Amnion Formation by Folds: This method of amnion formation takes place in the *marsupials, ungulates (pigs), lagomorpha (rabbit),* most *insectivores* and *lemurs.* In this method the amnion and chorion arise together as upwardly projecting folds of somatopleure (somatic mesoderm + trophoblast) called amniotic folds. The head and tail folds of somatopleure converge above the embryo and finally meet and fuse. The point of fusion is referred to as sero-amniotic connection. Fusion of the folds produces two foetal membranes over the embryo — the inner amnion and the outer chorion. The amnion consists of an inner *ectoderm* facing the embryo and an outer *somatic mesoderm.* The space enclosed between the embryo and the amnion is called the *amniotic cavity.* It gets filled with a fluid, the *amniotic fluid.* The chorion is made up of an outer *ectoderm* and an inner *somatic mesoderm.* The space between the amnion and chorion is called the extraembryonic coelom or exocoelom (Balinsky, 1970).

Differences in development between amnion, chorion of bird and mammal:

1. In the bird the *chorionic ectoderm* originates entirely from ectoderm of the extraembryonic blastoderm which grows out over the yolk. In the mammal, on the other hand, the ectoderm of the chorion is continuous with the remaining parts of the trophoblast in the extraembryonic area. The trophoblast thus becomes a part of the chorion. It actually forms the embryonic layer of the chorion over most of the extra-embryonic surface of the blastocyst.
2. *Inthehirdtheamniotic Head Fold Appears First : The tailfaid* arises by the third day of incubation and it grows slowly towards the amniotic head fold. Therefore, the

sero-amniotic connection lies behind the middle of the embryo's body. In the mammal, the *tail fold* often appears *earlier* than the head fold, and is, therefore, the longer of the two. The tail fold grows more rapidly than the head fold. As a result the point of final, fusion of the amniotic folds, the sero-amniotic connection lies above the anterior region of the embryo. In the pig, however, head and tail folds are virtually equal, and are continuous with the lateral folds which arise coincidently.

3. In the bird the head and tail folds of amnion have from the very start, their complement of somatic mesoderm. In the mammal, the head fold of amnion lacks mesoderm in the beginning for a short while.

Amnion Formation by Cavitation: In the *hedgehog, guinea pig, mouse* and other more advanced mammals the amniotic cavity arises merely as a space inside the inner cell mass or between the trophoblastic layer and the inner cell mass. The cells giving rise to the embryo proper sink deeper into the blastocyst, so that the formative cells do not appear on the surface. Therefore, the amniotic cavity can no longer be formed by the convergence of amniotic folds. Instead, the amniotic cavity is formed by a chink or small space appearing between cells in the future blastodisc area. This method of formation of the amniotic cavity is called cavitation.

Functions

1. The amnion protects the embryo from dessication. The embryo is fully immersed and bathed in the amniotic fluid which serves as an artificial swimming pool of the embryo.
2. The amniotic fluid serves as an efficient shock absorber. Being viscous and gelatinous, it protects the delicate embryo from external as well as internal mechanical pressures.

3. The amniotic fluid allows freedom of motion to the embryo.
4. The amnion protects the outer surface of the embryo from adhesion and abrasion.
5. In most mammals a part of the chorion forms finger-like outgrowths called chorionic villi that penetrate into corresponding crypts or depressions in the wall of the uterus. It is at this site where exchange of substances occurs between the embryo and the uterus in the body of the mother.

Yolk Sac Development and Functions : There is very little or no yolk in marsupial and eutherian eggs, yet a yolk sac develops in their embryos which points to their reptilian ancestory. In the mammals yolk sac begins to form during early gastrulation. In the blastocyst stage, the hypoblast endoderm cells found in the inner cell mass begin to spread along the inner surface of the trophoblast and surround the internal cavity of the blastocyst in the same way as the endodermal cells in reptiles and birds surround the mass of uncleaved egg. The cavity of the blastocyst within the enveloping endodermal layer is referred to as the yolk sac.

Yolk sac in Marsupials: In marsupials *e.g., Didelphys,* the Opossum, the yolk sac is well developed though it contains no yolk. However, a clearly defined area vasculosa is present on its upper surface. On the opposite side of the yolk sac, the endoderm comes into contact with the trophoblast of the blastocyst. During implantation the trophoblast is produced into folds which fit into corresponding crypts of the uterine wall. The crypts secrete a viscid fluid, the uterine milk, which is absorbed by way of the trophoblast and endoderm. Finally, it reaches the embryo, partly via area vasculosa.

Yolk sac in Pig: Although no yolk is present, a large yolk sac is initially established in the pig in a manner comparable to that in birds. The upper part of the yolk sac is highly vascularised and contains vitelline arteries and veins. The lower part of the yolk sac is not vascularised and it absorbs uterine milk from the uterine wall. The nourishing maternal secretion is then transported to the embryo by the vitelline circulation. Thus, although nutritive in function; yolk sac does not have a digestive role. But with the enlargement of the allantois and formation of placenta the yolk sac rapidly shrivels up and becomes insignificant.

Yolk sac in Rabbit: In rabbit, an area vasculosa is found in the upper part of the yolk sac. Its lower wall, which is in contact with the trophoblast of the blastocyst ruptures. Finally, the trophoblast also breaks up at this point and thus the interior of the yolk sac is placed in immediate communication with the uterine cavity. As a result, the nutritive secretions produced by the uterine wall diffuse into the fluid filling the yolk sac. From here, the uterine secretions are carried to the embryo by the vitelline blood vessels that develop in the Splanchnic mesoderm of the yolk sac in its embryo is only temporary and is soon replaced by a permanent attachment of the blastocyst to the uterine wall by means of a placenta.

Yolk sac is also supposed to assist respiration and haemopoiesis (formation of blood cells) in the embryo. The stalk of folk sac and that of allantois together with their blood vessels constitute the umbilical cord.

Allantois Development

The allantois arises as a ventral outgrowth of the hindgut before the sero-amniotic connection is formed. It is composed of splanchnopleure (endoderm + splanchnic mesoderm). The allantois grows very rapidly and soon spreads inside the extraembryonic coelom. The connection of the allantois of the hindgut is restricted to a narrow neck called allantoic stalk. The allantois soon develops umbilical or allantois arteries and veins which connect the embryo with the maternal part of the placenta. The free surface of allantois comes in close contact with the inner surface of chorion. In rabbit, the splanchnic mesoderm of allantois fuses with the somatic mesoderm of chorion over a small disc-shaped area to form a membrane called allantochorion.

Functions

(1) With the acquisition of viviparity in the massupials and the placental mammals, the original function of the allantois as a urinary bladder becomes altogether lost. The carbon dioxide produced by the embryo as well as the urea which is the end product of the protein metabolism, diffuse into the maternal blood and are excreted by the kidneys of the pregnant mother. As a result, the storage of the waste products in the allantoic cavity is no longer necessary and becomes greatly reduced.

(2) Blood vessels of the allantois supply the embryo with oxygen and nutrient substances from the maternal organism.

Male Reproductive Organs

Testes : The testes are extra-abdominal. These are suspended in a sac of integument called scrotum or scrotal sacs, situated on the sides of penis. Each scrotal sac is an extension of abdominal cavity and is connected with it by inguinal canal. The temperature of testes in scrotal sacs is several degrees lower than that of abdominal cavity. This is required for normal maturation of sperms.

Each testis is formed of large number of seminiferous tubules. Each seminiferous tubule is lined by a layer of germinal epithelial cells. The primordial germ cells of this layer produce spermatozoa. The large sertoli cells provide attachment to the spermatozoa during metamorphosis. According to CRAIGMYLE and PRESLEY (1975), sertoli cells can make androgens from precursors and thus provide androgenic environment within the seminiferous tubules independent of interstitial cells of Leydig.

The interstitial cells of Leydig are clusters of polyhedral cells with vacuolated cytoplasm. These secrete male sex hormones-testosterone.

Epididymis : The ends of seminiferous tubules unite to form a short straight tube, the tubuli recti, which opens into rete testis. It is a network of anastomosing ducts. A number of fine vasa efferentia from rete testis open into epididymis. Epididymis is an extremely long and highly convoluted tube. Its head region is called caput epididymis and tail region is cauda epididymis.

Epididymis stores spermatozoa. Its secretion contains certain biochemical substances like sialic acid, glyceryl phosphocholine, etc. which influence maturation of sperms.

Vas Deferens : Vas deferens arises from cauda epididymis. It enters the abdominal cavity through inguinal canal and opens into the seminal vesicle which is a small sac lying behind the urinary bladder. The secretion of seminal vesicles contains fructose, inositol, vitamin C and flavine derivatives. It serves as a vehicle for spermatozoa and provides an environment that activates and nourish them.

At the base of urinary bladder the vasa differentiate from two sides unite to form common ejaculatory duct. It runs through the prostate gland and opens into urethra.

Urethra and Penis : Urinary bladder opens in the urethra, which also receives opening of ejaculatory duct. Thus, it serves to convey both semen (sperm) and urine. Urethra passes through a muscular erectile intromittent organ, the penis. Its wall is spongy and vascular.

Accessory Glands : Associated with the male system are- (i) a large prostate gland situated at the base of seminal vesicle and (ii) a pair of Cowper's glands or bulbo-urethral glands. The prostatic fluid contains several lytic enzymes (citric acid, spermine and prostaglandins).

Female Reproductive Organs

Ovaries : A pair of ovaries are situated in the pelvis region. Each is a small structure and is attached to the broad ligament which extends laterally from uterus to ilium of pelvis. The cortex part of ovary encloses ovarian follicles in different stages of development. These are called Graafian follicles.

Fallopian Tube : In mammals, the oviduct is called Fallopian tube. Its anterior funnel-shaped opening is called infundibulum, that lies close to the ovary. It is surrounded by the finger-like processes of highly vascular tissue, called fimbriae. Fallopian tube is small and coiled and opens into uterus.

Uterus : Uterus is a brood pouch in which embryo is protected and nourished. It is lined with a heavy, mucous, glandular layer called endometrium. The uterus wall is formed of connective tissue and smooth muscle fibres. Endometrium and muscular portion are highly vascular.

In shape, mammalian uterus is quite variable. It is bicornuate in ruminants and perissodactyls; bipartite in most carnivores and uterus duplex in marsupials. In primates it is called uterus simplex.

Vagina : The two uteri unite mesially and open into vagina. Vagina is a wide tube. It opens to the exterior by a wide opening called vulva. In human beings the cervix of uterus projects into upper part of vagina. Vagina serves two functions- (i) acts as an organ of copulation and (ii) acts as a birth canal.

A pair of small Bertholin's glands are situated on the dorsal wall of vestibule. Their secretion lubricates vaginal passage during coitus.

Sexual Cycle in Mammals

Reproduction in mammals is an orchestrated process. It needs the co-ordinated preparation of many tissues in female starting from maturation of ovum, its release, its transportation, fertilization and also the preparation of uterine wall to receive developing egg and its implantation.

The preparations for reproduction are cyclic in mammals. The changes in structural and functional characteristics of both male and female reproductive tissue occur as a prelude to reproduction. These are mediated by hormones.

Estrous Cycle in Mammals

Sexual cycle is called estrous cycle. Sexual periodicity is much less developed in males than in females. In some mammals (deer family) there is a brief period of intense sexual activity at one particular season of the year and then a long period of cessation of spermatogenesis. More commonly male is sexually potent throughout adult life. A brief period of pronounced sexual activity is called 'rutting season'. It corresponds with the female's period of mating impulse (period of heat).

In mammals other than primates, the estrous cycle can be divided into following phases:

Estrous Phase : A short period when the male and female are fully prepared for reproduction and have strong sexual desire.

Post-estrous or Metestrum : A period during which the preparations made for pregnancy undergo regression due to failure of pregnancy.

Diestrum : A period of rest after regressive activities.

Proestrum : A period of active preparation for next estrous cycle.

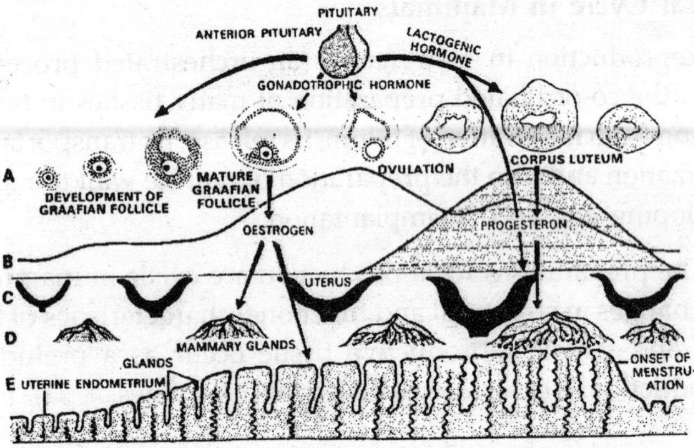

Menstrual cycle and changes occuring during this period in man.

Based on the number of estrous cycles in a year, the species can be :

(1) Monoestrous having one breeding season in a year. It is found in deer and sheep.

(2) Polyestrous having several breeding periods in a year. Majority of mammals are polyestrous.

Menstrual Cycle in Primates

In Primates the female sexual cycle is characterized by menstruation. Menstruation is the discharge of blood, mucus and cellular debris from the uterus during postestrous or metestrum phase. A menstrual cycle corresponds with one estrous cycle. In human females it occurs after about 28 days. The menstrual cycle is divided into three phases:

(i) Menses—the period of menstruation or discharge.

(ii) Follicular phase or proliferative phase—the period of restoration of uterine epithelium (when the endometrium of uterus regenerates).

Secretory or Luteal Phase : It is a preparatory phase, when uterine wall prepares to receive the fertilized egg. It becomes highly vascular and greatly thickened. Its glands are greatly distended. Its mucosa increases from 1mm to 4-5mm.

If implantation of fertilized egg does not occur, the activities of secretory phase end and menstruation follows.

Hormonal Regulation of Female Sexual Cycle

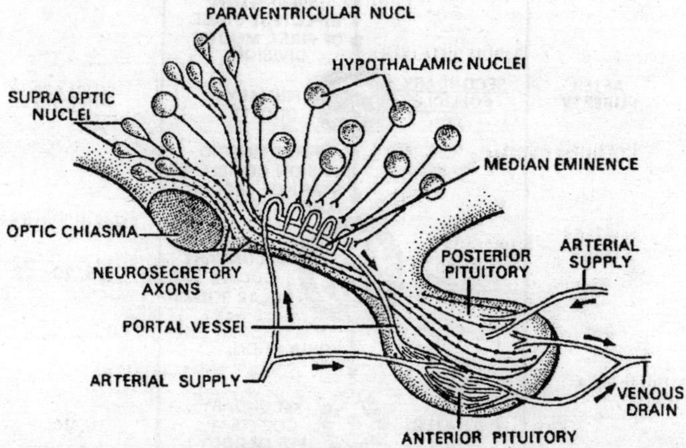

Control of pituitary by hypothalamus (feedback)

Hormones in female regulate maturation of gonads, their proper functioning and breeding rhythmicity or sexual cycle and also the attachment and parturition of foetus to uterine wall.

The primary hormonal activator is located in close association with the brain. It is pituitary gland or hypophysis. Its activity is in turn regulated by the hypothalamus.

Hypothalamus releases a number of chemicals, called the releasing factors which stimulate pituitary to secrete following gonadotrophic hormones :

Gonadotrophic Hormones Secreted by Anterior Pituitary Gland : The anterior pituitary secretes two gonadotrophic hormones. These are glycoproteins in nature.

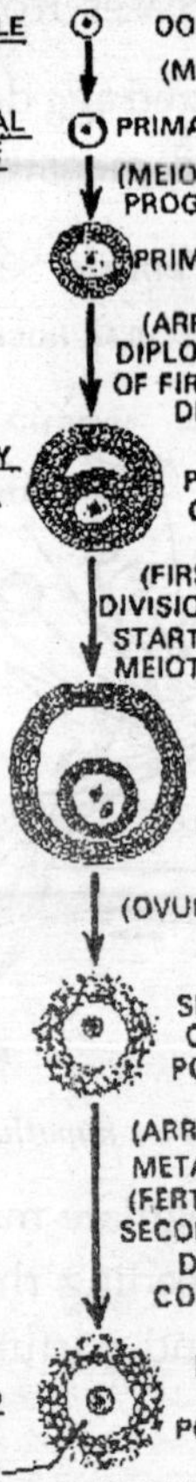

AGE	FOLLICULAR HISTOLOGY	MEIOTIC EVENTS IN OVUM	CHROMOSOMAL COMPLEMENT
FETAL PERIOD	NO FOLLICLE	OOGONIUM	2N, 2C
		(MITOSIS)	
BEFORE OR AT BIRTH	PRIMORDIAL FOLLICLE	PRIMARY OOCYTE	2N, 4C
		(MEIOSIS IN PROGRESS)	
AFTER BIRTH	PRIMARY FOLLICLE	PRIMARY OOCYTE	2N, 4C
		(ARRESTED IN DIPLOTENE STAGE OF FIRST MEIOTIC DIVISION)	
AFTER PUBERTY	SECONDARY FOLLICLE	PRIMARY OOCYTE	2N, 4C
		(FIRST MEIOTIC DIVISION COMPLETED, START OF SECOND MEIOTIC DIVISION)	
	TERTIARY FOLLICLE	SECONDARY OOCYTE + POLAR BODY-I	1N, 2C
		(OVULATION)	
	OVULATED OVUM	SECONDARY OOCYTE + POLAR BODY-I	1N, 2C
		(ARRESTED AT METAPHASE II) (FERTILIZATION SECOND MEIOTIC DIVISION COMPLETED)	
	FERTILIZED OVUM	FERTILIZED OVUM + POLAR BODY-II	1N, 1C SPERM
	SPERM		

Summary of events in the reproductive cycle of a mammal.

Follicle Stimulating Hormone (FSH) : It increases the size of Graafian follicles, and causes their ripening. It also induces the secretion of esterogens, formation of ovum and the phenomenon of oestrus.

Luteinizing Hormone (LH) : It is responsible for final maturation of ovarian follicles, ovulation and the initial formation, growth and persistence of corpus luteum and its secretion of progesterone. Indirectly it stops oestrus cycle and helps the implantation of ovum and thereby the further proliferation of corpus luteum. It maintains the normal pregnancy phase.

Prolactin (earlier called Luteotrophic Hormone-LTH) : It is also secreted by anterior pituitary. It controls a wide variety of regulatory functions.

Sex Hormones Secreted by Ovary

These are known as Estrogens.

Estrogens : These are estrone, α-estradiol, β-estradiol and esteriol. These are secreted from the Graafian follicles of the ovary. The estrogens control the development of secondary sexual characteristics, like onset of menstruation, development of breasts, growth of axillary and pubic hair. These induce growth of uterus, external genitalia, increased musculature of fallopian tubes, their contractibility and motility. These regulate the oestrus or menstrual cycle. During pregnancy these initiate growth of mammary glands.

Sex Hormones Secreted by Corpus Luteum

Progesterone : It induces mucus-secreting activity of the endometrium. It prepares the uterine wall to receive the fertilized egg *i.e.* it is responsible for the premenstrual growth phase in the non-pregnant uterus. It promotes implantation of fertilized egg in the uterine wall and the development of placenta.

Relaxing : It is produced both by corpus luteum and the placenta. It stimulates relaxation of pelvic ligaments towards the end of pregnancy.

Oestrous Cycle : In the early phase of oestrous cycle the ovary is stimulated by follicle stimulating hormone (FSH) secreted by the basophilic cells of anterior lobe of pituitary gland. It controls the development and progressive growth of ovarian follicles inside the ovary. Luteinizing hormone (LH) secreted by anterior lobe of pituitary assists the response of ovary to FSH and thus is said to have a synergistic effect.

Follicular Phase : Estradiol, the steroid sex hormone (esterogen) secreted by the ripening Graafian follicles, affects the secondary sex organs and secretory activity of pituitary. It stimulates the growth of uterus. The myometrium and endometrium increase in thickness and become more vascular and the secretory glands of endometrium grow in length. It stimulates the fallopian tube and vagina. The epithelium of vagina thickens and cornifies. Esterogen initiates increase in the size of mammary glands. Increase in the concentration of estradiol in blood inhibits FSH secretion and at the same time stimulates the production of luteinizing hormone.

Luteal Phase : Luteotrophic or lactogenic hormone of the pituitary gland aids in bringing about rupture of Graafian follicle, ovulation of ovum and formation of corpus luteum from empty- ruptured Graafian follicles. It also stimulates the production of progesterone from corpus luteum.

Oviparity, Ovo-viviparity and Viviparity—Oviparity: It is a form of reproduction in which all or most of the developments of the embryo in the egg takes place after the egg has been laid. Most fishes, amphibians, reptiles and all birds are oviparous. The eggs are shed to the outside, either in an unfertilized or a fertilized state. Among vertebrates, many fishes are oviparous with external fertilization, whereas all birds are oviparous with internal fertilizin. In oviparity, the eggs develop on their own, independent of the parents.

The food is obtained from yolk within each egg. The developing eggs ultimately hatch as larvae or as small, immature adults. If development proceeds in water, the zygotes are often surrounded by layers of jelly *(i.e. frog)*. Zygotes that develop on land are usually protected against dessication by cocoons (e.g., earthworm, spider and insects like cockroaches) or shell (e.g., reptiles and birds).

Ovoviviparity **:** The bearing of youngones developed from the eggs which have been retained in the female reproductive system, but without the maternal organism providing additional nourishment to the embryo, is known as ovoviviparity. The fertilization is internal. The young are born rather than hatched, and the females release fully formed animals instead of eggs. The examples are some of the fishes *(e.g. Mustelusvulgaris)*, amphibia, reptiles and mammals *(e.g. Echidna)*.

Viviparous **:** In this reproductive pattern, fertilization is internal. Zygotes are retained inside the female and the embryo establishes a direct connection with the maternal body, so that nutrients can pass from mother to the embryo. The female in this case is said to be pregnant and the young are born as developed animals.

Examples of viviparity among the anamniotes (lacking the extraembryonic membranes including amnion) are found in chondrichthyes. In some sharks, the highly vascular yolk sac lies in close contact with the inner surface of the uterus, with a resultant transfer of metabolic products from mother to foetus. In some amphibians *e.g. Pipa americana*, the Surinam toad, the females have small pits on their back in which eggs are carried till hatching. In others, connection between the mother and the embryo is established through a special organ, the placenta. It is an outgrowth of the embryo joined to the uterus of mother. Placentae are found in the protracheates *(e.g, Peripatus), in* the tunicates *(e.g. Salpa)*, in several elasmobranchs *(e.g., Mustelus laevis)* and in eutherian mammals. However, the mode of origin and the structure of placenta is different in each group. In reptiles, although egg laying is the common practice, some snakes and lizards are viviparous, certain of them utilize the yolk sac in association with the lining of the uterus, while others utilize rough chorion.

Evolution of Viviparity in Mammals : Paleontological evidences indicate that the mammals are derived from ancestors which were closely related to the early reptiles. It is expected, therefore, that they must have had large yolky eggs and their developmental history must have resembled with that of the reptiles. At some stage of their evolution some of the mammals switched from oviparity to viviparity.

In such cases, embryo received sufficient supply of nourishment from the mother while it was retained in the uterus; and the yolk supply of the egg becomes unnecessary. As a result, there was a progressive decline in the yolk supply and eventually its disappearance altogether. In this respect, there is a distinct gradation in the three sub-classes of the class Mammalia.

Subclass Prototheria : Mammals of this subclass are mostly oviparous as they lay eggs that develop outside the maternal body, *e.g., Omithorhynchus.* However, some of them are ovoviviparous, *i.e.,* though developing in the maternal body, they are not supplied with nourishment, *e.g. Echidna.* The eggs, therefore, have a large amount of yolk. They are meroblastic and develop in a reptilian pattern (FLYNN and HILL, 1939).

Subclass Metatheria (the Marsupials) : The quantity of yolk in the egg is insignificant and it is insufficient for the development of the embryo. Nevertheless, even this amount is ejected at the beginning of cleavage. Although the developing embryos receive nourishment from the mother in the uterus, the adaptations for this procedure are not much advanced and the young ones are born poorly or incompletely developed.

Subclass Eutheria (placental mammals) : The microlecithal egg is devoid of yolk right from the very beginning. Therefore, the embryos of these mammals develop inside the uterus and draw their nutrition from the maternal body through a 'physiological bridge' the placenta.

Ovulation

Fully mature Graafian follicle comes to the surface of ovary. The discuss proligerous breaks and ovum is set free. The ovum floats freely in the follicular fluid present inside Graafian follicle. The Graafian follicle ruptures and ovum is released near the ostium of Fallopian tube. It is drawn into the infundibulum. In some mammals only one Graafian follicle matures at a time as in man, cattle, etc. but mammals which produce litre, a number of ova are released at one time. In rabbit, Graafian follicle ruptures only following copulation. At the time of ovulation, the ovum is in secondary oocyte stage and its nucleus in metaphase.

Egg or Ovum

Mammalian egg is minute with little or no yolk (alecithal type). Its centre is occupied by a large single nucleus called germinal vesicle. The egg is in secondary oocyte stage. It is protected by following two membranes (the true vitelline membrane is absent).

Zona Pellucida or Zona Radiata : formed of thick transparent substance, perforated by fine canals. (ii) Corona radiata — formed of follicle cells.

Fertilization and Maturation

Fertilization usually occurs in the upper part of Fallopian tube. But, since both ova and sperm can survive for a day or even more the encounter of ova and sperm may occur in any part of oviduct. After coitus, sperm are introduced in the vagina of female. These ascend into the uterus and up in the oviduct. Within few hours, these reach the upper end of the oviduct where fertilization takes place.

The first maturation division generally occurs before ovulation. The germinal vesicle is in second metaphase stage when ovulation occurs. With the exception of a few mammals *e.g.* moles, rabbit and man, the second maturation division is completed after sperm penetration.

Early Development

The development in mammals is greatly complicated and usually occurs inside the body of female. The egg is small i.e. about 1mm. in size and contains little amount of yolk, distributed uniformly. It is enclosed in an outer covering of corona radiata and inner thick membrane of zona radiata. The corona radiata disappears after fertilization occurs in the anterior part of oviduct. After fertilization it gets surrounded by a thick covering of albumen..

Segmentation

Segmentation starts about fourteen or fifteen hours after fertilization and is holoblastic. The first cleavage is vertical, the second is also vertical but at right angles to the first one. The third cleavage is horizontal but slightly above the middle line. The subsequent cleavages are irregular and a ball of cells is formed. It is known as morula. In morula two types of cells are differentiated—

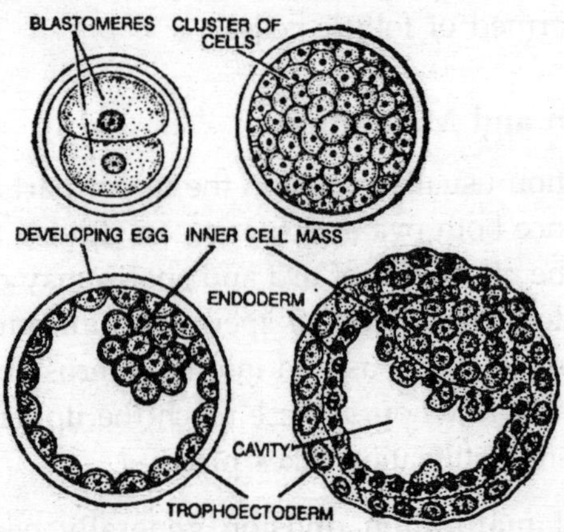

Early cleavage in the mammalian egg.

(i) Outer layer of small flattened epithelial cells. It gives rise to Trophoblast or trophoderm.

(ii) Central mass of large, spherical cells with granular cytoplasm. It gives rise to inner cell mass.

Blastocyst and Blastulation

At about 70 to 75 hours after mating a cavity appears inside the compact cell mass of the morula. The cavity is formed of crevices which appear between the inner cell mass and the cells of trophoderm. It is called blastocoel. But in no way it is homologous to blastocoel of frog. Fluid passes from the uterine cavity through the zona pellucida and begins to accumulate between the cells. The enveloping layer of cells gets lifted off the inner cell mass on most of its inner surface and remains attached on one side only. This side, later on, gives rise to the dorsal side of the embryo. The morula now becomes blastocyst or blastosphere. It corresponds to the blastula of lower forms. The cavity of blastocyst may be compared to the blastocoel. As subsequent development exhibits, the inner cell mass lying above the fluid virtually plays the role of blastoderm.

By further divisions in the cells of inner cell mass, the blastocyst increases in size. The inner cell mass remains attached to the blastoderm or trophoblast of the blastocyst at animal pole by cells, that form embryonal knob. The cells of trophoblast overlying the embryonal knob are called 'cells of Rauber.'

Gastrulation

After a short interval the cells from the lower surface of embryonal knob proliferate into the blastocoel immediately below the knob. These form the embryonic endoderm or hypoblast. The embryonal knob forms the embryonal ectoderm or epiblast. Later on, the cells of hypoblast form an almost complete layer lining the subgerminal cavity. After the formation of hypoblast the embryonal knob flattens forming the embryonal disc and the cells of Rauber disintegrate. Later on, zona radiata and albumen layer also disappear. The embryo at this stage represents the seventh day of development. It is exposed at the surface of blastodisc.

Primitive Streak and Mesoderm Formation : In the centre of the embryonal disc an opaque pear-shaped embryonal area appears. It is broad in front and narrow behind. Posteriorly, it is marked by an opaque long line, the primitive streak. The anterior end of the primitive streak swells up into primitive knot or Hensen's node or primitive node. All these changes occur due to active proliferation of cells. Active migration of cells from the primitive streak results in the appearance of a groove or channel in the primitive streak. It is known as primitive groove. These cells accumulate between the ectoderm and endoderm. Few cells also migrate forward, those from the upper part develop into the neural plate and the lower ones into the notochordal process.

Formation of Notochord and Medullary Tube : The formation of notochord and neural tube is quite similar to that in chick.

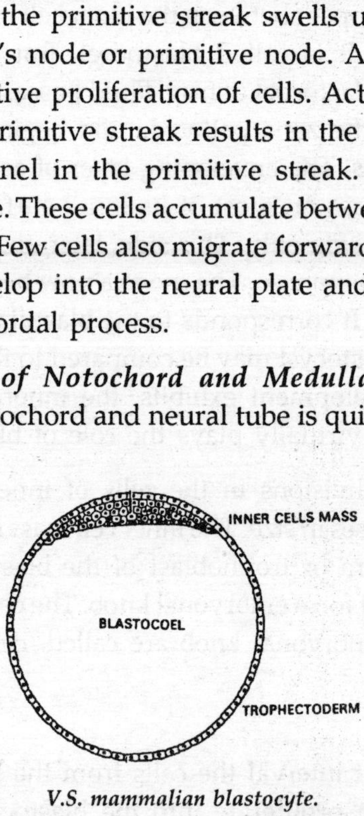

V.S. mammalian blastocyte.

(1) The notochord develops by the proliferation of cells from primitive knob. The area similar to proamnion of chick embryo is missing.

(2) The neural plate or medullary plate develops in front of primitive knob by the migration of cells from the

upper part of primitive streak. Neural tube is formed by the rolling up of the neural plate.

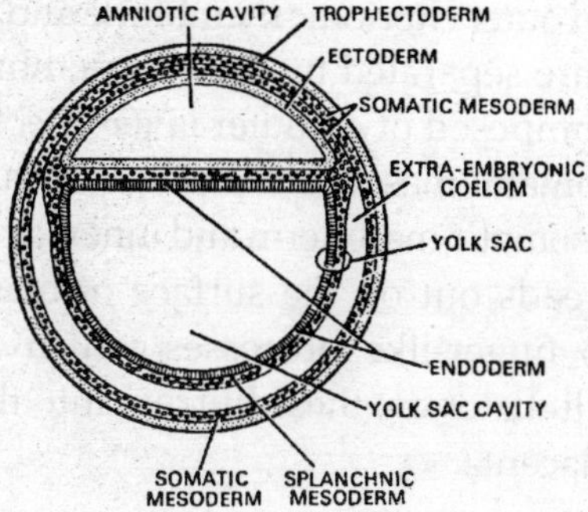

V.S. Embryo at the end of Gastrulation

With the formation of head, tail and lateral folds of mesoderm, the embryo becomes distinct from rest of the blastodisc. The mesoderm of the embryonic disc is called the infra-embryonic mesoderm. It gives rise to mesodermal structures of embryo.

Implantation

By this time the embryo becomes attached to the uterine wall. The process of attachment is known as implantation.

Development of Foetal Membranes

Development of Amnion and Chorion : The foetal membranes are amnion, chorion and allantois. The development of amnion and chorion starts simultaneously. Soon after the appearance of primitive streak, a fold of ectoderm arises from the rim of flattened embryonal disc both from the anterior as well as the posterior ends. These folds are respectively known as head fold and tail fold. These are soon invaded by the somatic layer of mesoderm and the coelom. The tail fold is comparatively longer and grows more rapidly than the head fold. Both the folds increase in size in the opposite direction and approximate each other slightly towards the head end. Later on, they get fused together and the connection is known as seroamniotic connection. The connection disappears afterwards and layers of two folds become continuous. Each fold consists of an outer chorionic membrane and inner amniotic membrane and are separated by the extra-embryonic coelom. The chorion is composed of an outer layer of ectoderm and an inner layer of somatic mesoderm and the amnion consists of an outer layer of somatic mesoderm and inner layer of ectoderm. The chorion spreads out on the surface of blastocyst, and is thrown off into finger-like processes which are known as trophoblastic villi. Later on, these burrow into the uterine wall and form the placenta.

Before the establishment of sero-amniotic connection, the endoderm from the hinder part of the embryo is thrown out into the extra-embryonic coelom in the form of a sac. It is surrounded externally by the splanchnic layer of mesoderm. It is known as allantoic sac. The sac increases in size and

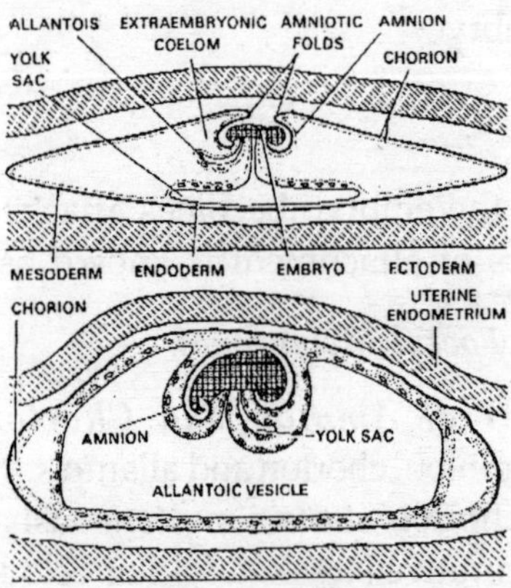

Development of foetal membrane in mammals.

extends in the space between chorion and amnion and later on fuses with them. With the chorion it forms allanto-chorion which consists of outer ectoderm, somatic mesoderm, splanchnic mesoderm and endoderm. The allanto-chorion is the most important layer which plays chief part in the embryonic respiration, excretion and nutrition by developing into a placenta.

Differences in Development between Amnion, Chorion of Bird and Mammal

1. In birds the chorionic ectoderm originates entirely from ectoderm of the extraembryonic blastoderm. It grows out over the yolk. In mammals, on the other hand, the ectoderm of the chorion is continuous with the remaining parts the trophoblast in the extra-embryonic area. The trophoblast thus becomes a part of the chorion. It actually forms the embryonic layer of chorion over most of extra-embryonic surface of the blastocyst.
2. In bird, the amniotic head fold appears first. The tail fold arises by the third day of incubation and it grows slowly towards the amniotic head fold. Therefore, the sero-amniotic connection lies behind the middle of the embryo's body (*i.e.*, towards tail). In mammals, the tail fold often appears earlier than the head fold, and is, therefore, longer of the two. The tail fold grows more rapidly than the head fold. As a result the point of final fusion of the amniotic folds, i.e. the sero-amniotic connection lies above the anterior region of the embryo.

   In pig, however, head and tail folds are virtually equal, and are continuous with the lateral folds which arise coincidently.
3. (a) In birds the head and tail folds of amnion have, from the very start, their complement of somatic mesoderm. In a mammal, the head fold of amnion lacks mesoderm in the beginning for a short while.

(b) Amnion formation by cavitation. In hedgehog, guinea pig, mouse and other more advanced mammals the amniotic cavity arises merely as a space inside the inner cell mass or between the trophoblastic layer and the inner cell mass. The cells giving rise to the embryo proper sink deeper into the blastocyst, so that the formative cells do not appear on the surface. Therefore, the amniotic cavity can no longer be formed by the convergence of amniotic folds. Instead, the amniotic cavity is formed by a chink or small space appearing between cells in the future blastodisc area. This method of formation of the amniotic cavity is called cavitation.

Functions

1. The amnion protects, the embryo from dessication. The embryo is fully immersed and bathed in the amniotic fluid which serves as an artificial swimming pool for the embryo.
2. The amniotic fluid serves as an efficient shock absorber. Being viscous and gelatinous, it protects the delicate embryo from external as well as internal mechanical pressures.
3. The amniotic fluid allows freedom of motion to the embryo.
4. The amnion protects the outer surface of the embryo from adhesion and abrasion.
5. In most mammals a part of the chorion forms finger-like outgrowths called chorionic villi that penetrate into corresponding crypts or depressions in the wall of the uterus. It is at this site where exchange of substances occurs. There is very little or no yolk in marsupial and eutherian eggs, yet a sac develops in their embryos which points to their reptilian ancestry.

In mammals yolk sac begins to form during early gastrulation. In the blastocyst stage, the hypoblast endoderm cells found in the inner cell mass begin to spread along the inner surface on the trophoblast and surround the internal cavity of the blastocyst in the same way as the endodermal cells in reptiles and birds surround the mass of uncleaved egg. The cavity of the blastocyst within the enveloping endodermal layer is referred to as the yolk sac.

Yolk sac in Marsupials : In marsupials *e.g., Didelphys, Opossum,* the yolk sac is well developed, though it contains no yolk. However, a clearly-defined area vasculosa is present on its upper surface. On the opposite side of the sac, the endoderm comes in contact with the trophoblast of the blastocyst. During implantation the trophoblast is produced into folds which fit into corresponding crypts of the uterine wall. The crypts secrete a viscid fluid, the uterine milk, which is absorbed by way of the trophoblast and endoderm. Finally, it reaches the embryo, partly via area vasculosa.

Yolk sac in Pig : Although no yolk is present, a large yolk sac is initially established in pig in a manner comparable to that in birds. The upper part of the yolk sac is highly vascularised and contains vitelline arteries and veins. The lower part of the yolk sac is not vascularised and it absorbs uterine milk from the uterine wall. This nourishing maternal secretion is then transported to the embryo by the vitelline circulation. Thus, although nutritive in function, yolk sac does not have a digestive role. With the enlargement of allantois and formation of placenta the yolk sac rapidly shrivels up and becomes insignificant.

Yolk sac in Rabbit : In rabbit, an area vasculosa is found in the upper part of yolk sac. Its lower wall which is in contact with the trophoblast of blastocyst ruptures. Finally the trophoblast also breaks up at this point and thus the interior of the yolk sac is placed in immediate contact with the uterine cavity.

As a result, the nutritive secretions produced by the uterine wall diffuse into the fluid filling the yolk sac. From here, the uterine secretions are carried to the embryo by the vitelline blood vessels that develop in the splanchnic mesoderm of the yolk sac in its upper part. But this arrangement of conveying nutrient to the embryo is only temporary and is soon replaced by a permanent attachment of the blastocyst to the uterine wall by means of a placenta. Yolk sac is also supposed to assist in respiration and haemopoiesis (formation of blood cells) in the embryo. The stalk of yolk sac and that of allantois together with their blood vessels constitute the umbilical cord.

Development of Allantois

The allantois arises as a ventral outgrowth of the hindgut before the seroamniotic connection is formed. It is composed of splanchnopleure (endoderm + splanchnic mesoderm). The allantois grows very rapidly and soon spreads inside the extra-embryonic coelom. The connection of the allantois to the hindgut is restricted to a narrow neck called allantoic stalk. The allantois soon develops umbilical or allantoic arteries and veins which connect the embryo with the maternal part of the placenta. The free surface of allantois comes in close contact with the inner surface of chorion. In rabbit, the splanchnic mesoderm of allantois fuses with the somatic mesoderm of chorion over a small disc-shaped area to form a membrane called allanto-chorion.

Functions

(1) With the acquisition of viviparity in the marsupials and the placental mammals, the original function of the allantois as a urinary bladder is altogether lost. The carbon dioxide produced by the embryo as well as the urea which is the end-product of the protein metabolism, diffuse into the maternal blood and are excreted by the kidneys of the pregnant mother. As a

result, the storage of waste products in the allantoic cavity is no longer necessary and it becomes greatly reduced.

(2) Blood vessels of allantois supply the embryo with oxygen and nutrient substances from the maternal organism.

Placentation in Mammals

The placenta may be defined as a structure produced by the apposition or fusion of the extraembryonic membranes with the uterine endometrium for the purpose of physiological exchange (Torrey, 1962). Endometrium (Gr. *endon,* within ; *thetra,* uterus) is the mucous membrane lining the uterus. It is composed of a simple columnar secretory epithelium overlying a broad lamina propria. Long tubular glands, the uterine glands are present in the lamina propria. Interglandular stroma is abundant. The placenta, from the point of view of origin, consists of two parts : *(i) a foetal placenta,* and (ii) a *maternal placenta.*

Foetal Placenta: This is formed by extraembryonic membranes. Chorion is the principal component of foetal placenta as it establishes a vascular link between the embryo and the maternal tissues. In mammals there are two possible sources of chorionic vascularization ; (a) the *vitelline circulation* provided by the *yolk sac,* and (b) the *allantoic circulation* provided by the allantois.

Maternal Placenta: It is furnished by a single component, the uterine endometrium.

Placentae are not found exclusively in mammals but appear also in animals belonging to diverse groups of the animal kingdom such as in Protracheatas *(Peripatus),* Tunicata *(Salpa),* Elasmobranchia *(Mustelus laevis)* and certain lizards. The mode of origin and the structure of placenta, however, is different in each case.

The mammalian placentae are classified into different types according to four major criteria. These are as follows :

Types of Placentae According to the Nature of the Foetal Membranes taking Part in the Formation of Placenta

Chorio-vitelline or "Yolk sac" Placenta: It is a primitive type of placenta found in some of the marsupials, *e.g., Didelphys* (opossum) and *Macropus* (kangaroo). In this type of placenta the allantois remains relatively small and never makes contact with the chorion, whereas the yolk sac becomes very large and fuses broadly with the chorion. The latter gets its blood supply from the vitelline blood vessels, *i.e.,* from the yolk sac. The foetal placenta in this case is said to be of the chorio-vitelline type. However, in marsupials the greatly expanded yolk sac bears vascular mesoderm over a restricted area only.

Chorio-allantoic Placenta: In this type of placenta, the yolk sac remains rudimentary. The connection is established between the uterine wall and the embryo by chorion lined by allantois with the allantoic blood vessel system. Thus, allantois furnishes the chorionic circulation. Since the foetal placenta is formed of chorion and allantois, it is called chorio-allantoic placenta. This type of placenta is found in all the Eutheria as well as in some marsupials *(Parameles, Dasyurus).*

In the case of chorio-allantoic placenta the surface of the blastocyst forms finger-like outgrowths known as the chorionic villi that penetrate into depressions or crypts in the wall of the uterus. Such outgrowths are initially formed by the trophoblast, *i e.,* the epithelial layer of chorion, but connective tissue and blood vessels later enter the villi. These blood vessels are ramifications from the allantoic blood vessels. Thus, a vascular chorio-allantoic membrane (allanto-chorion) is established which can be compared to that in the bird embryo, except that in this case, instead of being applied to the inner surface of an egg shell, it lies against the uterine wall.

Chorionic Placenta: The chorionic placenta consists essentially of a greatly thickened layer of trophoblast or chorion containing lacunae or sinuses filled with maternal blood. Chorionic processes or "villi" containing foetal connective tissue and capillaries extend into and across the trophoblastic lacunae. These "villi" are not homologous with the true villi described in connection with the chorio-allantoic placenta. Blood flows into the lacunae, and in this way nutritive substances contained in the blood becomes available to the foetal tissues over a very large surface of the reticulated trophoblast. This type of placenta is found in *human beings.*

The portion of the trophoblast which is nearer to the embryo is known as the cytotrophoblast. The more external lying part of the trophoblast is called syncytiotrophoblast as it is a syncytium of irregular strands with interstices in between. This part of the uterine wall to which the placenta is attached is known as the decidua basalis. The portion of uterine mucosa and epithelium which is reflected over the blastocyst, forming a cover or capsule for it, is called decidua capsularis. The remaining part of the uterine wall with which the thin chorion finally comes in contact, is known as the decidua vera.

Types of Placentae according to the Degree of Connection and the Minute Histological Relations between the Maternal and Foetal Tissues

The foetal placenta has allantoic blood vessels (in the case of chorio-allantoic placentae) or the vitelline blood vessels (in the case of chorio-vitelline placentae). These blood vessels run to and from the foetus whereas maternal vessels run to and from the maternal placenta, furnished by the uterine endometrium. By virtue of this arrangement, the two circulations are brought very close together. However, there is *no fusion of the foetal and maternal blood systems.* Foetal blood does not circulate in the mother ; nor maternal blood circulates in the foetus. All food materials, oxygen, carbon dioxide and urea pass from one circulation to the other through tissue barriers lying between the blood of the mother and of the embryo. The thickness of the partition between the foetal and maternal blood may be decreased by the removal of some of the layers of tissue or barriers lying between. Depending on which layers have disappeared, several types of placentae may be distinguished. The names given to the various histological types indicate the two tissues—one foetal, the other maternal which are in immediate contact with each other.

Epithelio-chorial Placenta: When the chorionic epithelium makes a contact with the uterine epithelium, the placenta is designated as an epithelio-chorial placenta. During their growth, the chorionic villi push in the wall of the uterus and later lie in pocket-like crypts of the uterine wall. This type of placenta is found in *all marsupials* and in the *ungulates (horses, asses, pig).* In the case of an epithelio-chorial placenta six layers of tissue or barriers lie between the foetal and maternal blood streams. A molecule of oxygen, for example, in diffusing from the blood of the mother to that of the embryo, would pass through in the following order :

1. The endothelial wall of the maternal blood vessel.
2. The connective tissue around the maternal blood vessel (endometrial connective tissue).
3. The uterine epithelium.
4. The epithelium of the chorion.
5. Connective tissue of the chorion.
6. The endothelial wall of the blood vessel in the chorion.

The epithelio-chorial placenta, presenting apposition of foetal and maternal components and six tissue barriers between the two blood streams, is supposed to be the primitive type from which other have been derived. These derivations indicate a changeover from apposition to some degree of fusion of the two halves of the placenta.

Syndesmo-chorial Placenta : In this type of placenta, the foetal and maternal components are fused so intimately as to result in a destruction of the uterine epithelium. As a result, chorion comes into contact with the endomaterial connective tissues (desmose). Only five barriers, therefore, intervene between the two blood streams. Syndesmochorial placenta is found in the *ruminant* (cud- chewing), *ungulates, e.g., camel, giraffe, goat, sheep, buffalo, cow* and *reindeer.*

Endothelio-chorial Placenta: If the destruction involves the uterine epithelium and the underlying connective tissue which is reduced, the chorionic epithelium comes into direct contact with the endothelial walls of maternal blood vessels. A placenta is then formed which is called an endothelio-chorial placenta. In this case the number of barriers between foetal and maternal blood streams is reduced to four. A placenta of this type is characteristic of the carnivores, *e.g., dog,* all "cats" including *house cat, lion, tiger,* etc. *fox, bear, mongoose, walrus.*

Haemo-chorial Placenta: A reduction of the barriers to three is found in the primates *(e.g.,* lemur, apes, women) many insectivores, bats and rodents. This type of placenta is called the haemo-chorial placenta in which the endothelium of the maternal blood vessels also disappears and the chorionic villi are bathed directly in maternal blood. Actually, the chorionic villi are surrounded by sinuses into which maternal blood enters through the arteries of the uterus and from which the blood flows into the uterine veins.

Haemo-endothelial Placenta: In this type of placenta all the three maternal tissues and two foetal tissues, *i.e.,* chorionic epithelium and chorionic connective tissues are completely eroded so that the foetal blood vessels dip into blood lacunae of the uterus. The number of barriers between the maternal and foetal blood streams, therefore, is reduced to just one. This type of placenta is found in higher rodents, *e.g., rat, guinea pig* and in the *rabbit.*

Types of Placentae According to the Fate of Uterine Endometrium at Parturition : The process by which the foetus is expelled from the body of the mother to terminate the period of gestation is called birth or parturition. Depending on the nature of contact between maternal and foetal components, three types of placentae may be recognized.

Non-deciduous Placenta or Semiplacenta: In the case of epithelio-chorial placentae, at parturition the chorionic villi are simply drawn out from the crypts in the wall of the uterus. Thus maternal and foetal tissues are separated without any damage to the uterine wall and no bleeding takes place. This type of placenta is also called a semiplacenta as there is a mere apposition of the foetal and maternal components. Non deciduous placenta is found in all marsupials and in odd-toed ungulates *e.g.*, horse, ass, zebra and tapir.

Deciduous Placenta or Placenta Vera: In other mammals the union of the maternal and foetal tissues is so intimate that at parturition not only the foetal component of the placenta is shed, but a variable amount of maternal tissue is torn away as well. An open would is left on the wall of the uterus and bleeding inevitably occurs. Placentae of this type are known as deciduous placentae, and the uterine wall participating in the formation of such a placenta is called the decidua. This type of placenta is also called placenta vera or true placenta because the chorionic villi fuse with the eroded uterine endometrium. The bleeding at parturition is normally stopped by the contraction of the muscular wall of the uterus which constricts the blood-vessels. It slows down the flow of blood, until clotting of the blood stops the haemorrhage altogether.

Contra-deciduate Placenta: In *Parameles* and *Talpa* (mole) that develop a non- deciduous placenta, even the foetal part of the placenta is not passed out at parturition. Instead, it is retained in the uterus where it is broken down and absorbed. This type of placenta is called contra-deciduate placenta.

Types of Placentae According to the Arrangement of Villi on the Blastocyst : In different mammals the placenta is further classified into six types according to the distribution and arrangement of villi on the surface of chorion.

Diffuse Placenta: The villi are uniformly distributed all over the surface of the chorion except the extreme ends. It is found in the ungulates, *e.g., pig, mare* etc.

Cotyledonary Placenta: *In cattle, sheep and goat,* the villi are found in groups or patches called cotyledons while the rest of the chorion surface is smooth. The placenta of this type is known as the cotyledonary placenta.

Intermediate Placenta: In this type the isolated villi are scattered between the "cotyledons." Thus the blastocyst is provided both with the villi and the cotyledons, *e.g., camel* and *giraffe.*

Zonary Placenta: In carnivores, *e.g., dog, cat, lion, tiger, fox, mongoose* etc., the villi are developed in the form of a belt around the middle of their blastocyst which is generally elliptical in shape.

Discoidal Placenta: The villi are restricted to a small disc-shaped area of the blastocyst. The functional placenta therefore, has the shape of a disc and is known as the discoida placenta. Example are *insectivores, bat, bear, rodents* (rat, guinea pig, porcupine) and *rabbit.* In the *monkeys,* the placenta consists of two discs and is, therefore, called a bidiscoidal placenta.

Metadiscoidal Placenta: The metadiscoidal placenta is found in *human beings* and the anthropoid *apes.* The early blastocyst is at first all covered with villi but later they disappear from its free surface, persisting on a small disc-shaped area attached to the uterine wall. This secondarily discoidal placenta is known as the metadiscoidal placenta.

The important details of the various types of placentae are summarised in Table.

S. No.	*Placenta (Histological types)*	*Maternal component (Uterine endometrium)* Endo-thel.	Conn. Tissue	Epi-thel.	*Foetal component* Epi-thel.	Conn. Tissue	Endo-thel.	*Arrange-ment of the villi.*	*Fate of Endo-metrium*	*Common Examples*
1.	Epithelio-chorial	P	P	P	P	P	P	Diffuse	Non-deciduous	Pig, Horse, Marsupials
2.	Syndesmo-chorial	P	P	A	P	P	P	Cotyle-donary	Transi-tional	Sheep, Cow
3.	Endothelio-chorial	P	A	A	P	P	P	Zonaryto Discoidal	Deciduous	Cat, Dog
4.	Haemo-chorial	A	A	A	P	P	P	Metadis coidal or Zonary	Deciduous	Apes, Women Rodents
5.	Haemo-endothelial	A	A	A	A	A	P	Discoidal	Deciduous	Guinea pig, Rabbit

P = Tissue present; A = Tissue absent.

Physiology of the Placenta

A. Positive Role

1. The placenta provides nourishment and oxygen to the embryo. *Water, oxygen* and small moleculed substances such as *monosaccharides, salts* of sodium, potassium and magnesium *diffuse* through the placenta from the maternal blood into the foetal blood. Some substances, e.g., *vitamins* pass by active transport. Passage of the proteins is effected by pinocytosis at the surface of the trophoblast.

2. It serves as an excretory organ of the foetus. Foetal metabolic wastes like urea and carbon dioxide pass from foetal to maternal blood through placenta.

3. The placental barrier existing between the maternal and the foetal blood prevents a direct contact of the two blood streams. This is very important for the foetus because the pressure of the maternal blood is far two high for the foetal blood vessels.

4. The placenta acts like a semipermeable membrane, blowing some substances to pass through but keeping out others. It prevents the passage of harmful materials (blood proteins, sex hormones etc.) from the maternal blood into the foetal circulation.

5. The placenta confers immunity upon the foetus against certain diseases, such as diphtheria, scarlet fever, smallpox and measles. The protein antibodies which have developed in the blood of a mother who has acquired immunity against these diseases are passed to the foetus through the placenta. Thus, the foetus becomes passively immunized against the said diseases in the first period afterbirth.

6. The placenta stores fat, glycogen and iron for the embryo, before its liver is developed.

7. The placenta functions as an endocrine gland. It secretes four important hormones in human female and most placental mammals. They are *estradiol, progesterone, chorionicgonadotropic hormone* and *placental lactogen.* These hormones help in maintaining pregnancy, abortion or premature birth. In some mammals such as rabbit, guinea pig and cow it also produces *relaxin* that relaxes public symphysis and thus facilitates birth of the young one.

B. Negative Role

1. Certain pathogenic Organism and viruses can penetrate through the placenta. They infect the foetus if the mother is infected. This is known to happen in infections with syphilis, smallpox, chickenpox and measles.
2. Certain drugs used medicinally may cross the placental I barrier and could harm the embryo. For example, the drug I *thalidomide,* which was used as a sedative, when taken by women in early pregnancy, caused non-perforation of the anus, and serious defects in the development of limbs and the heart.

6

Development of Fowl

Development of Chick

The Chick or fowl *(Gallus domesticus)* belongs to order Galliformes of superorder neognathae of class Apes (Vertebrata). The study of its development has been connected with such pioneers as Malpighi (1672), Wolff (1759), and Von Baer (1828). The hen's egg has long been a favourite cleidoic egg for development study because of the following reasons : (*i*) the eggs are large, easily available throughout the year and easily incubated artificially; (*ii*) its developmental purposes; (*iii*) the Chick embryo possesses certain very significant extra-embryonic membranes and appendages which also occur in the mammals, though in a somewhat modified condition; and *(iv)* the general development of chick is more nearly mammalian than that of reptiles and amphibians.

Nature of the Fertilized Egg

The fully formed and newly laid fertilized *egg* of hen is elliptical in shape with one end broader than the other. It is about 7 cm long and 5 cm broad. Since the egg is surrounded by a waterproof, calcareous shell, it is called cleidoic egg. Cleidoic means box-like. Such eggs are fully laden with rich, nourishing yolk and become, self-sufficient, but for the gaseous exchange. The avian egg contains enormous amount of yolk, hence called macrolecithal or megalecithal or polylecithal. Again, since the yolk occupies the largest portion of the egg except a small disc-shaped area of the cytoplasm (blastodisc), the egg is called a discoidal egg. The polarity of the egg is well-marked ; the ovum contains a nucleus placed in the blastodisc which always floats at the animal pole of the ovum.

The Ovum

The actual ovum of a bird is the part of the "egg" that is commonly spoken of as "yolk". The term egg, therefore, includes not only the ovum proper *i.e.*, the "yolk" but also all its tertiary membranes. Food resources, make up the bulk of the ovum ; the cytoplasm of the cell is confined to a small plate, termed the blastodisc. It is approximately 3.0 mm in diameter and occupies the animal pole.

At first the nucleus occupies the centre of the ovum, and the yolk granules begin to be formed in the cytoplasm around it. This yolk is of a light colour and termed white yolk. The central mass of the white yolk thus deposited is known as the latebra. After this, the peripheral layer of the protoplasm starts depositing around the latebra a darker coloured yellow yolk. The deposit of yellow yolk is interrupted by intermittent, generally thinner, layers of more white yolk. As a result the latebra becomes surrounded by alternate concentric rings of yellow and white yolk.

The ovum gradually enlarges in size due to a sustained increase in the yolk deposit. Concomitantly, the nucleus leaves its central location and takes a peripheral position. As a result, the yellow layer gets everywhere interrupted along the path which the nucleus has taken. There is a continuous deposit of white yolk along this path which extends from the latebra almost to the surface. It is known as the neck of the latebra. Just beneath the blastodisc, the mass of white yolk spreads slightly to form a plate, the nucleus of Pander.

Most of the yolk of bird's egg is liquid, but about 23% is in the form of solid yolk spheres. According to Romanoff and Romanoff (1949), the general chemical composition of the yolk is as follows :

(i) Water : 48.7 per cent

(ii) Proteins : 16.6 per cent

(iii) Phospholipids and fats : 32.6 per cent

(iv) Carbohydrates : 1 per cent.

The proteins of the avian yolk are *phosvitin* and *lipovitellin*. Part of lipovitellin is bound to phosvitin; this part of the yolk protein is insoluble in water. The residual part of the lipovitellin, referred to as "Livetin" (Flickinger, 1961), is water soluble. About 50% of the fatty protein of avian yolk is *neutral fat*, and the rest comprises *phosphatides* and *cholesterol*. The carbohydrates of the yolk are free *glucose* and *polysaccharides*.

The entire ovum or "yolk" including the blastodisc is invested by a plasma membrane.

Fertilized and Meiosis

During ovulation, meiosis, and fertilization the nucleus of the oocyte greatly enlarges and is known as the germinal vesicle. The first maturation division and the extrusion of the first polar body occurs about 4½ hours previous to ovulation. Completion of maturation and the formation of the second polar body take place after sperm penetrate the ovum. In birds, polyspermy prevails ; some three to five spermatozoa may enter the chicken's ovum. Only one of these, however, completes fertilization by fusing with the egg nucleus; the remainder are shunted into the yolk wherein they shortly degenerate. The oocyte is fertilized in the upper part of the oviduct before the deposition of the albumen around it.

The Application of Accessory Layers around the Fertilized Ovum

Following fertilization, as the ovum ("yolk") passes down the oviduct, it acquires, enroute layers of albumen, shell membranes, and shell. The oviducal journey is completed between twenty four to twenty five hours. During this period cleavage takes place and germ-layer formation is initiated.

Beside the plasma membrane, the yellow of the egg, which is the true egg cell, is enveloped by primary and secondary egg membranes. In all, these are five in number.

Vitelline Membrane: It is the innermost egg membrane that covers the surface of the yellow of the egg. This is a primary egg membrane which is actually double in its origin. The inner layer of the vitelline membrane is produced in the ovary, in the space between the oocyte and the follicle cells. This layer is made up of very rough fibres. An outer layer which is more finely fibrous, is secreted around the inner layer when the egg enters the upper portion of the fallopian tube (Bellairs, 1963). The vitelline membrane serves to separate the yolk from the albumen and to preserve differences in water content and osmotic pressure. It is to be remembered that the yolk contains about 50 per cent water, while the albumen has about 85 per cent.

The remaining egg membranes *i.e., layers of albumen* ; inner the outer *shell membranes;* and calcareous *shell* are tertiary in their origin.

Albumen or White of the Egg: Following the vitelline membrane is the white of egg or the albumen. It consists of 85% water and the remaining 15% is a mixture of several proteins, mostly albumen. The albumen is deposited in four layers namely, (*i*) a chalaziferous layer, (*ii*) and inner thin albumen, (*iii*) a middle dense albumen, and an outer thin albumen.

The innermost layer of albumen called the chalaziferous layer surrounds the ovum proper. It is made up to very viscous albumen, a glycoprotein. At each side of the yolk opposite each end of the shell this layer is spirally twisted into cords, the chalazae. 1 hey are produced by the rotation of the egg in the oviduct. The chalazae keep the rotation of the egg in the oviduct. The chalazae keep the blastodisc up always in whatever direction the egg is turned. The *chalazae* and the *chalaziferous layer* are products of uterus.

There occurs a very narrow layer of thin watery albumen immediately outside the chalaziferous layer. This part of thin albumen is secreted by uterus.

The middle layer of dense albumen is relatively dense and wide. Its density is apparently due to the presence of mucin threads. All of the dense albumen is secreted by magnum part of the oviduct through which the fertilized egg passes in a duration of about three hours.

The outer thin albumen is a fair wide layer of thin watery albumen that surrounds the dense albumen. A small fraction of thin albumen is said to be secreted in the isthmus part of the oviduct but it is in the uterus where practically all of the thin albumen is differentiated.

Besides providing protection, the egg white serves also as an additional source of nourishment and is gradually used up during the development of the embryo.

Outer and Inner Shell Membranes: The egg white or albumen is bounded externally by two layers of shell membranes. The two membranes adhere closely over most of the surface of the egg but are separated by an air space at the blunt end of the egg. The inner membrane adheres to the albumen whereas the outer membranes adheres to the shell. The shell membranes consist of fibres of keratin matted together. The egg passes through isthmus part of the oviduct in about 74 minutes wherein it receives the shell membranes.

Calcareous Shell: It is the outermost egg membrane consisting chiefly of calcium carbonate ($CaCO_3$), about 5 gm. in a hen's egg. The white or fawn-coloured shell is pierced by about 7000 fine pores which are filled by an organic substance related to collagen. Shell is entirely secreted by the uterus. Here the egg remains for about 20 hours. The shell is soft and flexible in a newly-laid egg, but soon becomes hard and brittle.

Cleavage and Blastulation

While the egg is passing down the oviduct and receiving its outer coverings, cleavage becomes practically completed. As the mass of inert yolk is very great, a macrolecithal condition prevails, and the yolk itself does not become subdivided. Segmentation involves only the blastodisc, which at the time of the first cleavage is about 3 mm in diameter and 0.5 mm thick. Cleavage is, therefore described, as being meroblastic (partial), in contrast to the holoblastic (total) cleavage seen in eggs containing moderate or small amounts of yolk. In birds, the cleavage is also said to be discoidal, as it is confined only to a disc of cytoplasm, the blastodisc. By the time the "egg" is laid the embryo is in the blastula stage. It takes place in the following manner :

The First Cleavage: The first division appears as an irregular furrow in about the middle of the blastodisc. The furrow not only falls short of the margin of the disc, but also fails to cut completely through the depth of the disc. This results in two incompletely separated blastomeres whose cytoplasmic contents are continuous around the ends of and beneath the furrow. The first cleavage is completed during the passage of the magnum of oviduct.

The Second and Third Cleavage: The second cleavage furrow is approximately perpendicular to the middle of the first furrow, and is of about the same depth. Like the first cleavage furrow, the second furrow neither reaches the margin of the blastodisc nor cuts entirely through its depth. The second cleavage furrow begins to form as the egg enters the isthmus part of the oviduct. There thus arise four cells, into each of which the furrow of the third cleavage soon appears.

The third cleavage furrows are formed roughly at right angles to the second. Showing considerable variability, however, these divisions produce eight incomplete separated blastomeres. From here onwards the pattern of cleavage becomes very irregular.

The Central and Marginal Cells: Following the third cleavage, further furrows soon appear, which result in the production of approximately sixteen cells. As seen from the surface, the blastoderm becomes differentiated into two groups of blastomeres : (1) completely bounded central cells formed by the cutting off of the inner ends of the original incomplete cells, and (2) incompletely bounded marginal cells produced by furrows running in a radial direction. As the process of cleavage goes on these marginal cells are constantly cut off and added to the central cells. Mean while, beyond them more marginal cells arise by peripheral, radial divisions that ultimately reach the margin of the disc. In this manner the central segmented area continually increases in diameter. A peripheral rim of unsegmented cytoplasm surrounding the central region of the blastoderm is known as the periblast. It is slightly darker in colour than the central portion, and is about 0.5 mm wide.

The Blastoderm and the Subgerminal Cavity: The third set of cleavage furrows, although originally shallow and vertical like the first two, soon curve so as to run horizontally and parallel to the surface. In this manner, the third cleavage furrows undercut the cytoplasm and separate it from the yolk. This process is repeated as the central cells increase in number. As a result the area of central cells becomes free from the underlying yolk while the marginal cells remain in contact with the yolk. Two other events take place at the same time : (1) the yolk underneath the central area liquefies, and (2) divisions of the blastomeres in planes parallel to the surface bring a stratification of cells. The result is a compact plate, acquiring a thickness of several cells, which is called the blastoderm.

The freeing of the central cells from the yolk creates a subgerminal cavity that is filled with the liquefied yolk. The subgerminal cavity at this stage may be regarded as the equivalent of the blastocoel, and the embryo is now in the blastula stage. The blastula of chick is in the form of a disc, hence called a discoblastula.

The Area Pellucida and Area Opaca: Seen from above by transmitted light, the blastoderm at the discoblastula stage shows two distinct areas : (1) a relatively clear area, the area pellucida, lying centrally, and (2) a narrower, darker zone surrounding it, the area opaca. The translucency of the area pellucida is due to the presence of the subgerminal cavity under the layer of central blastomeres while the area opaca corresponds to the extend of the marginal cells still in contact with the opaque yolk.

During the later course of development the embryo will be formed entirely within the area pellucida. On the other hand, the area opaca is involved with the digestion of yolk and, ultimately, with the formation of extraembryonic membranes and blood vessels.

Fate Map of Chick Embryo (Discoblastula): The blastoderm in birds consists of two parts : the area pellucida and the area opaca. The area opaca does not take any part in the formation of the body of the embryo. Instead, it gives rise to the extraembryonic ectoderm which during later developmental stages forms extra-embryonic membranes and blood vessels of area vasculosa. Therefore, the fate map, in so far as the parts of the embryo are concerned, is restricted to the area pellucida. Furthermore, the blastoderm is bilaminar, consisting of epiblast and hypoblast which have different fates in the course of their embryonic development. As a result, fat maps have to be made out for each of the two layers separately. Reconstruction of the fate map in avian embryo consisted of marking the blastoderm by vital staining (Watzel, 1929 and Pasteels, 1940), or of marking with carbon particles (Spratt, 1946). The marking was done either on blastoderms cultivated in vitro, or in situ in the egg, after a piece was cut out from the shell.

The Fate Map for the Epiblast gives an indication of prospective ectoderm and mesoderm.

1. The anterior half of the epiblast area of the pellucida is prospective epidermis. It also contains material for the extra-embryonic membranes.

2. A crescentic area occupying the rear of the epidermis and lying almost in the middle for the area pellucida is presumptive embryonic neural system.

3. Behind the neural tissue, in the middle, lies the presumptive notochord.

   Neural tissue and the presumptive notochord do not extend to the sides.

4. According to Waddington, 1952, the area containing somitic mesoderm (presumptive somites) is situated in the midline behind the notochordal area. Most of the posterior half of the area pellucida is occupied by the material giving rise to the mesodermal lining of the body cavity (ventrolateral mesoderm). It also includes the extraembryonic mesoderm which does not contribute to the formation of the embryo proper.

According to Torrey, 1962, just behind the notochord lies the prechordal mesoderm. This is flanked on each side by the somitic mesoderm. The lateral mesoderm destined to produce embryonic and extraembryonic parts, is present at the rear of the area opaca.

The epiblast also contains some prospective endoderm cells but they are very few in number and are not concentrated as a separate area. These cells are derived from the midline of the posterior part of the area pellucida.

The Fate Map for the hypoblast points out that the latter is Mainly prospective endoderm, though only a small part of it actually gets incorporated into the alimentary canal of the embryo. The remaining part gives rise to the lining of the yolk sac.

Gastrulation

The process of gastrulation in the Chick was studied by Chen, Hunt, Rawles, Rudnick, Woodside, Pasteels, Peter and Spratt. It is separable into three distinct phases : (1) *laying down of the embryonic endoderm* ; (2) *formation of the primitive streak* and *mesoderm* ; and (3) *formation of the embryonic axial* and *paraxial structures*.

Formation of Endoderm. The first step in gastrulation is marked by the appearance within the subgerminal cavity of a second cell layer, the hypoblast which, with later additions from the primitive streak, becomes the embryonic *endoderm*. After the formation of the hypoblast the upper layer is called the epiblast which encompasses prospective *ectoderm* and *mesoderm*. The space between the hypoblast and the underlying yolk then becomes the archenteron. There are different theories regarding the origin of hypoblast. They are as follows :

(a) *Theory of Involution:* This theory was proposed by Patterson (1909). According to this theory the hypoblast originates by involution of marginal cells through a temporary incontinency in the zone of junction along a small part of the blastoporal ring. At present, this theory is not accepted.

(b) *Theory of Invagination:* According to this theory, proposed by Jacobson (1938), the posterior end of the blastoderm invaginates into the subgerminal cavity to form a small pocket. The cavity of the pocket is the archenteron and the floor and roof become the endoderm. This theory is also not entertained now-a-days.

(c) *Theory of Infiltration:* This theory was proposed by Peter (1938). According to this theory, the individual cells detach themselves from the surface layer near the *posterior end of the blastoderm.* These cells then wander in within the subgerminal cavity and grow forwards as a new layer, the endoderm. Peter was of the opinion that the process of infiltration took place mainly toward the future posterior side, with a subsequent forward movement. According Pasteels (1945), it takes place more or less all over the area pellucida. Later, this sheet of embryonic endoderm becomes continuous with the extra embryonic endoderm around the margins of the blastoderm.

(d) *Theory of Elimination:* This theory was proposed by Spratt (1946). According to this theory, the many-celled thick blastoderm splits into two layers, an upper epiblast which includes future *ectoderm* and *mesoderm,* and a layer hypoblast which with later additions becomes the *endoderm.*

In birds the endoderm has a double origin: some of the cells are derived from the hypoblast whereas other endodermal cells are derived from the primitive streak. Some of the endodermal cells arising from the hypoblast are used for the formation of the alimentary canal of the embryo. Most of these cells, however, become the endodermal lining of the yolk sac. The endodermal cells derived from the primitive streak join up with the endodermal cells arising from the hypoblast after a process of invagination. These cells remain in the median strip of the endodermal layer which is used up for the formation of the walls of the alimentary canal.

Formation of the Primitive Streak and Mesoderm: After the separation of the endoderm, the next phase in gastrulation is concerned with the inward migration of the mesoderm and part of the endoderm in a special region inside the area pellucida. This region is a narrow strip of blastoderm which begins to appear at the posterior edge of the area pellucida. It gradually extends forward along the midline of the embryo and occupies about 3/5th of the entire length of the area pellucida. This strip of blastoderm becomes thickened during the stages of gastrulation and known as the primitive streak. The thickening of the blastoderm is brought about by a convergence of the upper-layer cells towards the midline. This results in a heaping up of prospective mesodermal and notochordal cells along the midline. The accumulation of cells is seen on the surface of the blastoderm as a dark or opaque streak, the primitive streak. It first becomes visible in the hindmost part of the area pellucida and is called the short primitive streak.

The early primitive streak is broad and its edges are vaguely indicated. The streak now elongated by the concentration of more and more material from the parts of the epiblast lying farther out laterally and anterolaterally toward the midline. Cells from these regions swing in a curve backward and inward to take the place of parts of the epiblast shifting toward the midline. The mature primitive streak becomes narrower and quite sharply delimited. This is called the definitive primitive streak.

When the primitive streak is fully developed, there runs a narrow furrow, the primitive groove along the middle of the streak. At the anterior end of the primitive streak there is a thickening, the primitive knot or Hensen's node. It is formed of cells from the prospective notochordal area and those which will form the floor of the neural tube. The centre of Hensen's node is excavated to form a funnel-shaped depression. The sides of the primitive groove are sometimes designated as the primitive folds.

During gastrulation in the birds, the cells move downward singly, though there are many cells moving in the same direction. As a result, the regular epithelial arrangement of cells found in the epiblast becomes lost. This type of gastrulation movement is called inunigration. Soon the migrating cells reach the hypoblast and join with the cells of this layer. The direction of movement is mainly downward from the surface of the blastoderm toward the hypoblast, but the migrating cells also spread out sideways and forward from the anterior end of the primitive streak. The formation of a furrow (the primitive groove) along the midline of the primitive streak and the funnel-shaped depression in the centre of Hensens node are due to immigration of cells from the surface of the blastoderm into the interior.

Formation of Embryonic Axial and Paraxial Structures

Head Process or Notochord Process: The association of prospective notochord with the anterior end of the primitive streak is manifested by a noticeably thickening, the primitive knot or Hensen's knot. Hensen's knot is indicative of a special type of movement: the midline movement of cells. The prospective notochordal cells start moving as a dense mass in the midline straight forward from Hensen's knot underneath the surface of the epiblast. The tongue of notochordal cells is called the head process or the notochordal process. It can be easily distinguished from the surrounding (mainly mesodermal) cells. The establishment of the head process marks the completion of the elongation of the primitive streak.

The head process actually consists of a thicker *central mass of cells* and more diffuse *lateral wings.* The thinker central portion alone gives rise to the definitive notochord, whereas the lateral wings contribute to the paraxial (somatic) mesoderm that comes to flank the notochord.

The Somites: The area of prospective somites lies in the anterior part of the primitive streak. From this part of the streak, the somite material (dorsal mesoderm) invaginates into the interior and becomes distributed in a strip on each side of the notochordal process. After formation of the notochord, the dorsal mesoderm becomes subdivided into segments—the somites. The segmentation proceeds from the anterior to the posterior end. It has been observed that one pair of somites is formed for every hour after 20 hours of incubation and the process continues upto about 40 hours regularly. Therefore, an embryo with 4 pairs of somites is 24 hours old; an embryo with 16 pairs of somites is 36 hours old and so on. Thus, the total number of somites present at a given stage of the embryo is added to 20 to determine the age of Chick embryo.

The fully formed Chick gastrula has three germ layers : ectoderm, mesoderm and endoderm.

Differentiation of Mesoderm (Intermediate and Lateral Plate) : The mesoderm is formed as two sheets of cells, one on either side of the notochord. It is divided into three regions : *(i)* a dorsal mesoderm that gives rise to somites as mentioned in the previous section, *(ii)* an intermediate mesoderm and *(iii)* the lateral plate mesoderm.

Intermediate Mesoderm or Nephrotome: It is also segmented and give rise to the excretory organs of the embryo. The intermediate mesoderm is represented by a narrow strip of cells that unite a somite to the lateral plate mesoderm.

Lateral Plate Mesoderm: Prospective lateral plate mesoderm is contained in the posterior part of the primitive streak. From here, cells of the prospective lateral plate mesoderm migrate downward, outward and forward. Later on, they are found as sheets on each side of the embryo as a lateral continuation of the dorsal mesoderm.

The lateral sheets for a time remain connected with the somites by means of the nephortomes. After this, the mesoderm of the lateral plate splits into two layers; the external somatic or parietal mesoderm and the internal splanchnic or visceral mesoderm. The somatic mesoderm together with the ectoderm constitutes somatopleure, whereas the splanchnic mesoderm together with the endoderm is called splanchnopleure.

The Coelom

The space enclosed between the somatic and splanchnic layers of mesoderm is known as a coelom. Since it is formed by a splitting of the mesoderm, it is called a schízocoel. The coelom present within the embryo is known as inter-embryonic coelom. Later, it spreads peripherally in the extraembryonic region where it is called the extraembryonic coelom.

Disappearance of the Primitive Streak : The over-all-elongation of the primitive streak during gastrulation is accompanied by a change of the area pellucida from a circular shape to a pear-shaped outline. The elongation of the primitive streak is, however, only temporary. As the prospective notochordal and mesodermal cells migrate into the interior of the embryo, the material of which the primitive streak consists becomes gradually exhausted. But the end of gastrulation, the whole primitive streak shrinks. The residue becomes partly incorporated into the tailbud, and partly into the coccal region of the embryo.

Development of Neural Tube (Neurulation) : The neurulation proceeds in an anteroposterior direction. The ectoderm above and along each side of the head process gets somewhat thickened and is called the medullary plate. A depression appears running down the middle of the medullary plate and on each side of this depression, the lateral parts of the plate rise up as two parallel ridges. The depression is called the medullary or neural groove, while the ridges are known as the medullary or neural folds. The anterior parts of the neural folds converge toward the mid-dorsal line until they meet and fuse. It results in the formation of a thick-walled tube, the neural tube which encloses a large cavity, the neural canal.

The neural tube remains open at the anterior end for sometime. This opening is called the neuropore which is closed during the first day of incubation. After the fusion of the neural folds in the mid-dorsal line, the neural tube separates itself completely from the overlying epidermis. As the neural tube is being separated from the ectoderm, a few loose cells are liberated into the space between the dorsal part of the neural tube and the surface ectoderm. These cells arrange themselves in the form of two bands on the dorsolateral wall of the neural tube. These bands are the neural crests which develop into the branchial skeleton, nerve ganglia, sensory nerves and adrenal medulla.

Development of Chick According to the Hours of Incubation

I. Summary of the Condition at the end of the First Day of Incubation (4-somite Stage)

Gastrulation is over by the end of the first day of incubation. The developments completed by this period are summarized below :

1. The dark peripheral area opaca and central translucent clear area pellucida are distinctly visible.
2. A primitive streak with a primitive groove bound by

primitive folds runs in the middle of the posterior half of the area pellucida.

3. At the anterior end of the primitive streak is present a thickening, the Hensen's node or primitive knot having a small depression in centre which is called the Hensen's pit.
4. Four pairs of somites are present, lying in front of the Primitive knot. They are connected with the mesoderm of the respective lateral plates by the longitudinal nephroto mal bonds.
5. The neural folds have appeared in the region in front of the Primitive knot. They have fused for a short space at their anterior ends forming the neural tube. The first part of the neural tube represents prospective forebrain.
6. In the anterior most part of the embryo, the ectoderms has given rise to the head fold.
7. The endoderm underlying the ectoderm is also transformed into a pocket like structure, the foregut.
8. Beneath the fore-gut, the walls of the amino-cardiac portions of the *coelom* meet each other at the end of 24 hours. These represent the rudiment of the pericardial cavity.
9. Proamnion is a small and comparatively more translucent region of the area pellucida lying in the anterior region. It lacks mesoderm.
10. Blood vessels and corpuscles have started to appear in the inner part of the area opaca, transforming it into the area vasculosa. The latter is beginning to be bounded by a blood vessel, the sinus terminalis.

II. 48 Hours Chick Embryo (25 Pairs of Somites)

Flexures: The embryo at this stage is like an inverted 'J'. This shape is due to two bendings or flexures in the head region of the embryo. One of the bendings, called carnial flexure lies at the level of the mesencephalon. By this flexure the anterior region of the brain is directed backwards. The second flexure, called cervica flexure is seen at the level of rhombencephalon. On account of these bendings, a transverse section of the embryo at the anterior end exhibits two neural tubes, two notochords and two foreguts.

Torsion: Former to this stage, the embryo lies with its ventral surface in contact with the yolk. But now the embryo is partially turned with the result that the anterior part of the body is twisted to the right side. This process of twisting of the entire embryo along the antero-posterior axis is referred to as torsion. This is quite apparent in somites 10 and 11.

Nervous system: The *neural folds* have met along the mid-dorsal line and the *neuropore* is closed. The brain is differentiated into three distinct divisions, namely, *prosencephalon*, *mesencephalon* and *rhombencephalon*.

Eye: The optic vesicle invaginates to form *optic-cup*. The ectoderm facing the optic vesicle thickens to form a *lens*.

Ear: There are *two auditory vesicles*, one on each side of the hind brain. In this stage, the mouth of the auditory vesicle is seen to be reduced to a small aperture.

Heart: The heart is tubular in shape. It has two *auricles*, a distinct *ventricle* and a *truncus arteriosus*. Two *aortic arches* are present. *Vitelline arteries* lie between somites, eighteen and twenty.

Alimentary Canal: The foregut is well formed and shows three divisions *viz.*, the *preoral gut*, the *pharynx* and the *oesophagus*.

The pharynx develops three pairs of lateral outpocketings called *visceral pouches*. These are separated from each other by solid bars known as *branchial arches*. The pharynx is closed ventrally by a double layered membrane called *pharyngeal membrane.* The hind gut begins to appear.

Excretory System: The pronephric tubules and ducts develop but they are solid in nature and hence non-functional. The mesonephric tubules begin to appear.

Foetal Membranes: The somatopleure grows over the head as folds to form the amnion and chorion. The *seroamniotic connection* becomes thin.

Tail Bud: It begins to develop posterior to the hind gut.

III. 72 Hours Chick Embryo (35 Pairs of Somites)

Flexures: In addition to the cranial and cervical flexures which were formed in the 48 hours embryo, two more new flexures appear. These are : (a) dorsal flexure in the lumbar region and (b) caudal flexure in the tail region. Caudal flexure causes tail to be at an angle of 90° to the body. As a results of flexure, the embryo acquires a typical shape of the mirror image of a question mark (?).

Torsion: The process of torsion continues throughout the development of the embryo as a result of which the entire embryo lies on its left side in the yolk.

Nervous System: The regions of the brain are well-demarcated. The cerebral hemispheres bulge outwards, the wall of the mesencephalon thickens to form crura cerebri and the *corpora quadrigemina* develop in the roof of the mesencephalon.

The posterior end of the brain passes into the *spinal cord.*

Sense Organs: Two olfactory pits lie near the tip of the head. The eyes exhibit well developed optic cup and lens. Due to flexure, they lie well posterior to the ears. The auditory vesicle is pear-shaped with a narrow ductus endolymphaticus.

Heart: The heart is S-shaped, the vascular area develops extensively and almost covers the yolk.

Alimentary Canal: The mouth forms by rupturing of the oral plate. Four pairs of visceral pouches are formed in the pharynx. An invagination in the floor of the pharynx develops into thyroid gland. Midgut is still incomplete. The hind gut terminates in a tail gut. The latter begins to degenerate in the hours to follow.

Excretory System: Pronephric tubules start degenerating. Mesonephric duct increases in length and acquires connection with cloaca.

Foetal Membranes: Amnion and chorion are well developed. Allantois develops as an outgrowth from the hindgut of the embryo. Yolk sac encloses about half of the yolk.

Limb Buds: The anterior and posterior limb buds are quite prominent and begin to exhibit nipple-shaped apices.

Extraembryonic Areas

Area pellucida of the avian blastoderm gives rise to the parts of the embryo. The area opaca is completely excluded from the formation of the body of the embryo. This portion of the blastoderm around the embryonic area is called the extraembryonic area. It gives rise to the extraembryonic structures like foetal membranes which degenerate at the time of hatching.

Area Vasculosa and Area Vitellina: During the second the third days of incubation, a network of blood vessels develops in the inner part of the area opaca and it is now referred to as the area vasculosa. The outer part of the area opaca becomes the area vitellina. The adjacent blood vessels in the area vasculosa establish communications among themselves and the whole mass is transformed into an irregular network. All the vessels of the area vasculosa are joined together on the periphery by an encircling blood vessel, the sinus terminalis. The sinus terminalis serves as a boundary line between the area vasculosa and the area vitellina. The blood vessels of the area vasculosa soon begin to extend into the area pellucida and eventually establish connection with the embryo proper. This connection is formed at two points : *(i)* with the venous system, by way of right and left vitelline veins, and (ii) with the arterial system, by means of right and left vitelline arteries, which arise from the dorsal aorta.

Blood Islands: Groups of densely packed cells from the postero-lateral margins of the mesoderm in the area pellucida wander into the area opaca. These groups of cells are known as the blood islands. The cells of blood islands becomes differentiated into two types :

(i) The cells on the periphery join up to form the endothelium of the future blood vessels.

(ii) The central cells become separated from each other and are differentiated as blood corpuscles.

The cavity of the blood vessel develops the fluid plasma when circulation begins. In this manner each blood island ultimately becomes transformed into a minute blood vessel.

Embryology of Chick

Reptiles, birds and mammals can be distinguished in their embryology from cyclostomes, fishes and amphibians in:

(i) laying their eggs on land, and

(ii) development of special embryonic envelopes called foetal membranes or embryonic membranes around the developing embryo. These membranes are — amnion, chorion, allantois and yolk-sac.

Based on the presence of amnion the vetebrates are classified as:

(i) Amniota (with amnion) *e.g.* reptiles, birds and mammals.

(ii) Anamniota (without amnion) *e.g.* Cyclostomes, fishes and amphibians.

It is believed that some amphibious ancestors of reptiles were the first vertebrates that laid their eggs on land.

Necessity of Laying Eggs on Land : During that period, the sea was a battle field where numerous invertebrates and vertebrates including numerous varieties of fishes were competing to exist and maintain their races. To avoid competition, some aquatic forms tried to invade the land which was unhaunted at that time and was thickly covered with vegetation. Laying of eggs on land was of great survival value as the embryos had following advantages-

(i) these had no danger of predators on land,

(ii) the eggs and embryos were neither subjected to water currents not to the deficiency of oxygen.

Necessity of Developing Foetal Membranes : Though advantageous, laying of eggs on land posed threat of rough and dry surroundings. This necessitated the following changes in the structure and development of egg.

Nourishment : The young animal that hatches out of the egg must be able to crawl on land and to defend itself from enemies. This requires a longer period of development and a large storage of nutrients. Therefore, amniotes have large yolky eggs and yolk sac.

Protection : On land the eggs and the embryo had to endure dry and harsh surroundings. Therefore, the eggs have developed a watery envelope of albumen, tough outer-membranes and often a hard shell.

Avoid Dessication : The delicate embryo also needs protection from the dry atmosphere and from shocks. This is possible by the development of a fluid-filled amniotic cavity and the amnion around the embryo. The amniotic cavity acts as a pool and keeps the embryo moist and protects it from dessication and shocks.

Respiration and Excretion : Embryo needs special

adaptations to carry on respiratory exchange of gasses with the surrounding air and structure to retain the nitrogenous excretory wastes, which if accumulate, within the embryo would be poisonous. To serve these two functions, the embryo has developed allantois and chorion. The eggs which meet the above requirements and self-sufficient are known as cleidoic eggs (NEEDHAM J. 1931). Cleidoic eggs are characteristic of reptiles, birds and monotreme mammals.

Gonads and Gametes

Testes and Sperm : In male fowl (cock or rooster), the testes are paired ovoid structures, suspended from the dorsal body wall by mesorchia. Sperm maturation occurs inside the seminiferous tubules of testes. A vas deferents arising from each testis carries sperms into the cloaca. The coccal opening lies on a genital papilla. A mature sperm of fowl is about 50 µ in length. Its head is short and cylindrical with a pointed acrosome. The tail is long tapering and vibratile.

Ovary and Ovum

The female fowl (hen) has only one functional ovary and a single oviduct. It is present on the left side. The right ovary

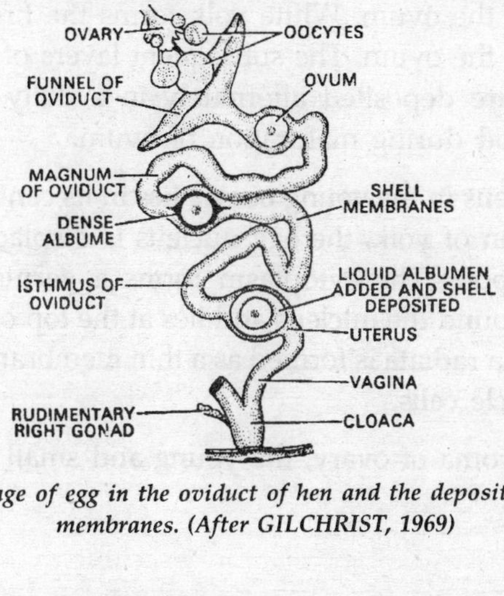

The passage of egg in the oviduct of hen and the deposition of egg membranes. (After GILCHRIST, 1969)

and oviduct are present in the young. In adult these are represented by streak. Ovaries are suspended from the dorsal body wall by mesovarium.

Significance of one Ovary

In all flying birds only one ovary of the left side is functional. The right ovary and oviduct degenerate. It is advantageous for the birds because:

1. Bird's eggs are large and megalecithal. The development of eggs in both the ovaries and their passage through both the oviducts would adversely affect the size of the eggs and put a limitation on the amount of reserve yolk.
2. Absence of one ovary and oviduct makes the body lighter and more efficient for flight.

The primordial germ cells differentiate in 5 days old chick embryo but the sex cells are alike in the two sexes.

The ovary consists of bundles of ovarian follicle, embedded in the stroma. Each ovarian follicle has a large central oocyte, surrounded by a peripheral layer of small follicle cells. Oocyte grows in size by the accumulation of yolk. The yolk is drawn from the maternal blood stream by the follicle cells and is deposited in the ovum. White yolk forms the first sphere in the centre of the ovum. The subsequent layers of yellow and white yolk are deposited alternately in a daily cycle for a specific period during maturation of ovum.

The nucleus in the young oocyte lies in its centre. But with the deposition of yolk, the egg nucleus is displaced towards the animal pole. The cytoplasm forms a germinal disc or blastodisc around the nucleus and lies at the top of yolk mass. Later on, zona radiata is formed as a thin membrane inside the layer of follicle cells.

In the stroma of ovary, the young and small follicles are

present in the centre and larger and older ones on the periphery. The fully- grown follicles bulge into the coelom.

Ovulation and Maturation

The fully-developed oocyte breaks through the ovarian wall, ruptures the follicle and comes out into the coelom near infundibulum. During ovulation the muscle fibres surrounding the mature follicle contract and egg bursts out of the capsule.

At this stage the nucleus of the oocyte enters first maturation division. Second maturation division occurs after ovulation , when secondary oocyte has reached the anterior end of oviduct.

Copulation and Oviposition

During copulation, the rooster crouches on the back of hen. While the hen elevates her tail turning the cloaca upward, the rooster turns his tail downward. Therefore, their cloaca get opposed. The spermatozoa are then transferred into vagina of hen. These ascend up and reach the anterior part of oviduct.

Fertilization

Fertilization occurs in the anterior part of oviduct. Although, a number of spermatozoa enter the ovum. Only one sperm nucleus fuses with the egg nucleus. The abortive nuclei or merocytes of the supernumerary spermatozoa can be seen in the cytoplasm of zygote. These degenerate subsequently.

Formation of Accessory Layers around the Fertilized Egg : As the fertilized egg moves down, the convoluted and glandular part of oviduct (magnum) deposits a thick layer of dense albumen around the egg. It adheres to the vitelline membrane and extends as cords at the two ends of the egg. These cord become spirally twisted due to the rotation of egg causes by the spiral folds in the wall of magnum. These spiral strands of albumen are known as chalazae.

Additional albumen is deposited in concentric layers as a colourless fluid, while the egg moves down in the oviduct. The shell membranes are secreted around the egg albumen by the wall of isthmus part of oviduct. The porous calcareous egg-shell is formed while the egg moves down through the shell gland portion of the oviduct or the uterus part.

Structure of Hen's Egg

Hen's egg is macrolecithal and strongly telolecithal. The yolk-free egg cytoplasm is represented by a small disc that forms a cap on the yolk at the animal pole.

A newly-laid hen's egg is a large elliptical structure with one end broader than the other. It consists of following parts:

Egg Shell

The egg-shell is the outermost protective covering. It is a white, hard but porous structure, formed of C_aCO_3. The pores have a diameter of 0.04—0.05mm and are about 7000 in number. These are more numerous at the broad end of the shell and are filled with some proteinaceous substance related to collagen. The pores permit diffusion of oxygen and carbon dioxide. The shell is secreted by shell gland portion of the uterus.

Shell Membranes

Inside the shell are two shell membranes. These are formed of keratin fibres matted together and are deposited by the isthmus part of oviduct. The outer shell membrane is thick and tough while the inner one is thin. The two membranes are in close contact throughout the inner surface of the shell except at the broad end, where they are separated by a wide air-space. The air-space is filled with air and is formed when the egg is about to be laid down. It helps the developing embryo in breathing.

In the fresh egg the air space is very small. It increases in size with the age of egg due to evaporation of water through porous shell.

Albumen : The space between the shell membranes and vitelline membrane of the ovum is filled with albumen or 'the white of egg'. It contains 85% water and 15% proteins. Albumin (protein) constitutes 94% of the total protein mixture. The egg albumen provides nutrition to the developing embryo, serves as a water store and provides envelope protecting embryo from mechanical and chemical injuries.

The egg albumen is separated into two parts. The outer part is watery and is known as light albumen. It is secreted partly by the isthmus of oviduct and partly by the uterus. The inner part of albumen is thick, gelatinous and semisolid and forms a close sac around the ovum. It is secreted by the glandular wall of magnum part of oviduct. The albumen at the two poles of the egg is twisted and forms two spirally-twisted strands, called chalazae. The chalazae help in keeping the ovum in the centre of albuminous mass.

Ovum : The ovum is a large spherical body embedded in the egg albumen. It is surrounded by a plasma membrane and a vitelline membrane. The vitelline membrane is a modified zona radiata and has a double origin. Its inner layer is formed in the ovary and is composed of very rough fibres, while the outer layer is formed in the upper portion of fallopian tube and is formed of fine fibres.

Yolk : The major portion of ovum is formed of yolk. It is differentiated into yellow and white yolk. The white yolk is represented by a central flask-shaped mass below the blastodisc and is known as latebra. It is surrounded by alternate concentric rings of yellow and white yolk. The outermost part of latebra just beneath the blastodisc is known as nucleus of pander.

Chemically, yolk contains 48.7% water, 32.6% phospholipids

and fats, 16.6.% proteins, 1% carbohydrates and 1.1% other chemicals. The proteins occur in the form of phosvitin (phosphoprotein) and lipovitelline or levitin (lipid protein).

The blastodisc or germinal disc is a small disc of active protoplasm situated at the top of yolk. It represents the living portion of ovum and contains the zygote nucleus which undergoes cleavage. It is whitish in colour and circular in outline. The somewhat darker area around the white blastodisc is known as periblast or marginal area.

Fertilization

Fertilization occurs in the upper part of oviduct. Several sperm surround the oocyte, but only one succeeds to penetrate the egg membranes and fertilizes the ovum.

Cleavage or Segmentation

Cleavage in hen's egg begins while it passes down the oviduct even before it is surrounded with albumen and other membranes. Because of much larger amount of inert yolk, the cleavage furrows never cut through the entire ovum but remain restricted to the small whitish blastodisc leaving the yolk uncleaved. The type of cleavage is known as partial or meroblastic. The cells formed by meroblastic cleavage are not completely demarcated but represent protoplasmic areas with separate nuclei, being isolated by cleavage furrows. Moreover, the cleavage furrows do not extend the whole area of blastoderm but are restricted to the centre of blastodisc. This results in the demarcation of central cells surrounded on the periphery by a rim of unsegmented cytoplasm. This unsegmented area is known as periblast or marginal zone.

The First Cleavage : The first cleavage is initiated by the formation of a small incision extending meridionally near the centre of the germinal disc. The furrow passes through both animal and vegetal poles. It is very superficial, as it does not extend even upto the lower portion of the blastodisc where the cytoplasm is filled with coarse yolk granules. Thus the two blastomeres thus formed, have incomplete wall and remain unseparated from the underlying yolk.

The Second Cleavage : The cleavage is also meridional. It begins while the egg passes through the isthmus. Its furrow is laid at right angles to the first cleavage furrow.

The Third Cleavage : The cleavage furrows of third cleavage are vertical cutting across the second set of cleavage furrows. These furrows tend to be parallel to the first cleavage furrow but are usually irregular. Third cleavage results in the formation of eight blastomeres.

The Fourth Cleavage : Its cleavage furrows are also vertical but not synchronous. These divide each of the eight blastomeres produced by third cleavage forming eight central blastomeres and eight marginal blastomeres.

Central and Marginal Cells

After fourth cleavage, the planes of further cleavage furrows become irregular, rapid and involve both central and peripheral cytoplasm and result in the formation of:

(1) The central cells that lie in the centre of the blastodisc. These cells have complete cell boundaries but are still continuous with the underlying yolk.

(2) The marginal cells that lie on the periphery of central cells. These have incomplete cell boundaries being connected with the marginal periblast on the sides and with the yolk on the under surface.

Morula and Periblast Formation : After 32-cell stage, the horizontal or latitudinal cleavage furrows are laid down first in the region of central cells and later in the marginal zone. This establishes a superficial single layer of cells completely separated from the egg cytoplasm beneath. This layer forms the blastoderm. Its cells rest upon a layer of cells which are continuous on their deep faces with the underlying yolk.

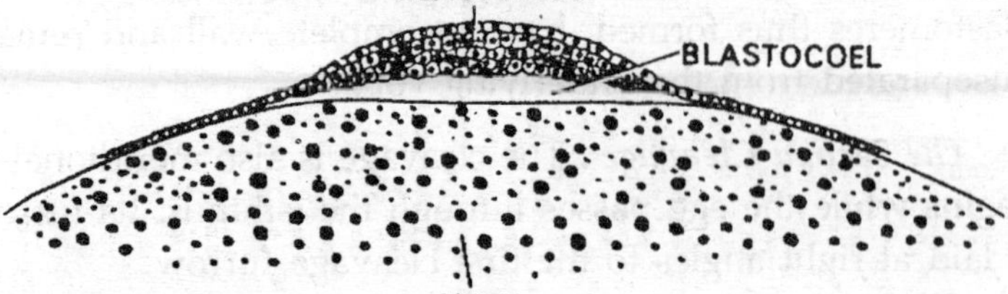

V.S. Blastodisc of Hen's egg in blastula stage showing blastoderm and sub-germinal cavity

The lower layer of incomplete cells is called central periblast. The marginal cells which are present along the margins of blastodisc remain continuous with each other around their outer edges are also continuous with the underlying yolk. These form marginal periblast.

The blastoderm of central area further divides by many vertical and horizontal divisions forming a 4-5 layer thick central area. It appears as a disc-shaped mass of cells and is called blastodisc. It is homologous with the morula stage.

Segmentation Cavity or Subgerminal Space : Once the blastoderm is formed, it gets separated from the central periblast by the appearance of a slit-like space. It marks the beginning of subgerminal cavity or primary segmentation cavity or blastocoel. The cells of central and marginal periblast lose their dividing furrows and form a syncytial mass. Thus, the subgerminal cavity has:

(i) roof formed of cells of blastoderm and

(ii) floor formed of central syncytial periblast with yolk underneath.

Periblast (both marginal and central) acts as trophoblast tissue. It helps in breaking down of yolk and its transportation to the developing embryo. Due to utilization of yolk and gradual increase in the number of blastoderm cells, the subgerminal cavity increases.

Discoblastula

In chick the fully formed or mature blastula is a discoblastula. It consists of:

1. A central multi-cellular multi-layered blastoderm free from the underlying yolk and central periblast. It forms area pellucida.
2. Underlying blastocoel or subgerminal cavity' that separates blastoderm from the underlying central periblast and yolk.
3. *Marginal Periblast Tissue:* It is present on the periphery of central blastoderm.

It is called germ wall. It may be differentiated into.

(i) Inner zone of distinct cells, which divide rapidly and contribute cells to the peripheral of growing cellular blastoderm.

(ii) Outer peripheral zone of syncytial germ cells, which is also called zone of junction. It lies in intimate contact with yolk.

Area Pellucida and Area Opaca : The peripheral area of discoblastula is opaque because the large yolk-laden blastomeres rest directly on the underlying yolk. This outer peripheral zone is known as the area opaca (Fig.). The cells of the central mass of blastomeres, overlying the fluid-filled subgerminal cavity, are smaller and relatively free from yolk and appear translucent. They constitute the area pellucida.

Fate Maps of Discoblastula

The blastoderm in discoblastula of chick consists of two parts: the area pellucid and area opaca. The area opaca (area vitellina) does not form any part of the embryo proper. It forms non or extra embryonic ectoderm which during later developmental stages forms extra-embryonic membranes and blood vessels (area vasculosa) to involve in the digestion of the yolk. Hence, the fate map is restricted to area pellucida. Moreover, fate map of both epiblast and hypoblast are to be made out separately.

The epiblast has material for ectoderm , mesoderm and also for endoderm, the hypoblast is formed exclusively of endoderm material.

(i) The anterior 2/3rd of area pellucida is prospective ectoderm consisting of prospective epidermis and extra-embryonic ectoderm.

(ii) A crescentric area is prospective neural area.

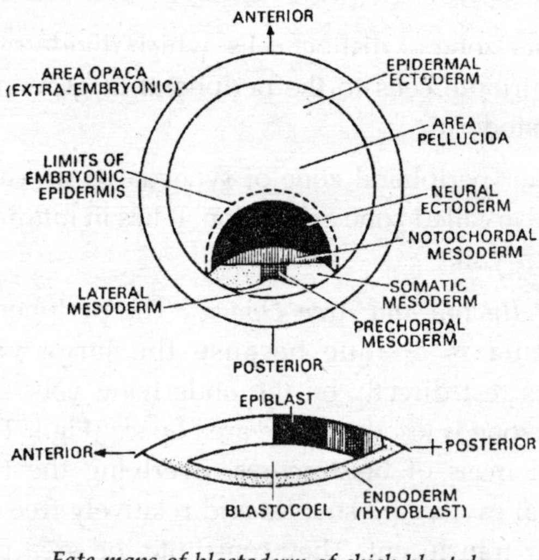

Fate maps of blastoderm of chick blastula

(iii) Next to neural area is the prospective notochord.

(iv) It is followed by prechordal mesoderm.

(v) On the side of prechordal region is the lateral plate mesoderm.

Gastrulation

Hen lays egg while the embryo is preparing for gastrulation. In chick, the process of gastrulation is prolonged and highly modified due to the presence of yolk. The gastrular movements responsible for the establishment of embryonic membranes are convergence, streaming, involution, epiboly and elongation.

Gastrulation is separated into three distinct processes or phases which occur in a chronological sequence. These are: (i) Formation of endoderm (ii) Formation of mesoderm (iii) Formation of embryonic axial structure primitive streak.

Separation of Endoderm or Hypoblast : Presumptive endoderm or hypoblast is formed during gastrulation by the elimination of large yolky cells from the inner surface of epiblast. These form a distinct layer in the subgerminal cavity above the yolk. A number of theories have been proposed. The important ones are:

(i) By the involution of marginal cells through a temporary pore present in the zone of junction.

(ii) According to JACOBSON (1938) hypoblast is formed by the invagination of epiblast at the posterior margin of blastoderm.

(iii) According to PETER (1938) hypoblast is formed by the infiltration of cells from the epiblast. The individual cells detach and get arranged within the subgerminal cavity. The layer thus formed is hypoblast or presumptive endoderm.

(iv) SPRATT (1946) suggested that elimination of cells from epiblast is responsible for the formation of hypoblast.

A number of processes appear to be responsible in the formation of hypoblast. Site of Origin of Hypoblast Cells -

There are different views as regard to the site from which hypoblast cells arise. According to PASTELES (1945) the hypoblast cells arise from all over the area pellucida of blastoderm. But PETER believed that cells arise from future posterior side and near the margin of blastoderm. Hypoblast gives rise to the gut lining.

Formation of Mesoderm

The cells of embryonic epiblast consist of prospective notochord, mesoderm and ectoderm. The cells of notochord and mesoderm migrate inward and form a layer in between the epiblast and hypoblast. These movements are evident in the form of primitive streak. Thus, the three embryonic layers are established. The uppermost or the epiblast now forms the ectoderm, the median layer mesoderm "and the lower one endoderm.

Formation of Primitive Streak : The prospective endoderm having migrated to the definite position, the central area of blastoderm is left with prospective somatic mesoderm, prospective prechordal mesoderm, neuroectoderm and the epidermal ectoderm.

Next formative movements are concerned with the segregation and 'carrying in of prospective mesodermal and chordal material. These cells begin to leave the under surface of the blastoderm, and converge in the middle line between epiblast and hypoblast (convergence) at the posterior end in the area pellucida. This mass movement is initiated at about 6th-7th hour.

Formation of Initial Primitive Streak : The lateral place mesoderm begins to converge towards the middle line from a point about a quarter of the way from the anterior end of the area pellucida (epiblast) towards the growth centre in the posterior quadrant (Fig.), to initiate in the formation of a thickening called the primitive streak. The next material to converge in the middle line is the somatic mesoderm followed by prechordal and notochordal materials which are rolled in

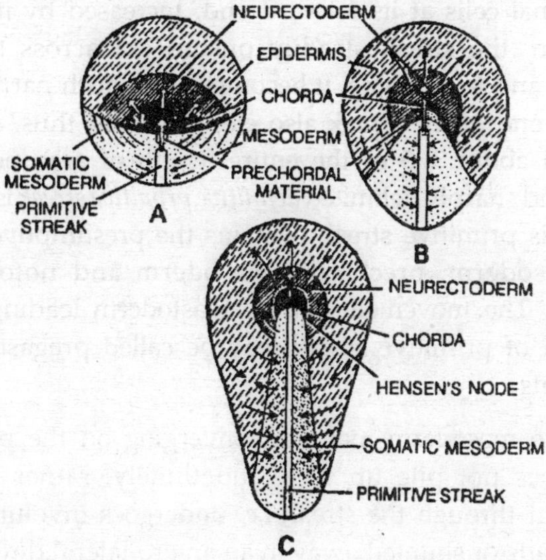

Stages of the gastrulation in chick (dotted arrows indicates movements beneath the surface).

and are incorporated in the primitive streak in the last. These cells swing backward in circular orbits. At the same time the posterior radius elongates in a forward direction. By the *eighth* hour the cells of the posterior radius have begun to heap up and form a short broad longitudinal strand, which is thicker than the rest of the epiblast of area pellucida. This is the initial primitive streak. This marks the first sign of differentiation of the embryo which will be formed along its axis. The initial primitive streak grows in its length along its anterior end, partly by proliferation but mainly by the growth of cells which come to it from the sides. By the twelfth hour the *intermediate streak* formed is about one-half the length of the circular area pellucida. It continues to grow in length, elongating backward at its posterior end. The oval area pellucida becomes pear-shaped to accomodate the lengthening streak.

Formation of Definitive Primitive Streak : By the 19th hour of incubation there is forward streaming or stretching in the primitive streak, owing to the addition of more and more mesodermal cells at its forward end. Increased by its active elongation, the streak steadily pushes out across the area pellucida and in so doing, it becomes very much narrow. The posterior end of the streak also elongates and thus, a much-elongated about 3/5 of the entire length of area pellucida, narrow and sharply delimited *definitive primitive streak* is formed (Fig.). This primitive streak contains the presumptive lateral plate mesoderm, prechordal mesoderm and notochordal materials. The movements in the blastoderm leading to the formation of primitive streak may be called pregastrulation movements.

As the mesoderm material converging on the primitive streak does not pile up there indefinitely, rather it turns downward through the streak *i.e.* undergoes involution and then spreads or shunted away in an antero-lateral direction as a separate sheet of mesoderm between the hypoblast and the surface layer. Most of the mesodermal cells entering the streak from one side move out again on the same side, but some cross over to emigrate on the opposite side. The rate at which cells leave (involute) the lower lateral borders of the primitive streak is greater than at which the cells converge over it from the upper layer. This results in the formation of a groove along the entire length of the streak and is known as the primitive groove, and the primitive ridges that flank the groove.

Similarly, the presumptive somatic mesoderm is also soon shunted laterally and forward to become continuous with the extra-embryonic mesoderm. Therefore, two distinct movements, one of convergence and other of divergence are involved in the process.

Homology of Primitive Streak : Formation of primitive streak in the middle line is considered homologous to the formation of lateral lips of blastopore in amphibian gastrula. It means primitive streak of chick is homologous with the closed blastopore. The reasons for such a homology are as follows :

(i) Both primitive streak and lateral lips of blastopore develop by the migration of presumptive chorda mesodermal and mesodermal elements.

(ii) The head process is equivalent or homologous to the notochord and axial mesoderm of amphibian embryo.

(iii) The neurentric canal in amphibian embryo originates by the fusion of neural folds over the anterior part of blastopore. In chick, though the neurentric canal is absent, a pit occur at this point, corresponding to blastopore. It is covered with neural folds. In some birds the neural pit opens into the archenteron.

(iv) In some birds, something like neurenteric canal is formed at the anterior and of streak. It shows similarity to frog where neurenteric canal is formed at the closed blastoporal end. In both anus arises at the posterior end of the neurenteric canal.

(v) Cells about the dorsal lip of early blastopore possess remarkable inductive capacity and induce formation of nerve cord, etc. Primitive streak also possesses similar power of induction.

However, because of the following differences embryologists disfavour the concept of homology between primitive streak and blastopore..

(i) The primitive streak never develops a communication with archeteron, but blastopore in frog's gastrula is basically opening of archenteron to the exterior.

(ii) In primitive streak cells migrate from one side to the other but not in case of blastopore.

(iii) In chick the primitive streak is without ventral lip.

Functional Relation of Primitive Streak : Following structures develop from the primitive streak:

Differentiation of Ectoderm, Mesoderm and Endoderm

(i) The primitive streak is formed by the accumulation of cells from different regions of the embryo, which are destined to develop into different organs. The cells of mesodermal layer migrate out of the streak and arrange themselves between epiblast and hypoblast. Thus, the primitive streak consists of cells of

(a) Epiblast or ectoderm — above

(b) Hypoblast or endoderm — below and

(c) Mesoderm — in between the two.

(ii) Convergence now centres in the anterior part and in the region of the prospective neuro-ectoderm. This material is carried towards the middle line and with simultaneous extension of the embryonic axis (head process and primitive streak) in the antero-posterior direction, it becomes extended lengthwise just above the notochord to from the neural plate.

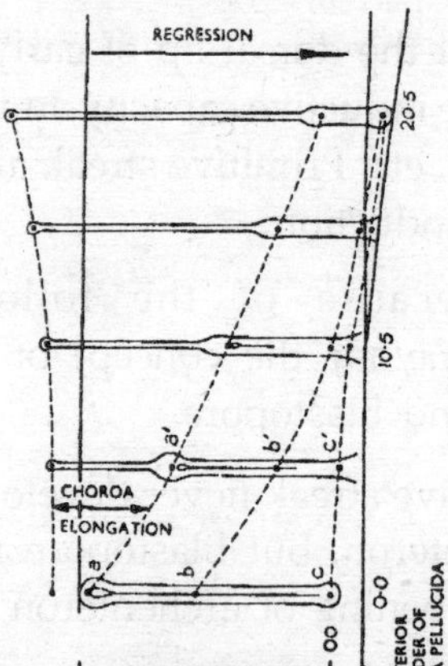

Diagrammatic representation of gradual regression of primitive streak in chick embryo.

(iii) *Disappearance of Primitive Streak* : The establishment of the head process marks the completion of the elongation of the primitive streak. Henceforth, the lengthwise streaming movements within the streak are directed rearward. Hensen's node in a sense travels backward *i.e.* the streak gradually shortens and ultimately becomes reduced to a fragment in the tail-bud and finally disappears, signifying that the development of mesoderm is complete. The entire embryo, thus, develops anterior to the streak.

(iv) *Development of Head Process* : As the node and streak move posteriorly, the head process and prechordal mesoderm stretch out anteriorly in accompaniment to the forward elongation of the blastoderm as a whole. Closer examination of the head process reveals that it consists of a thick central mass of cells which provides the definitive notochord and more diffused lateral wings which contribute to the somatic mesoderm that flank to the notochord. With its differentiation, the notochord becomes detached from the hypoblast yellow, except for fusion at the extreme anterior end.

Post-gastrular Development

Post-gastrular development comprises the differentiation and development of embryonic structures from the embryonic materials, and the formation of *embryonic membranes* from the extra-embryonic materials.

Organogenesis Phase I (Tubulation) : In chick, the process of tubulation occurs in the same way as in amphibians- (i) The ectoderm differentiates into neural ectoderm and epidermal ectoderm. The neural ectodermal plate is converted into neural tube; (ii) the chorda-mesoderm differentiates into notochord and mesoderm. The latter further differentiates into its different sub-kinds; (iii) the endoderm develops into primitive gut.

Neurogenesis : During post-gastrular development the neural tube formation proceeds in antero-posterior direction.

The neural plate appears in the anterior region from the prospective neuroectoderm and lies just dorsal to the notochordal process. As Hensen's node recedes farther, the farther parts of the neural plate become differentiated. The median portion of the neural plate sinks down as the neural groove and its edges rise up as neural folds (Fig.). The folds approach each other at about 5-somite stage, above the median neural groove and meet to convert the groove into the neural tube. Eventually, a neural tube forms throughout the embryo, except in the area of primitive pit and primitive streak, where the neural folds fan out to create a rhomboid-like depression called sinus rhomboidalis (Fig.). For some time, neural tube opens to the outside by the neuropore.

Notogenesis : While the neural plate is being converted into the neural tube, the chordamesoderm is also differentiating. Its anterior part, the prechordal mesoderm gives rise to much of the mesenchyme of the head behind it lies the notochord. The notochordal cells become separated from rest of the adjoining sheets of mesoderm and differentiate into a rod of cells (notochord) which becomes compact and is surrounded by the sheath that develops from the materials of sclerotomes.

Mesogenesis : Mesoderm is present between ectoderm and endoderm throughout the embryo. It consists of loose mesenchymal cells derived from prechordal mesoderm and from the forward extension of axial mesoderm, together with some contribution from the neural crest.

On each side of the notochord are three longitudinal strands of mesoderm:

(i) The thicker medial strand or the *axial* or *somatic mesoderm* (epimere) which begins to differentiate after 21 hours of incubation as dark bands on each side of notochord. A cleft appears across each band, a short distance anterior to the primitive knot. It marks the division between 1st and 2nd mesodermal somites.

Approximately one hour later, a second cleft appears posterior to the 1st cleft and divides the second somite from the future 3rd somite. The process repeats itself approximately once an hour for 20 hours. After that the somites continue to appear at a somewhat slower rate. The most posterior somites are, of course, the youngest.

(ii) The *intermediate mesoderm* (mesomere) is less denser region, lateral to the axial mesoderm and medial to the lateral mesoderm. In cross section, it appears as "necks" of cells connecting the somites with the lateral mesoderm.

(iii) The *lateral mesoderm* (hypomere) is present farthest to the sides of the embryo and posterior to it. Its future is partly embryonic and partly extraembryonic. It lies as a sheet on the left and a sheet on the right of the longitudinal axis of blastoderm spreading between the ectoderm. The sheets occupy a considerable part of the area opaca and swing forward as right and left "horns", leaving a small area right in front of the notochordal process without mesoderm. This area is known as the proamnion. The mesodermal horns ultimately join in front of the embryo and later on completely surround the proamnion. As the Hensen's node retreats behind, more somites are differentiated in front of it.

Formation of Coelom : Initially mesoderm develops as a solid sheet of loosely-arranged cells, on either side of notochord. It soon splits up into an outer somatic layer and inner splanchnic layer. The space between these two layers is the coelom. It is called schizocoel because it develops by the splitting up of mesoderm. The somatic layer of mesoderm comes to lie along with ectoderm and the two together form somatopleure (ectoderm + somatic mesoderm). The splanchnic mesoderm lies with endoderm and forms splanchnoplure (splanchnic mesoderm + endoderm).

Enterogenesis : The primitive gut appears between the yolk and the raised endoderm. There is no cellular floor to the gut so far, except the yolk-bed. As the neurulation proceeds, the foregut appears at the head end of the embryo on the first day of incubation as a blind pocket of splanchnopleure . During early stages, the fore- gut remains open at its sides and posteriorly on the yolk by the opening called anterior intestinal portal. At about 40 hours of incubation, the hind gut appears as the cavity of the tail-fold. Its cavity remains communicated anteriorly to the future mid-gut (a space on the yolk mass) through the posterior intestinal portal. The two portals come to lie close together but do not meet.

The endoderm bounding the anterior end of the foregut fuses near its ventral surface with the ectoderm to form the oral plate. The anal plate is similarly formed at the posterior end of the hindgut. These plates become perforated to form the mouth and the anus respectively.

Further Development of Chick According to the Hours of Incubation : It is customary, when speaking stages beyond tubulation, to refer to the hour of incubation and in terms of somites. The regular addition of somites as embryo increases in age makes the number of somites a useful criterion of the stage of development. Therefore, to designate the stage of development on the basis of the number of somites they have formed in a particular time is an estimation of age of the embryo. The word "pairs", is usually omitted, thus a four somite embryo is one with 4 pairs of somites. The most widely used stages are the 24-hour, 33-hour, 48-hour, and 96-hour chick embryos.

Embryo at 24 hours (4-pairs of Somites)

(i) By the end of the first day of incubation embryonic and extra-embryonic regions of the blalstoderm become sharply defined.

(ii) The rapidly growing head rises above the blastoderm and projects forward as a cylindrical part of the embryo and overhangs the proamnion region.

(iii) In a zone of opaque area bordering the area pellucida are mottled masses of mesodermal cells, the blood island from which originate blood cells and some blood vessels which fuse into a definite network and develop into a distinct subdivision of area opaca to be called the area vasculosa, while the distal portion of area opaca is called area vitellina.

(iv) Simultaneously with the extension of the head, endodermal component of the original head fold is elongated as an internal tubular pocket. This is the primitive foregut. Cranially it is a blind sac and caudally where the yolk still constitutes the only floor is the midgut which opens out on the yolk through an arched aperture termed the anterior intestinal portal.

(v) The neural folds appear as a pair of dark bands first in about the centre of the head region and progress towards the head and caudal ends. At its cephalic end the neural folds are correspondingly more prominent and form a deep and broad neural groove. Dorsally, the component neural folds have approached and are ready to fuse. Caudally the folds diverge and become increasingly indistinct.

(vi) The notochord is now a definite rod, visible through the transparent ectoderm at the neural groove. The primitive groove runs along the length of the primitive streak and the primitive knot lies at the anterior end. The proamnion still exists.

(vii) Following the mesoderm from the middle line towards either side, the three zones can be made out: (a) The dorsal clearly defined block-like mesodermal somites; (b) a thin and narrow plate of cells, the intermediate mesoderm, connecting the dorsal and lateral mesoderm; (c) the lateral mesoderm which has splitted into somatic and splanchnic layer with a coelomic cavity between them.

Embryo at 33 hours (12 pairs of Somites) : Although a total view of a chick embryo at this stage much resembles the one last described, yet it does show certain distinct advances :

(i) The vascular area of the blastoderm is better organized and extends anteriorly but the proamnion is not yet invaded by the mesoderm.

(ii) At the level of optic vesicle, the head is thrust forward over the ectoderm and the space between it and the head is called the *subcephalic pocket.*

(iii) Except for an increase in size, the foregut is little changed. The midgut is fully defined, anterior intestinal portal persists and the hindgut appears as the cavity of tail fold.

(iv) The lips of the neural folds have fused throughout the cranial two-third of the embryo to form the neural tube which is open at each end; the cranial communication to the outside is called the anterior neuropore. Posteriorly, the neural folds flare out around the primitive streak, creating a rhomboid-like depression, the *sinus rhomboidalis.* The anterior region of the neural tube has begun to expand into three brain regions. From the prosencephalon the optic vesicles are bulging laterally. From its floor arises a ventrally-directed evagination, that forms infundibulum.

(v) The primitive streak is still prominent caudally and the notochord can be followed caphalad from the primitive knot.

(vi) Throughout most of the head region, the mesodermal germinal layer makes up a diffused meshwork of mesenchyme that fills in the space between the two epithelial layers. In the caudal part of the head and in the remainder of the body, the middle layer at this stage is organising into more compact mesoderm. Nearest the mid-plane, the epimere has divided, and approximately one pair of somites is added each hour after 21 hours. Thus the 33-hour chick has approximately 12 pairs of somites. Lateral to each somite is a plate of unsegmented mesoderm called the intermediate mesoderm, frequently called the nephrostomic plate. The somatic layers of mesoderm and ectoderm are closely associated, the two together are designated the somatopleure. It will make up the bodywall. Similarly, the splanchnic mesoderm and endoderm are jointly termed the splanchnopleure.

(vii) The heart is a straight double tube, lying in the mid-plane and ventral to the gut; it is continuous caudally with the omphalomesenteric veins, which serve to connect the yolk mass with the developing heart. From the cephalic end of heart are given off short ventral aortae. The coelom is already enlarged in the region of the heart anticipating its destiny as the pericardial cavity.

Embryo at 48-hours (35-pairs of Somites) : The period between 33 and 48 hours of development is very significant one. Due to torsion and flexure there is change in the over all appearance of the embryo. Instead of lying with its ventral surface in contact with the yolk, it is now partly turned so that the anterior portion of the body is lying with its left side to the yolk. In the head region the neural tube bends in the region of the mesencephalon so that the fore and hindbrains are nearly parallel. This is the cranial flexure, which marks the embryo f-shaped. Another slight flexure occurs in the posterior region of the brain. This is called *cervical flexure.* These two flexures give the anterior portion of the embryo a C-like appearance.

(i) The area pellucida is dumbbell-shaped. It develops a vascular network. The extraembryonic vessels of the area opaca are well differentiated and the vascular area ends in a bordering terminal sinus. Adjacent to the caudal end of the heart, the vascular network of the blastoderm converges and becomes continuous with the stem of the omphalomesenteric veins. The head is more prominent and the promniotic area is reduced to a small region in front of the head. The primitive streak is short and relatively inconspicuous.

(ii) *Central Nervous System and Sense Organs* : The neural tube is closed along most of its length. At the anterior end, the neuropore is closed. The three brain regions further differentiate into five regions-telencephalon, diencephalon, mesencephalon, faintly differentiating meten cephalon and the myelencephalon. The tuberculum posterior develops in the floor of the mid-brain. Anterior to the infudibulum, a depression, the recessus opticus is formed. Dorsally in the region of the dienception slight evagination occurs, this is the epiphysis which is the forerunner of the pineal gland. The elongated hindbrain (rhombencephalon) gradually passes into the spinal cord. It is now closed to its extreme end, and consequently the rhomboidal sinus no longer exists.

The ectoderm is thickened into a lens placode, where it overlies the lateral wall of each optic vesicle. The optic vesicle flattens at this point and will soon invaginate to produce to optic cup. Dorso-laterally, in the region of the hindbrain the ectoderm is also thickened into auditory placodes.

(iii) The broad foregut, folds inward and shows further differentiation. At the cephalic end, the pharynx is close ventrally by double-layered pharyngeal membrane, and an ectodermal deep pit external to it is the stomodaeum. In front of the pharyngeal membrane develops a ^-shaped median ectodermal sac, the Rathke's pocket, which will form the epithelial portion of the hypophysis. The pharynx bears three pairs of lateral outpocketings known as pharyngeal pouches. They occur opposite the three external branchial grooves, and here ectoderm of the groove and endoderm of the pouch are in contact, forming closing-plates.

The first pair of plates ruptures to form branchial clefts, corresponding to the gillclefts in lower aquatic vertebrates. Between the successive pouches lie solid, bar-like portions, branchial arches. At the level of the second pair of pouches, a broadly open pocket grows away from the median floor of the pharynx; it is the thyroid gland. Beyond the pharynx the fore-gut narrows and just before it, opens into the mid-gut. There it is budded off in a bilobed diverticulum which will give rise not only to the liver but also the gall bladder and various ducts, associated with these glands.

(iv) The tubular heart is enlarged and flexed to form a 'S'-shaped structure. Four regions can be distinguished: (i) the caudal end of the tube, where the vitelline (omphalomesenteric) and common cardinal vein open in the sinus venosus; (ii) a dilated, dorsal chamber, the atrium; (iii) a tubular ventral portion, bent in the form of a 'U' of which left limb is the ventricle and the right limb is auricle, (iv) the bulbus cordis. From the bulbus is given off the truncus and ventral aortae. The blood flows in a spiral course through the heart, beginning at the sinus venosus and passing through the atrium, ventricle, bulbus, arteriosus and into the ventral aorta. Three pairs of aortic arches connect the ventral and dorsal aortae.

(v) The formation of new somites and the progressive differentiation of older ones into sclerotome, myotome and dermatome continues. The nephrotome region (intermediate mesoderm) develops pronephric and mesonephric tubules. The mesonephros constitutes a functional kidney of the embryo. The lateral mesoderm persists as component of the somatopleure and splanchnopleure; the somatic mesoderm will give rise to the parietal walls of the pericardial, pleural and peritoneal cavities, while the splanchnic layer forms the epimyocardium, the visceral pleura, the mesenteries and the mesodermal layer of the gut.

The somatopleure, on each side of the head, folds over the dorsal surface of the head to form the chorion and aminon. The splanchnopleure forms the yolk sac.

Embryo of 72-hours (35-pairs of somites) : Several gross advances have occurred during the third day. The vascular area continues to spread over the surface of the yolk. A continued flexion has developed two more flexures—the lumbar flexure in the lumbar region and the caudal flexure in the region of the tail. The tail flexure has demarcated a definite caudal end of the trunk, which now terminates in a conical tail bud.

(i) The cervical flexure is now so pronounced that the hindbrain is the most cephalically situated part of the embryo, and the forebrain is made to point at the heart. The eyes lie much farther cauded than the ears. The limb buds make noticeable swellings along the trunk.

(ii) *Nervous System and Sense Organs :* The paired cerebral hemispheres, lined by lateral ventricles, bulge from the roof of the telencephalon. The diencephalon bears a dorsal evagination which is the epiphysis. The diencephalon bears a dorsal evagination which is the epiphysis. The mesencephalon sets off from the hindbrain, and the later subdivides into a thick-roofed metencephalon and a long thin-roofed myelencephalon. The caudal end of the brain passes into the spinal cord. The foreman of Monro connects the lateral ventricles to the diocoel.

An increased thickness of both the wall and floor of the mesencephalic region results in the formation of crura cerebri. The narrow cavity of the mesencephalon, the *cerebral aqueduct* or the aqueduct of Sylvius, will connect the third ventricle with the fourth ventricle. In the roof, the mesencephalon develops the corpora quadrigemina.

The roof of the metencephalon thickness to form cerebellum and its floor develops into the primordium of pons Varolii. The roof of the myelencephalon becomes extremely thin and vascular to form the posterior choroid plexus. The gray matter and white matter in spinal cord make their appearance.

Along the ventro-lateral border of the myelencephalon, paired masses of cranial ganglia occur. Similarly, in the region of spinal cord, the spinal ganglia begin to show as definite *segmental masses.*

The shallow olfactory pits lie near the tip of the head. The eyes develop completely, the auditory vesicles become pear-shaped and the pharyngeal cleft is ready to become middle ear.

(iii) *Digestive and Respiratory Systems* : The oral plate ruptures to form the mouth. A fourth pair of pharyngeal pouches has been added to the three previous sets. The first two pairs show partially-ruptured closing plates, so that there is temporary communication between these pouches and their corresponding branchial grooves. The laryngo-tracheal groove bifurcates posteriorly into lung buds surrounded by the pleural cavity.

The foregut is seen to differentiate into a short tube, the oesophagus and continues into a shortly-dilated stomach. Between the stomach and the anterior intestinal portal, the gut is referred to as the duodenum. From the duodenum, liver primordia are given off. The primordium of the pancreas also develops. In the duodenal portion, the ductus choledochus, the common duct for the pancreas, liver and gall bladder enters. There is further differentiation of gall bladder, bile duct, hepatic duct and also the cystic duct. Midgut opens into the foregut and hindgut by intestinal portals. The hindgut terminates in a short tail-bud.

(iv) *Mesoderm and Coelom :* By 72-hours as many as 35 pairs of mesodermal somites extend all the way to the tail-bud. At different levels there are various stages in the differentiation of the dermatome, myotome and sclerotome. Dorsal and ventral mesenteries develop and septum transversum separates the pleuropericardial cavity from the body cavity.

(v) *Cardiovascular System : The* truncus arteriosus lies in the floor of the pharynx and gives off by now four aortic arches. Interauricular septum has started developing external and internal jugulars lead into Cuvierian ducts. Vitelline arteries pass to the yolk sac and paired vitellines merge in the liver.

(vi) *The mesonephric ducts* increase in length and become connected with cloaca.

(vii) *Extraembryonic Membranes:* By now the splanchnopleure, spreading over the surface of the yolk has half enclosed it as a yolk sac. Allantois has appeared as a local bulge coming up out of the hindgut. The head fold and lateral folds of amnion close in and extend the aminon and chorion far down the embryo. The tail fold appears just caudal to the embryo and extends a short distance cephalad. Thus, amnion is still not a closed sac.

Embryo of 96-hours (41 pairs of somites) : By now the flexures and torsion are much more complete than they were at the 72-hour stage. Torsion which began at approximately 48 hours, has now reached a point at which the entire embryo lies with its left side toward the yolk. The body divisions *i.e.* head, trunk and tail are clearly demarcated.

The more increasingly pronounced flexion in the cephalic, cervical, lumbar and caudal regions gives to this embryo a C-shaped appearance, so that its head and tail approach each other. The limb which just make their appearance at 72 hours, are now extensive and paddle-like structures.

The somites which already had differentiated into dermatomal, myotomal and sclerotomal regions, now continue their internal differentiation.

The thyroid gland continues to push ventrally.

(i) *Nervous System and Sense Organs :* Cerebral hemispheres become prominent and esencephalon is more bulging. New nerves arise from the mesencephalon, metencephalon and myelencephalon respectively. These are the trochlear (IV), abducens (VI) and vagus (X). Accessory (XI) and hypoglossal (XII) nerves are just appearing. The olfactory pits are deep; eyes and ears increase in size; spinal ganglia are distinct. A chain of autonomic ganglia lie on each side dorsolateral to the aorta.

(ii) *Digestive and Respiratory Systems :* The region of the open gut above the yolk greatly reduced and forms a slender yolk stalk leading to yolk sac. The stomodaeum (mouth) becomes continuous with the pharynx by the rupture of pharyngeal membrane, but the coccal membrane is intact. The laryngotracheal groove has now further differentiated into a series of structures.

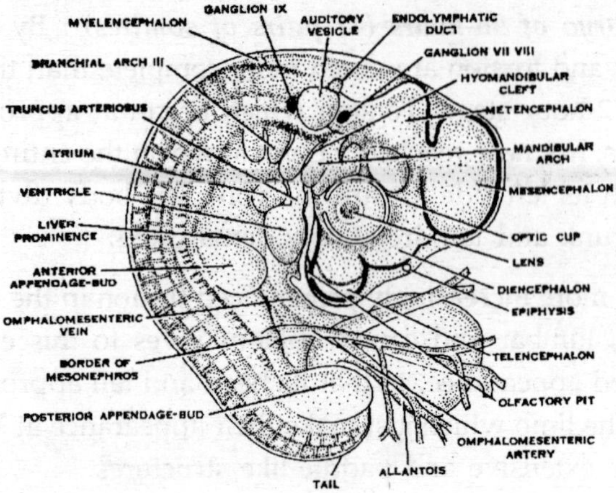

Dorsal view of 96-hour chick (xl7)

The opening from the pharynx into the respiratory passage is the glottis, followed immediately by the larynx and trachea. Posterior to the trachea are bifurcations representing the lung buds. The branchial arches are much thicker and more conspicuous. Derivative of the sixth arch, the pulmonary artery soon becomes intimately associated with the developing lung-buds.

The liver increases in length, and develops diverticulae and branching cords of cells which become the secretory units of the hepatic tubules. Blood sinusoids of the liver also develop . Dorsal and ventral pancreatic primordia start budding from the intestine and bile duct respectively.

(iii) *Cardiovascular System* : Sinus venosus leads antero-ventrally into the atrium which is separated from it by a faint constriction. The atrioventricular canal develops. Inter auricular and interventricular septa develop between the right and left side of the heart. V and VI aortic arches are added to the aortic series. The second arch degenerates. The first has already degenerated on 3rd day of incubation. Internal and external carotid arteries, vitelline veins, portal vein and also the inferior venacava have developed. Allantoic arteries and veins are also distinct.

(iv) *Urinogenital System* : The mesonephric tubules are still developing and differentiating and the metanephros is just making its appearance. Future gonads make appearance between mesonephros and mesentery.

(v) *Extra-embryonic Membranes* : The vascularized yolk sac continues through a narrow yolk stalk with the midgut. The *allantois* is now a prominent, stalked and highly vascularized bladder-like dilation. Amnion and chorion have completed their arching growth and have created a closed *amniotic sac* filled with amniotic fluid in which the embryo floats. The chorion formed by the same arching process, surrounds the embryo yolk sac and allantois.

Embryos of Seven and Ten Days : As a result of process of embryo formation in the chick more than one-half of the four day chick is head. This necessitates a different rate of growth during the last 17 days of development. Therefore, the body grows much more rapidly than the head during this period. The phenomenon of differential growth is referred to as heterogonic growth and the foetus becomes unmistakably bird-like in its external characteristics, even though the eye is disproportionately large. The original cervical flexure has been lost, and a distinct neck now separates head and thorax. The first branchial arch modifies into primitive jaws, which assume the appearance of a beak. The first branchial cleft is retained as the external acoustic meatus, about which no auricle develops. The other arches and clefts have disappeared. The ventral surface of the body bulges prominently as viscera becomes more protuberant. The limb buds, which arose at 72 hours continue to grow. As they do, the internal development becomes more apparent. The mesencymal cells lying in the central axis of the limbs begin to differentiate into precartilage or chondroblasts. These chondroblasts become organized into definite skeletal structures, and the limbs become jointed. The bones in the limb of chick from a proximal-distal direction are the humerus, radius and ulna, carpals, metacarpals and phalanges.

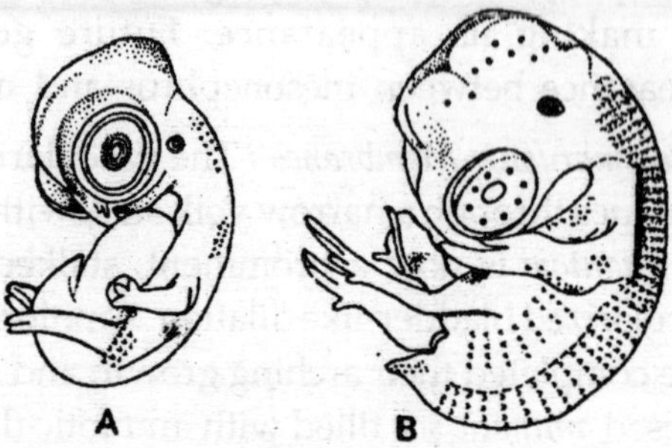

Advanced chick embryo viewed from left side A-Seven days old; B-nine days old..

Feather primordia appear in definite patterns. The contours of body, including the head become recognizably avian and the fore-limbs are wing-like. A condensation of blood vessel beneath the developing feather forms the feather pulp. The position of the feather is also genetically controlled and follows a well-established pattern.

The mesonephric duct is no longer utilised by the chick as the metanephros develops.

The amnion narrows to a tube, which contains the allantoic and yolk stalks and attaches to the lower body wall as a sort of umbilical cord. The yolk sac, which was so prominent in the early stages of development, is gradually absorbed as the developing embryo utilizes this yolk for its metabolic needs. At birth, the yolk sac is completely absorbed, and the ectoderm which originally surrounded it becomes the ventral body wall. The yolk sac absorption is shown in the figure.

Extra-embryonic Membranes in Chick

The history of the foetal-membranes in chick is correlated with the presence of an enormous mass of yolk and an embryonic life spent within a shell. Although the original blastoderm is a small disc, it spreads by peripheral growth and eventually covers the entire surface of the egg. But only the most central region is directly concerned with the formation of the embryo proper. All the remainder of the blastoderm is *extra-embryonic* and it is this portion that furnishes the *embryonic* or *foetal membranes.* These are auxiliary organs which have arisen partly for protection of the embryo, and more especially to provide for its nutrition, respiration and excretion until the independent existence is attained.

The fundamental set of embryonic membranes in chick and other amniotes includes the yolk-sac, amnion, chorion (serosa in mammals) and allantois which have been evolved with relation to the following structures that were already in existence: yolk-sac (gut); amnion and chorion (body wall) and allantois (primitive bladder).

All these extra-embryonic membranous sacs are composite structures and involves two germ layers. The amnion and chorion are composed of extra-embryonic ectoderm and somatic layer of mesoderm (somatopleure) while the yolk sac and allantois are composed of extra-embryonic endoderm and splanchnic layer of mesoderm (splanchnopleure), separated by a space which is *extra-embryonic coelom.* These components are continuous with their counterparts in the embryonic territory of the blastoderm.

The Yolk-sac

The yolk sac is the first of the extra-embryonic membranes to make its appearance. The splanchnopleure of the chick, instead of forming a closed gut, grows over the yolk surface as extra-embryonic extension and eventually encloses the entire yolk to form the yolk-sac. The primitive gut has a cellular wall dorsally only, with the yolk acting as a temporary floor (Fig.). However, concomitantly with the spreading of the extraembryonic splanchnopleure about the yolk, the intra-embryonic splanchnopleure is undergoing a series of changes which result in the establishment of a completely-walled gut in the body of embryo. The part of the gut which still remains open to the yolk is known as the midgut. But by the progress of the sub cephalic and sub-caudal folds, the foregut and hindgut are increased in extent at the expense of the midgut. The midgut is finally diminished until it opens ventrally by a small aperture which flares out like an inverted funnel into the yolk sac. This opening is the *yolk duct* and its wall constitutes the narrow *yolk stalk* through which the walls of yolk sac are still continuous with the wall of gut.

As the neck of the yolk sac is constricted, the omphalomesenteric (vitelline) arteries and omphalomesenteric (vitelline) veins are brought together and traverse the yolk-stalk side by side. The vascular network in the splanchnopleure of the yolk sac encompasses it. Apparently no yolk passes directly through the yolk duct into the intestine, rather endodermal cells lining the yolk sac secrete some appropriate digestive enzymes which make the yolk soluble at the spot. This soluble material then can be absorbed through the lining of the vitelline blood vessels to the circulating blood by which it is carried to all parts of the growing embryo. In older embryos the epithelium of the yolk sac penetrates deep into the yolk and forms a series of foldings which greatly increase its surface area for absorption.

During development the albumen loses water, becomes more viscid and rapidly decreases in bulk. The growth of the allantois, an extra-embryonic structure, forces the albumen toward the distal end of the yolk sac and the albumen is eventually compressed by the yolk sac. The yolk-sac absorbs and transfers, by way of the extra-embryonic circulation, to the embryo.

Towards the end of the period of incubation, usually on

the 19th day, the remains of the yolk sac are slipped through the naval into the belly cavity of the embryo. After its inclusion in the embryo, both the wall and the remaining contents of the yolk sac rapidly disappear, their absorption being practically completed in the first six days after hatching and the body wall closes behind it.

Amnion and Chorion

The amnion and chorion are so closely associated during their origin that they must be considered together. Both are derived from the extra-embryonic somatopleure. The first indication of amnion formation appears in chick at about 30 hours of incubation.

The head of the embryo sinks slightly into the yolk and at the same time the extra-embryonic somatopleure in front of the head is thrown into a fold, the head fold of the amnion. In dorsal aspect the margin of this fold is crescentic in shape with its concavity directed towards the head of the embryo. As the embryo increases in length, its head grows anteriorly into the amniotic fold.

At the same time growth in the somatopleure itself tends to extend the amniotic head-fold caused over the head of the embryo. By continuation of these two growth processes the head soon comes to lie in a double-walled pocket of extra-embryonic somatopleure which covers the head like a cap.

On the third day, the tail-fold of the amnion springs up similarly from the margin of a posterior limiting fold, but it grows in the opposite direction, its concavity being directed anteriorly and its progression being cephalad (anteriorly).

The lateral folds of amnion develop dorsomedian. The head and tail folds grow to meet over the back of the embryo and are soon joined mid-dorsally by similarly-formed lateral folds of the amnion to enclose the embryo in two sheets of somatopleure from all sides except the region of yolk-stalk. At the point where the folds meet, they become fused in a scar-like thickening termed the *sero-amniotic raphe* or the sero-amniotic connection. Since the tail-fold of amnion arises at the much later stage and at a time when the head-fold has already grown beyond the middle of the length of the embryo, the tail fold is smaller, and the sero-amniotic connection is behind the middle of the embryo.

The amniotic folds involve essentially the doubling of somatopleure upon itself. The outer wall of the somatopleure has an outer layer of ectoderm and an inner lining of somatic mesoderm; the two layers together form the chorion.

The inner wall of the fold has the layers reversed *i.e.* its outer layer is of somatic mesoderm and inner of ectoderm, the two together form the amnion. The cavity between chorion (serosa) and amnion (sero-amniotic cavity) is a part of the extra-embryonic coelom. However, when amniotic fold is first formed in front of the head of the embryo (the head fold), it consists only of part of the extra-embryonic ectodermal layer.

The lateral folds from the start consist of extra-embryonic ectoderm and extra-embryonic mesoderm. Mesoderm also secondarily penetrates the anterior portion of the fold, so the composition of the fold becomes uniform throughout.

As the folds of amnion meet, they enclose an amniotic cavity, over and around the embryo completely lined by ectoderm. This cavity is at first a very narrow slit between the embryo and the thinner wall of the amniotic fold, but soon a fluid is secreted into the cavity by the amniotic epithelium, which distends it. Thus the embryo, in a way lies in a pond, floating freely in the cavity, connected to extra-embryonic parts only by the umbilical cord.

The salty amniotic fluid does all that is necessary to prevent desiccation. Besides this, the fluid of the amniotic cavity is an efficient shock absorber and protects the embryo from possible desiccation. Unstriped muscle fibres develop in the mesoderm on the fifth day and produce waves of contraction, rocking the embryo gently, thus, preventing its adhesion to various embryonic membranes or to itself, or from friction against it.

The chorion (serosa) continues to grow and keeps pace with the growing blastoderm and exocoel. It carries the chorion about the yolk-sac, which it envelops. The albumen-sac is also surrounded by folds of chorion. The allantois, after its establishment, develops between it and the amnion. Thus, the chorion encompasses the embryo itself and all the other extraembryonic membranes. It provides an additional protective umbrella over the embryo.

According to BALINSKY (1970), formation of amniotic cavity has a slightly negative effect. It removes the embryo from the surface of egg and forms the source of oxygen.

The Allantois

This accessory organ was primarily evolved in reptiles and birds as temporary sac for urinary storage. It differs from the amnion and serosa because it arises within the body of the embryo. Its proximal portion remains intra-embryonic throughout development. Its distal portion, however, is carried outside the confines of the intraembryonic coelom and becomes associated with the other extra-embryonic membranes.

The allantois grows out late on the third day of incubation as a diverticulum of splanchnopleure from the ventral wall of the hind-gut just in front of the anal plate. During the fourth day of development, the allantois pushes out of the body of the embryo into the extra-embryonic coelom. Its narrow proximal portion, which is parallel and caudal to the yolk-stalk is known as the allantoic stalk and the enlarged distal portion as the allantoic vesicle. Fluid accumulating in the allantois distends it so the appearance of its terminal portion is baloon-like.

The allantoic vesicle enlarges very rapidly from the fourth to the tenth day of incubation. Extending into the sero-amniotic cavity, it becomes flattened and finally encompasses the embryo and the yolk-sac between the amnion and chorion. In this process the splanchnic mesoderm of the allantois becomes fused with the somatic mesoderm of the chorion to form the allanto-chorionic membrane.

In this double layer of mesoderm an extremely rich vascular network develops which is connected with the embryonic circulation by the allantoic arteries and veins. Through this circulation, the allanois carries its primary function of oxygenating the blood of the embryo and relieving it of carbon dioxide. This is made possible by the position occupied by the allantois, close beneath the porous shell, only separated from it by the shell membranes.

In addition, the allantoic cavity continues to act in its primitive capacity as a reservoir for the excreta of the kidney or rather the urinary bladder. The growth of the embryo involves the metabolism of protein with the formation of urea in the early stages of development and later the excreted material becomes chiefly uric acid. These wastes of the embryo, when formed are passed down into the hind-gut (cloaca) near its base by the Wolffian ducts, thence passed and stored in the allantois without ill effects.

The part of its wall also assists in the absorption of egg albumen. The allantoic-stalk becomes further narrow as development proceeds and is combined with the yolk-stalk in a single outer covering to form the *body-stalk* or *umbilical cord*. At the time of hatching the body-stalk is ruptured, the distal portion of the allantois with its contained excretory products is left behind as a shrivelled membrane adherent to the broken shell, and the place of umbilical cord is healed up.

Functions of Extraembryonic Membranes

Function of Yolk Sac : Yolk sac is the primary organ for nutrition (digestion and absorption) of the embryo. Its glandular wall secretes digestive enzymes which convert the yolk into soluble form. It is absorbed by the yolk-sac wall and is sent to the embryo.

Function Chorion : It acts as an organ of respiration and lies in association with allantois.

Functions of Amnion : Since the amniotic cavity forms watery pool around the embryo, it serves the following functions:

1. It protects the embryo from the danger of dessication.
2. It protects the embryo against external shocks.
3. It protects the embryo from adhesion with itself and the embryonic membranes.
4. It helps in the absorption of albumen.

Allantois : Allantois serves as a receptacle for excretory products. It is connected with the gut. The highly vascular allantochorion comes in contact with the shell membrane and forms the embryonic respiratory surface for the embryo.

Extraembryonic Membranes

The embryos of reptiles, birds and mammals are provided with a series of embryonic, foetal, or extraembryonic membranes that protect against dessication and shock and serve in respiration, excretion and other necessary functions during embryonic life.

They do not enter into the formation of the embryo itself, but are external to, and devoted in one way or the other to the care and maintenance of the embryo. Collectively, these structures are spoken of as *extraembryonic membranes*.

Types of Extraembryonic Membranes

During the embryonic development four types of extraembryonic membranes are formed. They are : (1) yolk sac, (2) amnion, (3) chorion, and (4) allantois.

Yolk Sac: It encloses a mass of yolk. In reptiles, birds and some mammals, it is nutritive in function.

Amnion: It surrounds the embryo. The aminotic fluid present in the amnion provides a kind of "private pond" to protect the embryo from dessication and mechanical shocks.

Chorion or Serosa: It is the outermost membrane which is protective and respiratory in function. In mammals, it participates in the formation of foetal part of the placenta and takes up the additional responsibilities of nutrition, excretion etc.

Allantois: Its main function is excretion but it also acts as an embryonic respiratory surface in reptiles and birds. In eutherian mammals it joins with chorion to form a composite membrane, the allantochorion (foetal placenta), which serves in nutrition, respiration, excretion and other functions of the embryo.

During neurulation of chick and other vertebrates, the lateral plate mesoderm becomes split into two layers, an external layer applied to the ectoderm known as the parietal or somatic layer, and an internal layer applied to the endoderm, the visceral or splanchnic layer. The space between the two layers is the coelom. It is customary to refer to *somatic layer of mesoderm* and adjacent body (somatic) *ectoderm* as the *somatopleure,* and to *splanchnic mesoderm* plus adjacent gut *endoderm* as *splanchnopleure.*

Yolk Sac

Development: In reptiles and birds the somatopleure and splanchnopleure develop from the periphery of the blastodisc which is differentiated as the area opaca. These gradually spread peripherally over the yolk mass. Soon afterwards, the embryo begins to be undercut by a series of folds which appear all around the body of the embryo. The folds involve all three germ layers, *i.e.*, the ectoderm, the mesoderm and the endoderm. Directed downward and inward, these are known as the *body folds.*

The extraembryonic splanchnopleure (splanchnic mesoderm + endoderm) continues to spread over the yolk mass and as a yolk sac eventually encloses the mass of yolk in a large measure. The yolk sac however, never surrounds the yolk fully. A small passage is left on the ventral side for the embryo to absorb the remains of albumen at a later stage.

Coincidentally with the formation of the yolk sac, the intraembryonic splanchnopleure is subjected to folds resembling with the more superficial body folds. The intraembryonic folds give rise to a walled digestive tract, or gut, in the body of the embryo. The middle of the embryonic gut remains open to the yolk beneath. At this level the yolk sac is connected to the digestive tract by a constricted yolk stalk.

The wall of the yolk sac is thrown into folds on its inner surface that penetrate the yolk mass. These folds are known as the yolk sac septa. A system of blood vessels is developed in the walls of the yolk sac, entering the heart by means of a pair of vitelline veins.

Functions: The function of yolk sac is to digest the yolk and to transfer the products to digestion to the embryo. Digestion is brought about through the mediation of appropriate enzymes secreted by the endodermal cells lying in contact with the yolk, particularly at the yolk sac septa. Although the yolk sac is connected to the digestive tract by the yolk stalk, the yolky food is not transported to the embryo by this route. Instead, the products of yolk digestion are picked up and carried to the embryo by the vitelline veins running in the mesoderm of the sac.

Amnion and Chorion

Development: The amnion and the chorion are developed together as upwardly projecting folds, the amniotic folds of the extra embryonic somatopleure. The latter is elevated over the embryo by a folding process consisting essentially of a doubling of the somatopleure upon itself.

The first to appear is the part of the fold just in front of the head end of the embryo. This section, which may be referred to as the head fold bends backward over the head and covers it with a double somatopleuric hood. Now the lateral ends of the fold are prolonged backward along both sides of the embryo.

The lateral folds come near each other over the body of the embryo and fuse from the front end backward, so that more and more of the embryo becomes covered by the folds. Eventually, a tail fold also develops behind the embryo. All these folds finally converge so as to encase the embryo in two sheets of somatopleure.

The inner somatopleuric sheet becomes the amnion, the outer, the chorion. The point where the head and tail folds meet is called the sero-amniotic connection. It lies somewhat behind the middle of the embryo's body.

The amnion consists of a layer of extraembryonic *ectoderm* on the inside and a layer of extraembryonic *somatic mesoderm* on the outside. The chorion is made up of a layer of extraembryonic *ectoderm* on the outside and a layer of extraembryonic *somatic mesoderm* on the inside. The latter is, however, continuous with the ectoderm and splanchnic mesoderm converging the yolk sac.

The cavity between the amnion and the embryo is termed the amniotic cavity. In between the amnion and the chorion is the chorionic cavity or extraembryonic coelom, which is continuous with the coelomic cavity in the embryo proper.

Functions of Amnion

(1) The primary function of the amnion is to protect the embryo from dessication. The embryo gets a special advantage by the development of a fluid-filled amniotic cavity. It becomes immersed in a container filled with fluid and thus can carry out its development in a fluid medium, although the egg is placed on "dry land".

(2) Muscle fibres differentiate within the mesoderm of the amnion. The amnion with its muscle fibres and contained fluid serves as an efficient shock absorber. It protects the embryo from mechanical shock resulting from the possible violent agitations of the whole egg caused by incubating hen sitting on it.

(3) The amnion provides a "private salty pond" to the embryo to buoy in at a time when its own soft, collapsible tissues do not have adequate skeletal support.

(4) The amnion separates the embryo from the shell of the egg. Thus it protects it from adhesion to the shell or from friction against it.

Functions of Chorion

(1) The fluid of the chorionic cavity, which is also called the extraembryonic coelom, provides further protection to the embryo.

(2) It provides space into which the allantois can expand itself at a later stage.

(3) The chorion joins with the allantois and plays an important role in gaseous exchange through the porous shell.

Allantois

Development: The allantois arises as a ventral outgrowth of the splanchnopleure from the hindgut. The outgrowth consists of endoderm with a layer of visceral or splanchnic mesoderm covering it from the outside. The allantois grows very fast and eventually penetrates into the extraembryonic coelom, into the space between the yolk sac, the amnion and the chorion.

The proximal part of the allantois forms a narrow neck or the allantoic stalk with which it remains connected with the hindgut of the embryo. The distal part of the allantois expands and penetrates between the amnion and the yolk sac on one side and the chorion on the other side. By the middle of the incubation period, the allantois spread all around the egg underneath the chorion.

The mesoderm on the external surface of the allantois fuses with that of the chorion forming a conjoined chorio-allantoic membrane. Actually, it consists of three layers :

(i) Ectoderm on the outside.

(ii) Mesoderm (splanchnic layer of allantois + somatic layer of chorion) in the middle.

(iii) Endoderm on the inside.

The chorio-allantoic membrane gets pressed against the porous shell. It becomes highly vascular by developing allantoic circulation.

Functions

(1) The cavity of the allantois serves as a urinary bladder. It stores the protein breakdown products in the form of water-insoluble crystals of uric acid inside the egg upto the time of hatching. As the storage goes throughout the time of incubation, the allantois increases to enormous proportions.

(2) The vascular "chorio-allantoic membrane" lies in a close proximity to the inner surface of the porous shell. It acts as an extraembryonic lung by supplying the embryo with oxygen. Gaseous exchange takes place between the blood circulating in the chorio-allantoic membrane and the external air through the porous shell. A network of blood vessels develops in this membrane and this network of blood vessels develops in this membrane and this network is in communication with the embryo proper by means of blood vessels running along the allantoic stalk.

The allantoic circulation is continued till the chick breaks the eggshell and begins to breath the air.

(3) Together with the chorion, the allantois also surrounds the albumen to form the albumen sac and thus assists in the absorption of nutritionally rich albumen.

7

Development of Frog

The embryology of the frog is generally taken up as the first example of the development of a true vertebrate. The frog is a valuable object for such study because its eggs and other developmental stages are easily accessible. During its development the frog shows the origin of all fundamental vertebrate systems. The living material is usually available at a particular time of year and it is easy to handle. The embryos are relatively straight and not twisted like embryos of other vertebrates. This makes their description easier.

Ovulation

The Indian bull frog, *Rana tigrina* breeds during monsoon *i.e.*, from July to September. The female discharges ova in the water by a process known as ovulation. Ripe ova are released into the body cavity of the female by rupture of the epithelial covering of the ovary. These ova are in the form of secondary oocytes. By the ciliary action of the peritoneum the eggs are conveyed to the ostia of the oviducts. These are also ciliated and the ova are drawn into the ducts. The oviduct are lined with ciliated cells interspersed with glandular cells. They dilate posteriorly into thin-walled ovisacs or uteri. Each uterus narrows down and opens into the cloaca. The eggs pass down the oviducts and accumulate in the uteri.

As the egg travels down the oviduct from the ostium to the uterus, the glandular walls of the duct secrete around it three layers of albuminous material (jelly) which constitute a tertiary egg membrane.

Spawning

Spawning is the act of expelling eggs from uteri of female frog stimulated by the male during *sexual embrace* or *amplexus.* In such a position, the male is always capable of discharging sperm over the ova as they emerge. Frog eggs are laid in a coherent mass or *spawn.* The number of eggs in a spawn varies in different species of frogs and in different individuals. A single spawn of *Rana tigrina* may contain 3000—4000 eggs. After spawning, the jelly, which surrounds the egg absorbs water and swells.

Functions of Jelly: Several functions have been assigned to the jelly-coat:

1. It protects the eggs from mechanical injury.
2. It serves to make the eggs adhere to each other and to submerged objects such as water plants. In this way they are not readily washed about.
3. The jelly is distasteful, hence it prevents the eggs from being eaten by water snails, aquatic insects and birds.
4. It prevents infection from bacteria and fungal spores.
5. The jelly serves as a lens to concentrate the rays of the sun upon the eggs. The jelly is thus able to keep the eggs warmer, phenomenon that speeds up the pace of development.

Organization of the Unfertilized Egg : The fully mature egg of a frog is a relatively large spherical cell, measuring about 2.0 to 3.0 mm in diameter. With respect to yolk content, the egg of frog is of mesolecithal type, *i.e.,* it contains a moderate quantity of yolk. The yolk is present in the form of small platelets or void granules. However, the distribution of yolk is unequal. It is collected eccentrically in the lower part (vegetal pole) of the egg. Accordingly, amphibian eggs are said to be telolecithal.

The unfertilized egg is spherical. It is surrounded by a thin, transparent vitelline membrane. It is released from the ovary in the primary oocyte stage. Nearly one-half of the surface of the egg is pigmented black. This part is called the animal hemisphere which contains a nucleus or germinal vesicle. The centre of the animal hemisphere is called the animal pole. It is that region of the egg where polar bodies are eliminated. The other half of the egg is white or pale yellow. It is known as the *vegetal hemisphere.* The centre of the vegetal hemisphere is called *vegetal pole.* It is the region of lowest metabolic rate. The line connecting the two pole of the egg is considered to be the *main* or *polar axis* of the egg.

Fertilization

The Penetration of the Sperm: Fertilization is external and takes place in water. It involves penetration of a sperm into an egg. As the eggs are laid by the female, the male frog immediately discharges over them the seminal fluid which contains thousands of spermatozoa. Many of these pierce the outer jelly, but usually one of them enters the egg. The entrance of sperm always occurs in the animal hemisphere.

Formation of Fertilization Membrane: Entrance of a sperm into the egg results in the elevation of the vitelline membrane away from the egg surface and its transformation into a fertilization membrane. The space that appears between the egg surface and the fertilization membrane is known as the perivitelline space. It is filled with a fluid, within which the egg is free to rotate.

Penetration Path: Usually the whole spermatozoon enters the ovum taking a minute or two for the complete invasion of the cortex. The tail piece may be broken off, but the head and middle piece travel steadily along a path determined by the direction of penetration. This path is generally approximately a radius of the egg and is referred to as the penetration path. As the head and middle piece move along the penetration path, the usual *rotation* of these parts occurs, thus placing the middle piece with centrosome ahead of the nucleus contained in the head of the spermatozoon. The nucleus, which is now referred to as the male pronucleus, starts swelling. The centrosome becomes surrounded by an aster. The sperm nucleus, together with the centrosome, moves through the egg cytoplasm toward the female pronucleus. Since the amphibian eggs are heavily pigmented, the spermatozoon takes along within some of the pigment granules of the surface layer to the interior of the egg. Therefore, the course of the sperm head may be marked by pigment granules trailing along its path.

Completion of Maturation of Egg: The activation of the egg by the spermatozoon incites the completion of the second maturation division of the egg nucleus which had paused in the metaphase stage. As the suspended mitosis is completed, the second polar body is given off into the perivitelline space. The female pronucleus withdraws from the surface of the ovum usually to a position in the polar axis. The male pronucleus then proceeds toward it.

Copulation Path and the Fusion of the Egg and Sperm Nuclei: Frequently, the sperm penetration path may not be directed exactly toward the egg nucleus. In these cases the sperm path makes a slight change in its course so that it will meet the egg nucleus. This new course is called the copulation path because it results in the copulation or fusion of the two nuclei. Like the penetration path, in the case of frog, it is also marked by a trail of pigment.

In the meantime the centrosome of the spermatozoon has divided into two and an achromatic spindle has been formed to which the chromosomes derived from the male and the female pronucleus become attached. This arrangement, making readiness for the first cleavage division, represents the completion of fertilization.

Simultaneously with sperm activation, the albuminous jelly swells to its maximum by imbibition.

Gray Crescent

After sperm penetration, the surface layer of egg cytoplasm starts contracting towards the animal pole. During this contraction, the pigmented cytoplasm covers up the gap in the pigment layer at the animal pole, where the first polar body had been pinched off. About 10 minutes later, practically the whole cortical layer of the egg is rotated in respect to the internal mass of cytoplasm (Ancel and Vintemberger, 1948). At the future ventral side of the egg the cortical cytoplasm moves downward towards the vegetal pole, and at the opposite, future dorsal side of the egg, the cortical cytoplasm moves upward towards the animal pole. (Fig. 11.6). As the edge of the darkly pigmented cortical cytoplasm rises above the equator on the dorsal side, the deeper lying ring of marginal cytoplasm is exposed. The marginal cytoplasm, although bearing some pigment, is much lighter coloured than the cortical cytoplasm. The result is that there appears on the dorsal side of the egg a lightly pigmented, crescent-shaped region known, because of its colour, as the gray crescent.

Symmetry of the Egg, Zygote and Future Embryo : *Before fertilization,* the egg is radially symmetrical about an axis passing through its poles. *After fertilization,* appearance of the gray crescent confers bilateral symmetry on the egg. Gray crescent is destined to be distributed to the right and left sides of the embryo. In other words, a plane bisecting the crescent will correspond to the median axis of the future embryo. The zygote can only be divided into two similar halves by a plane passing through the middle of the gray crescent and the poles. Commonly, the first cleavage plane coincides with the prospective median axis ; thus each of the first two blastomeres contains half the gray crescent and represents one side of the future embryo. Orientation of the future embryo can also be determined now, for the gray crescent is the forerunner of the notochord and as such it marks the dorsal side of the embryo. The animal pole represents the anterior end and the vegetal pole—the posterior end.

In the amphibian egg, animal hemisphere is much more pigmented than the vegetal hemisphere. This difference is so marked that while the animal hemisphere is black, the vegetal hemisphere appears clear white. Between the dark the light areas is always present a zone of intermediate, gradually fading, pigmentation which is known as the marginal zone.

Cleavage

Division of the egg is complete or holoblastic. After the second cleavage, it is unequal. Segmentation begins about 2 hours after fertilization.

The first cleavage is *meridional.* It runs from animal to vegetal pole through the middle of the gray crescent and point of sperm entry. The first two blastomeres are equal in size.

The second cleavage is also *meridional,* but at right angles to the first, producing four equal sized blastomeres. This second cleavage begins to appear about 1 hour after the completion of the first cleavage.

The third cleavage is *horizontal* or *latitudinal* and at right angles to both the first and the second cleavages. It forms slightly above the level of the equator. This shifting of the cleavage plane towards the animal hemisphere is due to the presence of more cytoplasm and relatively less yolk in that region. This *differential* or *discriminatory cleavage*, therefore, results in an eight-cell stage consisting of four smaller animal cells designated as micromeres and four larger vegetal cells called macromeres. The third cleavage, begins about 30 minutes after the second is completed.

The planes of the fourth cleavage are in general meridional, but henceforth the planes become more and more variable. Micromeres divided more rapidly and with greater frequency than the macromeres which are hindered by yolk.

Blastula

At about the fourth or fifth cleavage a small space, the segmentation cavity or blastocoel, appears within the cell cluster. The embryo in this stage is called a blastula. The presence of a cavity in the blastula distinguishes it as a coeloblastula. The blastocoel is formed as a result of the curvature of the inner surfaces of the blastomeres. It become infiltered by an albuminous fluid secreted by the surrounding cells. The blastocoel rapidly increases in size. Since the horizontal cleavages appear toward the animal hemisphere, blastocoel is formed in an eccentric position above the level of the equator. The blastocoel is covered by a relatively thin, multilayered roof of animal cells. On its floor are present large yolky blastomeres.

Fate Map of Frog Embryo

A fate map is simply a topographical chart of the blastula with respect to the ultimate fate of the various parts of the blastoderm. The fate maps of various blastulae have been worked out by many experimental embryologists among whom are Born, Butschli, Rhumbler, Spek, Vogt, Dalcq, Vintemberger,

Pasteels, Nicholas, Schechtman, Spratt, and Holtfreter. They have used various experimental methods such as natural marking by injury of cell areas, artificial marking with vital dyes and carbon particles.

Construction of Fate Map by Artificial Marking: An artificial marking of parts of the blastoderm to reconstruct the fate map was devised by Wather Vogt (1925). This is done by the use of so-called vital dyes (Nile blue sulphate, neutral red, Bismarck brown) which are retained by cells for considerable periods and do not interfere with normal development processes in any way. The method consists in soaking a block of agar in a vital dye and then pressing it against a chosen area of the blastoderm for a short time.

The dye diffuses from the agar into the cells of the embryo. By so marking, it is possible to follow the movements of gastrulation by continuous observation as the position of the stained cells in the differentiated embryo clearly shows the fate of the stained area. It has been experimentally established that the vital due remains restricted to the cells which had originally taken up the dye and to their descendants. Using different colours like red, blue and brown, several areas may be marked simultaneously on the surface of the same embryo. In this way the fate of many parts of the early embryo may be ascertained at the same time by a single experiment.

The entire surface of the blastula of frog may be roughly divided into three regions: (1) the animal region on and around the animal pole, (2) the marginal zone, going all around the equator of the blastula and (3) the vegetal region around the vegetal pole. Inside each region are found areas corresponding to the future organs of the animal.

Animal Regions

It consists of two main areas :

Neural Ectoderm: This area is found largely on the dorsal side. It develops into the nervous system of the embryo. Inside the nervous system area, a small sub-area may be traced which participates in the formation of the eyes of the embryo.

Epidermal Ectoderm: This is found on the antero-ventral side and is destined to become the skin epidermis of the embryo. The material for the nose and the ears and the ectodermal part of the mouth may be traced in the epidermal area.

Marginal Zone

This is the intermediate zone which contains the following prospective organ regions :

Notochord: It occupies a large area on the middorsal side of the blastula.

Prechordal Plate: Notochord is followed by an area containing the material for the prechordal connective tissue. Lying nearer to the vegetal pole, this area is called prechordal plate.

Endoderm Lining: Below the prechordal plate toward the vegetal pole, is present the endoderm material for the anterior parts of the alimentary canal. This is destined to become the endodermal lining of the mouth, and the pharynx of the future embryo.

Segmental Muscles: The parts of the marginal zone on both sides of the notochordal area on the dorsal side are taken up by the mesoderm for the segmental muscles of the body.

Ventrolateral Mesoderm: The lateral and ventral parts of the marginal zone give rise to the mesodermal lining of the body cavity and the kidneys etc.

Vegetal Region

It is composed of cells that are later found in the midgut and hindgut.

Gastrulation

The end of cleavage and the formation of blastulas followed by the next phase of development called gastrulation. This is a phase during which the materials comprising the blastula are redistributed in such a way as to create a stratified embryo termed the gastrula. The events by which the blastula is converted to a gastrula comprise gastrulation. These are essential movements of areas of the blastoderm.

Several processes occur simultaneously during gastrulation. It includes four kinds of morphogenetic movements (1) invagination and formation of blastopore, (2) involution, (3) epiboly and (4) rotation.

***Invagination and Formation of Blastopore* :** Gastrulation in frog is inaugurated by the formation of a depression or groove on the dorsal side of the embryo, at the boundary between the gray crescent and the vegetal region. This groove represents the blastopore. It is produced by the invagination of the endodermal and mesodermal material into the interior of the embryo. These cells assume the elongate shape of a bottle and stream into the interior of the embryo toward the blastocoel cavity. Their steadily elongating necks remain attached to the surface of the blastula, whereas the bulky cell bodies move inward.

As a result, a pull is exerted along their thin necks which creates an indentation at the surface. With continued multiplication and thinning out of the bottle cells, the indentation or invagination deepens. The area of the blastoderm immediately above the blastopore may be spoken of as the dorsal lip of the blastopore.

On the dorsal side of the embryo, a cavity is formed which leads from the groove on the surface into the interior of the embryo. Lined on all sides by the invaginated cells, this cavity is called archenteron. It is at first a narrow slit-like cavity, but later, as more cells invaginate, it expands at its anterior end. In the process, it pushes the yolk-filled megameres toward the blastocoel and the latter is eventually obliterated.

Involution and Closure of the Blastopore : In frog, invagination is always accompanied with involution. Involution can be described as the *rolling* of the superficial cells (future notochord and mesoderm) over the rim of the blastopore and into its interior while new portions of the blastopore approach the rim in their place. Thus cells are carried inside the gastrula, and locked in beneath the outer layer. Involution is most active on the dorsal lip of the blastopore.

The Prechordal Plate: In the blastulae lies just below the presumptive notochord. The prechordal plate is the first mesoderm which involutes over the dorsal lip of the blastopore and becomes a part of the archenteron roof. In the gastrula, it lies in front of an anterior end of the presumptive notochord.

The Notochord: The notochord involutes by rolling over the dorsal lip of the blastopore into the interior of the embryo. It becomes stretched along the dorsal side of the archenteron and forms the mid-dorsal strip of the archenteron roof. During the process, the prospective notochord elongates in the longitudinal direction. However, it also undergoes a corresponding contraction in the transverse direction.

The Mesoderm: Most of the mesoderm "turns the corner" and moves to the interior by rolling over the lateral and ventral lips of the blastopore. After entering the embryo, the mesoderm advances in an anterior direction in the form of a sheet of cells that penetrate between the ectoderm on the outside and the endoderm on the inside.

In the next phase of gastrulation the blastoporal groove begins to spread transversely. The area of cells rolling inwards increases laterally so that the dorsal lip of the blastopore grows downwards forming lateral lips.

The lateral lips of the blastopore meet ventrally to form a ventral lip so that the blastopore assumes the shape of a ring. The space enclosed by the rim of the blastopore is seen to be filled by yolk-laden macromeres of the vegetal region. These cells are called yolk plug. The rim of the blastopore, however, continue to contract and eventually almost covers the yolk-plug except for a narrow canal leading into the interior.

While the superficial cells are involuting over the rim of the blastopore, the rim itself does not remain at a fixed position. Instead, it gradually shifts over the surface of the vegetal region, moving away from the animal pole and toward the vegetal pole. As a result of involution, therefore, the material of the vegetal region disappears eventually into the interior of the embryo.

Epiboly

Epiboly is the overgrowth of the ectoderm-forming regions around the inwardly moving prospective mesodermal and endodermal regions. The presumptive epidermis and the presumptive nervous system that are present in the animal region, greatly increase in their surface during gastrulation. This increase of surface area takes place at the expense of a thinning out of the epithelial layer. The prospective epidermis expands in all directions, but in the case of the prospective nervous system the expansion is mainly in the longitudinal direction, *i.e.*, towards the blastopore. As a result of epiboly, therefore, the ectoderm covers the whole embryo after the mesoderm and the endoderm have disappeared inside at the end of gastrulation.

Rotation

Movement of the heavy yolky megameres from the posterior to the ventral position, reduction of the anterior blastocoel, and *the enlargement of the dorsal archenteron* together change the gravitational axis of the gastrula, shifting it about 90° away from the position of the blastopore. It causes the vegetal region of the embryo to be drawn into the interior and at the same time to rotate. Therefore, at the end of gastrulation, the vegetal region comes to lie in the ventral part of the archenteron, *i.e.*, the embryo swings round within the vitelline membrane to bring its antero-posterior axis in a horizontal plane. Further, the presence of the archenteric roof and the pre-chordal and notochordal cells above it cause the overlying ectoderm to thicken and the whole embryo becomes elongated in an antero-posterior direction.

The embryo is now called the gastrula. A completed gastrula is nearly 3-layered. Endoderm is lacking only in the mid-dorsal region, but soon the free edges of the endoderm approach each other in the midline and fuse, thus completely enclosing the midgut. In this way, the three primary germ layers *viz.* ectoderm mesoderm and endoderm are established.

Neurulation

After the closure of the blastopore, the ectodermal epithelium of the prospective nervous system, situated along the mid-dorsal axis of the embryo, becomes differentiated from the rest of the ectoderm in the form of a neural plate. The cells of the neural plate become thick and elongated. They arrange themselves into a columnar epithelium. In contrast, the cells of the epidermis remain more or less flat and are arranged as a stratified epithelium usually two cells thick.

The margins of the neural plate become thickened and elevated above the general level as neural folds. The midline of the neural plate is depressed, forming a shallow groove along the length of the body. Later, the neural folds become higher and meet dorsally in the median line forming a tube which subsequently separates from the parent ectoderm. This is the neural tube whose anterior portion will give rise to the brain with brain cavities. The remainder part of the neural tube will later become the spinal cord.

The formation and closure of the neural plate is known as neurulation. The embryonic stage which possesses a neural plate, is called a neurula.

Neural Crest: A certain number of cells on the sides of the neural plate are not incorporated in the neural tube or in the epidermis. After the separation of neural tube from the epidermis, these cells occupy the space between the neural tube and the overlying epidermis. This irregular flattened mass of cells is called the neural crest. It may be continuous across the midline at first, but later on the mass of cells separates into two halves, each lying dorsolaterally to the neural tube.

The neural crest cells play a special part in the development of the embryo. They give rise to the branchial skeleton, dorsal root ganglia, sensory nerves, sympathetic nervous system, and medullary part of the adrenal gland.

Development of Notochord

The median-dorsal region of the mesoderm segregates from its lateral parts lying on both sides. It is this median strip that rounds up and forms the notochord lying between the gut roof and the developing neural tube above. As the notochord is separated from the mesoderm, the strand of notochordal cells becomes converted into a cylindrical body, which is round in cross-section. The cells become vacuolated and soon a sheath develops around the notochord.

Differentiation of Mesoderm and Formation of Coelom : The dorsal part of the mesoderm lying on the sides of the notochord becomes subdivided into a series of mesodermal segments called Samites. The thinned out lateral and ventral parts of the mesoderm on each side do not become subdivided into segments. These parts of the mesoderm are known as the lateral plates. Concomitantly with the segmentation of the mesoderm in its dorsal part, the lateral plate mesoderm splits into two layers : (*i*) an external layer applied to the ectoderm known as the parietal or somatic layer, and (*ii*) an internal layer applied to the endoderm, the visceral or splanchnic layer. The narrow space between the two layers is the coelomic cavity or coelom. In later stages the cavity expands and becomes the body cavity of the adult animal.

According to *Torrey* (1962), the mesoderm on each side of the embryonic body becomes subdivided horizontally into three distinct regions : (*i*) a dorsal *epimere* *(ii)* an intermediate mesomere, and

(ii) a ventral hypomere. Mesodermal somites as described by Balinsky (1970), comprise an epimere and a mesomere per somite. Lateral plate mesoderm, however, represents the hypomere. Epimere is composed of three components : *(a)* a lateral dermatome, *(b)* a ventromedian *myotome* and a dorsomedian *sclerotome.*

Fate of the Primary Germ Layers : During gastrulation in animals, a single layer of cells, the *blastoderm,* gives rise to two or more layers of cells known as the germinal layers. The germinal layers are complex rudiments from which are derived the various organs of the animal's body. In frog and higher animal, the body consists of several layers of tissues and organs that may be traced back to 3 germinal layers, the ectoderm, the mesoderm, and the endoderm. The future fate of these germinal layers is given in an outline plan as follows :

Embryo		*Adult*
	—	Epidermis of skin
	—	Skin derivatives (glands, hair, nail, feathers, claws etc.)
	—	Olfactory organ (nasal epithelium)

Somatic Ectoderm	--	Lens of eye, Cornea and Conjuctiva
	—	Inner ear (Membranous Labyrinth)
	—	Enamel of Teeth
	—	Lining of Stomodaeum and Proctodaeum
	—	Anterior Pituitary
Neural Crest	—	Branchial skeleton
	—	Dorsal root ganglia and sensory nerves
	—	Sympathetic Nervous System
	—	Adrenal Medulla
	—	Pigment cells
	—	Brain and Spinal Cord
	—	Cranial and Spinal motor nerves
	—	Retina and optic nerve
		Posterior Pituitary
Neural Tube	—	Pineal body
Notochord	—	Reduced or obliterated
— Dermatome	—	Dermis of skin
— Empimere	—	Sclerotome
	—	Skull, Vertebral column
— Myotome	—	Skeletal muscle and Appendicular skeleton — Excretory organs
— Mesomere	—	Reproductive ducts
— Somatic layer	—	Parietal peritoneum
	—	Visceral peritoneum
	—	Muscles of Viscera
	—	Mesenterise
— Hypomere	—	Splanchnic layer
	—	Heart, Pericardium, Blood Cells and Blood vessels

		—	Spleen
	—	—	Gonads
	Coelom		Body cavities
		—	Lining of Digestive tract except Stomodaeum and roctodaeum
		—	Gastric and Intestinal Glands
		—	Liver, Pancreas, Bile and Pancreatic ducts
— Archenteron		—	Respiratory system
(Primitive Gut)		—	Urinary bladder
		—	Middle ear and Eustachian tube
		—	Certain endocrines like Thyroid, Parathyroids and Thymus
		—	Lining of vagina, urethra.

Post-neurular Development

Formation of Tadpole Larva: About four days after fertilization, the embryo is said to be at the tail bud stage of development when it is about 3 mm long. The tail bud larva undergoes a series of changes in its external and internal structure within the egg membranes to become the tadpole larva. The larva elongates in an antero-posterior direction and shows distinct differentiation into head and trunk. At the hind end appears a small outgrowth or tail bud indicating the beginning of the tail. Small swellings on each lateral side of the head indicate the position of the internally developing eyes. In front of each bulge is present a small nasal pit, and behind the nasal pit of each side lies the rudiment of the ear. A "V-shaped glandular pit, the adhesive organ or cement gland develops just below the prospective stomodaeum on the ventral surface of the head.

In the anterior part of the trunk, three pharyngeal pouches are formed as lateral outpushings of the fore-gut. These are the rudiments of first three gill clefts. The trunk bulges ventrally and laterally due to the presence of a large amount of yolk beneath and at the sides of the developing gut. A small depression, thc proctodaeum lies between the tail and the trunk on the ventral side. It will form the cloaca and the cloacal aperture. The larva also has a well-differentiated brain.

***Hatching*:** When the embryo is about 12 days old, it dissolves the egg membranes by *hatching enzymes* produced in the skin and emerges from the jelly envelope. This process is known as hatching and the hatched larva is called a young tadpole. It is a blackish, fish-like creature, about 7 mm long. The newly hatched larva swims for a short while, but soon fixes itself to some floating vegetation or moss-covered walls of the ponds by means of a sticky secretion of mucous glands present in the adhesive organ. It does not take any food due to the absence of mouth and is nourished from the yolk present in the ventral bulge of the trunk.

During the larval life of tadpole, following developments occur :

(1) The mouth forms.

(2) A pair of horny jaws, bearing papillae or horny teeth, develop around the mouth. The larva now beings to feed upon algae and other vegetable matter by the rasping action of the teeth.

(3) Three pairs of finger-like external gills project from the sides of head in the branchial region.

(4) The external gills gradually disappear under an opercular fold of the skin. Meanwhile, true or internal gills have been gradually developing by perforation of the pharyngeal gill pouches. The opercular chamber opens to the outside by an aperture called spiracle on the left side. The space between the body wall and operculum is called branchial or gill chamber.

(5) The tail elongates and becomes a powerful organ of locomotion. It acquires a dorsal and a ventral tail fin.

(6) Adhesive organ begins to degenerate.

(7) Lens and cornea are formed and the eyes become functional.

(8) Hind limb buds appear, one on each side of the cloaca.

The embryo is now a free-swimming, actively feeding tadpole larva, which has no resemblance with the fish-like tailed semi-terrestrial adult frogs.

Metamorphosis

The term metamorphosis is derived from a Greek work *metamorphoun*, which means "to transform". In embryology it is defined as transformation of the larva into adult during which many structural as well as physiological changes take place. Larval forays and accompanying metamorphosis are found in most groups of animal kingdom.

When about 8 weeks old, the tadpole larva undergoes a series of rapid changes, which, transform it into a young frog. This is called metamorphosis.

The metamorphic changes in frog tadpoles may be grouped into three categories : (A) changes in habits and habitat, (B) changes in morphology, and (C) changes in physiology.

Changes in Habits and Habitat

(1) In frog, metamorphosis is associated with a transition from an aquatic to a terrestrial mode of life. The metamorphosing larva comes frequently to the surface of water to breath air. Later, it beings to take short trips to land, *i.e.*, it becomes amphibious.

(2) The changes of environment during metamorphosis is associated with a change in feeding. The tadpoles are

herbivorous feeding upon algae and other vegetable matter—which they scrape off with the help of the horny teeth surrounding their mouths. Adult frogs, on the other hand, are carnivorous — living on insects, worms etc. Sometimes, they also devour larger prey, such as smaller frogs and even little birds and rodents which they overpower and swallow.

Changes in Morphology

Regressive or Destructive Changes: These include the reduction or complete disappearance of those organs or structures which are necessary during larval life, but not essential in the adults. The important changes of this nature are as follows :

(1) The long tail of the tadpole along with the fin folds is absorbed again during metamorphosis and disappears altogether at the end of the metamorphosis.

The reduction of the tail is affected by autolysis of the component tissues with active participation of amoeboid *macrophages.* These are rich in lysosomes that contain a proteolytic enzyme *catepsin.* The macrophages phagocytose the debris of the disintegrating cells. During metamorphosis, however, the tadpole is nourished by the substance of its tail.

(2) The gills are resorbed, the gill clefts are closed and the branchial cavities disappear. The resorption of gills also takes place by autolysis.

(3) The horny teeth of the perioral disc as well as the horny lining of the jaws are shed.

(4) The lateral line sense organs present in the skin of tadpoles, disappear during metamorphosis.

(5) The cloacal tube becomes shortened and reduced.

(6) Some blood vessels, including parts of the aortic arches, are reduced.

Progressive or Constructive Changes: These include the development of some organs which become functional only during and after metamorphosis.

(1) There is a progressive development of the limbs which increase in size and differentiation. The forelimbs, which in the tadpole develop under cover of opercular membrane, break through to the exterior. At the same time there is a great increase in the length and strength of the hindlimbs. Joints develop in them and the toes appear.

(2) The middle ear develops in connection with the first pharyngeal pouch. The tympanic membrane develops. It is supported by the circular tympanic cartilage and enables the frog to receive air-borne vibrations.

(3) The eyes bulge up on the dorsal surface of the head and develop nictitating membrane.

(4) There is development of the tongue and the vomerine teeth.

Remodelling of Some Structures: Some organs which function both in the larva and the adult, change their differentiation during metamorphosis so as to meet the requirements of the adult mode of life.

(1) The skin of the tadpole is covered with a double-layered epidermis. The number of layers of cells in the *epidermis* increases during metamorphosis. Surface layers become cornified. Multicellular *mucous* and *serous glands* develop in the skin. The *pigmentation* to the skin is changed : new patterns and colours appear.

(2) There is a widening of the mouth gap due to rotation of the quadrate cartilage backwards and the true jaws become functional.

(3) The tongue grows much larger and more muscular.

(4) The stomach and the liver enlarge.

(5) The eyes grow more prominent.

(6) In tadpoles, the intestine is very long and wound up into a spiral like a watch spring The intestine becomes greatly elongated due to a herbivorous habit because the vegetable diet contains less nourishment than the animal diet. Hence, a longer gut is required to extract most of the nourishment. During metamorphosis, the intestine is greatly shortened and most of the coils which it forms in the tadpole become straightened out. This change is apparently correlated with the carnivorous habits assumed by the adult.

(7) Two chambered heart of frog is transformed into a three chambered one.

(8) Lungs do not undergo major changes. They develop very gradually and become fully functional.

(9) The cartilaginous skeleton of tadpole undergoes ossification.

(10) The larval pronephric kidney is transformed into a mesonephros.

(11) The blood vascular system is modified with the disappearance of some aortic arches and increase of blood supply to the lungs and the skin.

Changes in Physiology

(1) The endocrine function of the pancreas starts at metamorphosis as it begins to secrete *insulin* and *glycogen* hormones. This is related to the increased role of the liver in the turnover of glycogen.

(2) A marked change takes place in the excretory function.

In the tadpole, the end product of nitrogen metabolism is ammonia which is easily disposed off by diffusion in water. After metamorphosis, however, the frogs excrete most of their nitrogen in the form of urea and only small amounts as ammonia. The latter is highly toxic and if accumulated in a terrestrial animal, it could become dangerous. This change over, occurring in the late stages of metamorphosis is due to a changed function of the liver, which begins to synthesize urea.

Physiological Control of Metamorphosis in Frog (Anura) : Metamorphosis in the anurans (frogs and toads) is initiated by the anterior lobe of the pituitary when it reaches a certain degree of differentiation and becomes capable of producing the thyrotropic hormone (TTH).

The thyrotropic hormone activates the thyroid gland, which builds up and releases the thyroid hormones. The most important of them are tri-iodothyronine (I3Thn) and tetra-iodothyronine (I4Thn) or Thyroxine. In both of these compounds two residues of the amino acid tyrosine are joined together, and to these are attached 3 (in I3Thn) or 4 (in I4Thn) atoms of iodine. The structural formulae of these hormones are as follows :

Of the two compounds, thyroxine is produced in much greater quantities and is thus the main action substance released by the thyroid gland, although the activity of tri-iodothyronine is three to five times as high as that of thyroxine.

The thyroid hormone is carried to the various body organs through the blood stream and affects the tissues directly. While it causes the degeneration and necrosis of some cells, it stimulates the growth and differentiation of others, thus causing the metamorphosis.

Organogenesis of Frog

During neurulation of frog, the three germinal layers, namely ectoderm, mesoderm and endoderm become tubulated and differentiated into *primary organ rudiments* of their respective organ systems. These primary organ rudiments, further subdivided into *secondary organ rudiments* which gradually develop and differentiate into organs of adult frog. These processes of organogeny occur during the conversion of neurula into tadpole larva, and metamorphosis of tadpole into the adult frog. The organogenesis of different organs of frog can be studied separately for each germinal layer as follows :

Development of Ectodermal Organs : The ectodermal tissue of neurula stage of frog have become differentiated into the *epidermal ectoderm, neural ectoderm*, and *neural crest cells*. During organogenesis, these ectodermal tissues form a variety of body organs as under :

Development and Differentiation of Epidermal Ectoderm : Following structures get differentiated from the epidermal ectoderm :

Skin : Major part of epidermis develops into skin.

Sense Organs : Olfactory organs, ears, lateral-line canal, lens and cornea of eye develop from epidermal ectoderm.

External gills, median-fins and adhesive organs (sucker) and frontal gland.

Development of Skin

The epidermal epithelium of young tadpole has two layers :

(i) outer, ciliated layer - the periderm, and

(ii) inner nervous layer - the stratum germinativum.

The cells of periderm loose cilia become flattened and form the outermost layer — the squamous epithelium epidermis. It contains pigment granules and unicellular glands.

The cells of stratum germinativum proliferate and form stratified epithelium, the epidermis. The basal layer forms the malpighian layer which keeps on dividing and adding layers to the epidermis.

The mesenchyme cells that originate from dermatome and neural crest, accumulate under the Malpighian layer and form dermis layer of skin. Its cells develop into connective tissue, blood vessels, nerve fibres, sensory receptors and pigment cells.

Development and Differentiation of Neural Ectoderm : The neural ectoderm gives rise to complete central nervous system, peripheral nervous system and eyes.

Development of Central Nervous System : The central nervous system develops a dorsal thickening of neural ectoderm. It is called neural or medullary plate. It extends from the dorsal lip of blastopore in an anterior direction as a median band of thickened ectoderm. It widens anteriorly to form the brain. Therefore, the development of brain can be studied under two headings:

1. Formation of neural tube.
2. Differentiation of anterior part of neural tube into different parts of brain. Formation of neural tube has already been studied.

Development of Brain

The primitive neural tube, when formed is of unequal diameter throughout. Its anterior end is expanded, the cavity is broader and the walls are thicker than the posterior part of the tube. This anterior expanded portion of neural tube marks off the development of brain while the remaining neural tube forms the spinal cord.

Differentiation of Primary Brain Vesicles : As the embryo increases in length, the neural tube assumes a slightly concave orientation. In the head region the floor of the embryonic brain vesicle bends ventrally around the top of the notochord. The process of bending is known as cranial flexure and the anterior part of the floor of brain which has undergone bending, is called tuberculum posterium or posterior tubercle.

It lies in line with the notochord and the anterior neuropore. It forms the floor of mesencephalon. Opposite to the tuberculum posterium, placed somewhat anteriorly in the roof of the brain is a thickened area. This is dorsal thickening. It lies just behind the closed anterior neuropore. The dorsal thickening marks the roof of mesencephalon.

Therefore, at this stage it is possible to differentiate the three primary parts of the embryonic brain. If a line is drawn from the point just anterior to tuberculum posterium to the point just anterior to the dorsal thickening and another line from the posterior end of the tuberculum posterium to the posterior end of dorsal thickening, the brain is divided into three distinct regions.

1. Prosencephalon
2. Mesencephalon
3. Rhombencephalon.

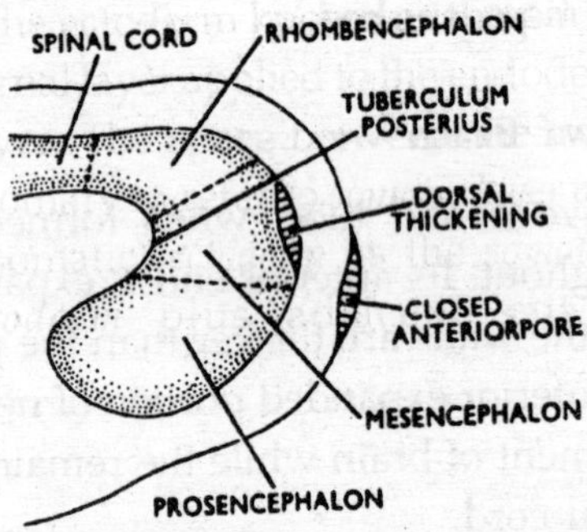

Sagittal section of head of frog embryo showing differentiation of three primary regions of the embryonic brain.

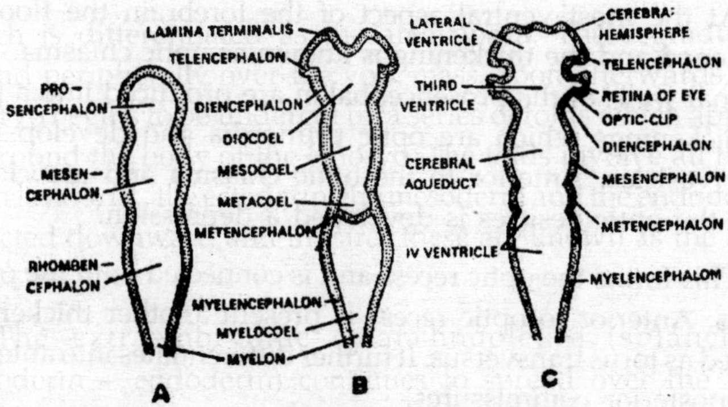

Development and formation of basic parts of frog's brain shown in V.L.S.

Derivatives of Prosencephalon or Forebrain : In the early embryo only forebrain differentiates into its constituent parts. Shortly after the differentiation of three regions of the brain a ventral evagination occurs in the floor of prosencephalon. This vesicular evagination forms the infundibulum. As the

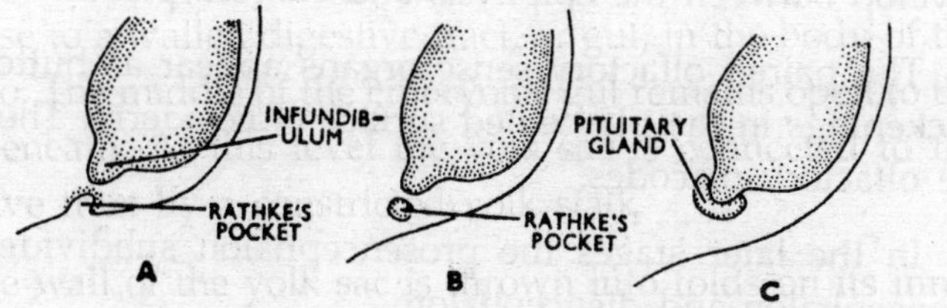

Diagrammatic representation of the development of pituitary in Frog.

infundibulum grows out, aninvagination from the roof of stomodaeum develops towards the infundibulum. This invagination is known as Rathke's pocket. It is formed of the foregut. Rathke's pockets soon pinches off from the roof of stomodaeum and forms a sort of vesicle. It moves towards the infundibulum and finally fuses with it to form the rudimentary pituitary gland. The infundibulum forms the pars nervosa or the posterior lobe pituitary gland whereas the Rathke's pocket forms pars distalis, pars intermedia and pars tuberalis of the adult pituitary gland (anterior pituitary).

At the most ventral aspect of the forebrain the floor is thickened and the thickening is known as optic chiasma. The internal walls of the prosencephalon are produced into a pair of thickenings which are optic primordia and develop into optic vesicles. Anterior to the optic chiasma and associated with the optic vesicles is developed a depression.

This forms the optic recess and is connected with the optic stalks. Anterior to optic recess is present another thickening named as torus transversus. It further differentiates into anterior and posterior commissures.

The roof of the forebrain evaginates slightly dorsal to the imaginary line drawn from the anterior end of notochord. This evagination is known as epiphysis. It represents the primordia of pineal body. Anterior to the epiphysis the roof of the forebrain becomes folded and vascular and forms the anterior choroid plexus. Later on, habenular ganglia and habenular commissure develop between the epiphysis and choroid plexus.

The paired olfactory sense organs appear as button-like thickenings in the pigmented surface of ectoderm. These are the olfactory placodes.

In the later stages the prosencephalon subdivides into telencephalon and diencephalon.

Telencephalon (Secondary Forebrain) : It is the anterior-most portion of the forebrain and its cavity is known a telocoel. It is the embryonic cerebrum. The telocoel expands laterally and gives rise to the right and left lateral ventricles and the thick-walled cerebral hemispheres.

The lateral ventricles are partially constricted off from each other and are connected together by foremen of Monro, which opens into the third ventricle. The third ventricle overlaps and connects the telocoel and diocoel. The torus transversus differentiates into anterior commissure and the anterior pallial commissure. Further development includes enlargement of the cerebral hemispheres and consequent reduction in the size of their ventricles.

A pair of olfactory lobes bud off from the cerebral hemispheres but soon become fused mesially except at the point of origin of olfactory nerve. The anterior choroid plexus develops in the roof of forebrain at the junction of telencephalon and diencephalon.

Diencephalon (or Thalamencephalon) : It lies immediately behind the telencephalon. Its cavity is known as diocoel. It extends anterodorsally beneath the epiphysis, anteroventrally into the optic recess, posteroventrally into the infundibulum and laterally into the relatively large optic vesicles. The optic primordia develop from the diencephalon.

The Derivatives of Diencephalon on the Dorsal side are : (i) posterior commissure, (ii) epiphysial recess, and (iii) the epiphysis. The epiphysis grows into the browspot of the adult which is homologous to pineal gland of higher vertebrates, (iv) Habenular ganglion and commissure develop in the roof of diencephalon between epiphysis and anterior choroid plexus, (v) Paraphysis is the dorsal outgrowth from the roof of diencephalon.

Optic chiasma, optic recess and the infundibulum are present on the floor of diencephalon. The latter forms a part of pituitary gland of the adult.

Mesencephalon : The mesencephalon develops extremely thick walls and the lateral thickenings are known as crura cerebri. These contain various nerve tracks which extend from prosencephalon to rhombencephalon. The original dorsal thickening is subdivided by a median fissure to form a pair of optic lobes or corpora bigemina. These do not reach the full development until the time of metamorphosis.

The cavity of mesencephalon *i.e.* mesocoel is narrowed

because of the thickening of lateral walls and roof. This forms the aqueduct of Sylvius or cerebral aqueduct. This connects and third and fourth ventricle of the brain.

Rhombenecephalon (Hindbrain) : The rhombencephalon is demarcated from the mesencephalon by a transverse constriction. A transverse thickening develops in the roof of rhombencephalon. It develops into the cerebellum. Just behind the cerebellum the roof becomes broad, thin and vascular and folds into the cavity of rhombencephalon (the rhombocoel). This specialized vascular area is known as posterior choroid plexus. The ventral and ventrolateral walls of rhombencephalon constitute the medulla oblongata.

The rhombocoel is known as fourth ventricle which communicates with the third ventricle and central canal of spinal canal cord.

Development of Sense Organs

Development or Eye

Development of Optic Cup : The eyes originate as a pair of lateral evaginations from the ventrolateral walls of the diocoel. Each evagination appears as a vesicle in the beginning but soon its dorsal wall grows faster towards the head ectoderm and makes a contact with it. On coming in contact with the ectoderm, it flattens and finally invaginates to form the double-layered optic cup.

The rim of the optic cup exposes the pupil and the thickening of the wall of optic cup between dorsal and ventral limits marks the region of presumptive retina. The thickening, later on, differentiates into the sensory cells, the rods and cones. The visual elements, rods and cones, appear at about 6mm stage and are fully formed by 11 mm stage. The outer wall of the optic cup finally develops pigment and is modified into choroid layer.

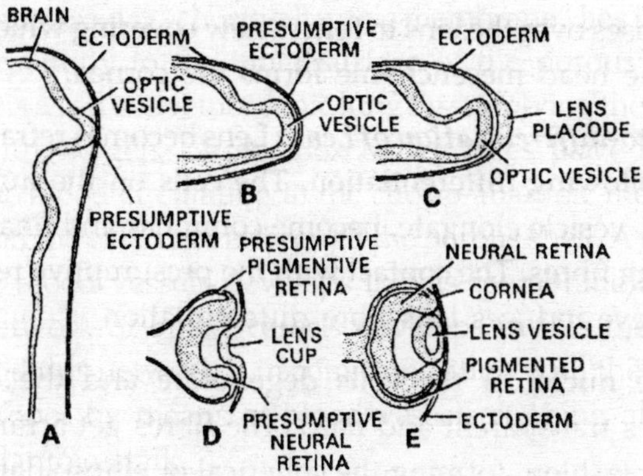

T.S. head of frog embryo showing development of eye.

The cup invaginates further and grows in thickness till it obliterates the original cavity of the optic lobe (the optocoel). As a result the retinal and inner pigmented layers of the optic lobe are brought together in close proximity. The original optocoel is now represented by a slit-like space.

In the beginning, the optic vesicle is connected with the cavity of diencephalon. But as the vesicle grows, it becomes constricted into a tubular optic stalk by the convergence of the surrounding mesenchyme. When the wall of the optic cup thickens to form retina, the optic stalk is displaced to a more ventral position. The optic stalk is traversed by an inverted groove, the choroid fissure, which serves as a passage for the nerve and blood vessels.

Development of Lens : The nervous layer of head ectoderm in the region of contact with the optic vesicle proliferates into the optic cup forming the lens placode. The placode invaginates to form the lens vesicle which pinches off from the head ectoderm and comes to lie within the cavity of optic cup and is supported by suspensory ligament. The outer wall of the lens vesicle is formed of cuboidal epithelium, whereas the cells of inner wall elongate to form lens fibres. The head ectoderm then closes over the lens to form a new covering which together with the head mesenchyme forms the cornea.

Cyto-differentiation of Lens : Lens becomes refracting body after following differentiation. The cells on the inner side of the lens vesicle elongate, become columnar and finally change into long fibres. The contact with the presumptive retinal layer of the eye induces lens fibre differentiation.

The nuclei of the cells degenerate and the cytoplasm becomes transparent and hard. The fibres get arranged in an orderly fashion, forming the spherical or ellipsoidal refracting body. Part of the lens epithelium remains unchanged and covers the sphere of fibres distally.

Cyto-differentiation of Retina : The inner-most layer of the retina, *i.e.* nearest the centre of the eye differentiates first and the sensory layer of rods and cones in the last. Once differentiation has begun, the intricate and inter-related processes leading to the final cyto-architecture comprise a self-directing and self-sustaining complex mechanism..

The step-by-step sequence of retinal cell differentiation is as follows:

Glial Cells : These develop Muller's fibres and envelop the retinal neurons. These develop cytoplasmic processes to connect the inner and outer surface of the sensory retina, the terminal ends of the processes combine to form the internal and external so-called limiting membranes.

Ganglionic Cells: These form the inner-most layer of the retina. These send out axons which constitute the optic nerve along the optic stalk. The dendritic processes of the ganglion cells form synapses with axons from the next layer to differentiate *i.e.* the inner nuclear layer that contains at least three kinds of neurons viz., amacrine, bipolar and horizontal cells.

The Outer Nuclear Layer : It is the outermost layer of the neural retina. It differentiates last, after the local cell division ceases. Their axons synapse with the dendrites of the bipolar cells of the inner nuclear layer.

Rod and Cones : These develop from the outer ends of the cells of the outer nuclear layer. In the process, each cell produces a cytoplasmic bud at its outer end that protrudes through a pore in the external limiting membrane. In this bud further differentiation occurs. The inner segments of the rods and cones are first formed and from them the outer segments arise. Several specialized cell organelles appear in the inner segment, the important being myoid, ellipsoid, paraboloid, and oil droplets. The myoid is a contractile region in the basal portion of the inner segment which positions the photo-sensitive elements. The ellipsoid, also called lentiform body, is tightly-packed aggregation of mitochondria.

The paraboloid is rich in glycogen granules and is derived from granular ER. The oil droplets are spherical globules of carotenoids generally confined to the cones. They appear between mitochondria of the ellipsoid and the tip of the inner segment. They serve as focussing lense and optic filters. Basal body (diplosome) also migrates into the inner segment. Its outer centriole eleborates a contractile cilium which participates in the development of outer segments of the rods and cones.

The peripheral doublets of the cilium lengthen and form the axial filament of the outer segment which when become of 1.0 to 1.5 μ in length is enveloped in a club-shaped cytoplasmic bud. Rows of ciliary vesicles extend from the tip of the ciliary tubules to the apex of the developing outer segment. At the point where ciliary vesicles touch the plasma membrane, the cell surface folds inward to form irregular large sacs. These sacs become flattened in a plane perpendicular to the long axis of the outer segment and soon become stacked like the stack of coins. As the stack grows, the outer segment elongates.

Finally, the melanin pigment granules accumulate in the cuboidal epithelial cells of the outer wall of the optic cup. These granules are manufactured by Golgi apparatus of the concerned cells. Soon numerous long fine cytoplasmic processes arise from these pigmented cells which interdigitate with the outer segments of the rods and cones, thus lacking the two layers together.

Development of Cornea: The cornea originates partly from mesenchyme and partly from epidermal epithelium. The epidermal epithelium gives rise to external cornea which remains continuous with the skin, while mesenchyma gives rise to internal cornea which remains continuous with the sclera. A narrow space lies between these two cornea. During metamorphosis the two cornea fuse and become transparent.

The fully-formed cornea consists of all kinds of cells, nerve fibres, collagen fibrils, and mucopolysaccharides. According to Cops (1965) all these components are so assembled that the cornea develops a characteristics that contribute to its refractory power and transparency.

Development of Choroid Coat and Selera : The choroid coat and the sclerotic coat develop from mesenchyme which accumulate around the eye ball. The inner layer of mesenchyme cells develops network of blood capillaries surrounding the pigmented retinal epithelium. This is the choroid coat. The outer layer of mesenchyme forms the fibrous coat. This is called sclerotic coat or sclent.

Role of Organizers in the Development of Eye : In the development of eye, the whole chain of inductors can be briefed as below:

(i) The roof of the archenteron (primary organizer) induces the neural plate and therefore the eye cup which is the part of the former.

(ii) The eye cup rudiment (secondary organizer) develops into the optic vesicle which induces the epidermis to form a lens.

(iii) The lens (tertiary organizer) induces the neuro-sensory layer of optic vesicle to invaginate and then develops into lens, the later induces the epidermis and mesenchyme for the formation of cornea, choroid coats and sclera.

The space between the lens and retina fills with a viscous fluid secreted by the retinal cells. This is vitreous humor. The head mesenchyme forms a coat of connective tissue around the optic cup and forms the middle layer of eye ball, the choroid. It lies outside the pigmented layer of retina. Outside the choroid coat the mesenchyme forms a tough coat of sclerotic.

Summary of the Source of Different Parts of Eye Ball

(1) Neural Ectoderm of Diencephalon	-	Sensory layer of retina, non-sensory pigment layer of retina optic nerve.
(2) Epidermal Ectoderm	-	Lens, and cornea.
(3) Mesoderm sclerotic, cornea	-	The choroid, vascular tissue, connective tissue, and eye muscles.

Development of Olfactory Organs

The rudiments of a pair of olfactory organs appear just after the closure of neural tube. These appear as epidermal thickenings, the olfactory placodes, at the antero-lateral sides of presumptive telencephalon. Each placode invaginates in the centre forming an olfactory sac. Its opening to outside is called external nare or external choanae. The cells of dorsal and lateral walls of olfactory sac form olfactory epithelium. Its cells become sensory and their basal ends join to form the olfactory nerve. The olfactory nerve joins the telencephalon of the brain.

The ventral wall of each olfactory sac grows out into an elongated, tubular nasal canal. It grows down to open into the buccal cavity. Their apertures are called primitive choana or internal nare.

Development of Auditory Organ (Ear)

Development of Internal Ear : Development of ear begins as a pair of thickenings in the sensory ectoderm of head against the sides of hindbrain. These are called auditory placodes. Each auditory placode separates from the epidermis and invaginates forming a closed otic vesicle or ear vesicle. It marks the rudiment of internal ear.

The ear vesicle is roughly pear-shaped. Its pointed end is directed upward and later develops into endo-lymphatic duct. The ear vesicle enlarges and pushes the surrounding loose mesenchyme. At places the wall of ear vesicle becomes very thin with its epithelial cells almost flattened. This membranous area of vesicle is called labyrinth or membranous labyrinth. Its media-ventral becomes thick. Its cells become columnar and in it develop patches of sensory epithelium. These sensory patches form maculae of internal ear.

At places the ear vesicle bulges out and assumes a complicated shape. Its lower part differentiates into sacculus and utriculus. The utriculus gets drawn into three mutually perpendicular folds, the rudiments of three semicircular canals. A hollow outgrowth from sacculus forms rudiment of lagena.

Development of Middle Ear : After the development of internal ear is completed, the development of middle ear starts as an invagination in the dorsal region of first branchial pouch. An elongated club-shaped mass of cells appears from the hyomandibular gill cleft. This cell mass soon develops a cavity with rounded outer and tubular inner ends. The rounded outer end forms the tympanic cavity and tubular inner end develops into eustachian tube. The outer opening of typanic cavity gets covered by a circular fold of epidermis and forms tympanic membrane or tympanum Collumella auris is formed from the roof of tympanic cavity.

Development of Mesodermal Organs : From mesoderm develop muscles, endoskeleton, heart, blood vessels, kidneys, reproductive organs and their ducts, connective tissue, coelom, etc.

Development of Heart

The first rudiment of heart develops early in the embryonic development in the region beneath the pharynx. The lateral plate mesoderm of the body of the embryo extends in the body ventral to the pharynx as mesenchyme. This mesenchyme gets arranged into sheets and slits into two layers which correspond to the somatic and splanchnic layers of the mesoderm. The space in between these two layers forms the pericardial cavity, whereas the outer layers of mesenchyme corresponding to the somatic layer of body mesoderm will form the pericardial membrane and the inner one corresponding to splanchnic layer of body mesoderm will form the myocardium or heart muscles. The endocardium or the lining of the heart arises from other group of cells which accumulate in between the pharynx and developing pericardium.

Development of Pericardium : Under the inductive influence of the floor of archenteron the cells from the mesenchyme grow ventrally in the middle line just below the pharynx. These aggregate and arrange into sheets. Finally, they organize into a pair of spaces which are known as anterior coelomic spaces. These converge mesially and fuse together in the mid-ventral line below the pharynx. As a result of fusion two tubes are formed one inside the other. The wall of the inner tube forms the myocardium, whereas that of the outer one is the pericardium. The space between the two is the pericardial cavity.

Development of Heart : Isolated endothelial cells organize themselves into sheet in the space between the pharynx and the developing pericardium. These cells are known as endocardial cells. These may be derived from the splanchnic mesoderm or may be remnants of the invaginating cells of the ventral lip of the blastopore. In either case, these form a complete tube and form the lining of the heart, the endocardium. It lies in close approximation with the myocardium. The myocardium gets thickened and gives rise the striated, syncytial and involuntary muscles of the heart.

The pericardial cavity is separated from the peritoneal cavity of the embryonic coelom by septum transversum. The heart is attached both anteriorly as well as posteriorly by means of double-layered suspensory membrane, known as the dorsal mesocardium and the ventral mesocardium. Both of them soon rupture and disappear to provide space for the growing heart. This is accomplished in part by the rapid growth and expansion of the heart itself. The heart at this stage is in the form of a tube which finally lengthens and divides to form the coiled, folded and three-chambered heart of the adult.

Differentiation of Different Parts of Heart : The cells of the heart continue to divide mitotically at a very fast rate so that the tube increases in length. But the anterior and posterior attachments do not permit its increase in anteroposterior direction and the body organs provide a limited space to grow. The increase in size is accomplished by a folding of the original straight tube into S-shaped coiled tube. The posterior part become folded dorsally and anteriorly and the anterior part is folded ventrally and posteriorly. At this stages it is possible to identify the presumptive regions of the adult heart. The posterior most part of the heart tube is the sinus venosus. Just anterior to it is the thin-walled atrium, followed by a large thick-walled ventricle. The most anterior part of the tube is bulbous arteriosus which bifurcates into two trúncus aortae.

Before the development of heart has progressed to this stage, a pair of blood vessels appear in the ventro-lateral splanchnic mesoderm. These are the vitelline veins and are derived by the separation of yolk endoderm and ventral mesoderm. The two vitelline veins are connected with the sinus venosus. Further growth and enlargement results in more pronounced curvatures and foldings. Ventricle becomes folded caudally and ventrally to the atrium. Truncus arterious becomes partially subdivided by a vertical and longitudinal septum giving rise to paired aortae. Even prior to that a longitudinal sheet of endocardium grows down from the roof of atrial chamber and forms interatrial septum. This divides the atrium into right and left auricles. The sinus venosus comes to lie dorsally and opens into the right auricle. The left auricle gets connected with the pulmonary veins. With further changes in form and growth in size the heart of the adult frog is formed.

Development of Blood Vessels

The blood and blood vessels develop from the mesenchyme early in the development and form the so-called blood islands of mesenchyme cells. These specialized cells are called angioblasts or vasoformative cells. The outer cells of these islands flatten and form the endothelial lining of vitelline blood vessel. The inner cells of blood islands become haemocytoblasts. The haemocytoblasts differentiate into erythroblasts and leucoblasts that mature into RBCs and WBCs respectively.

The blood capillaries develop first, and arteries and veins later. The mesenchyme cells surrounding the blood vessels form the musculature. Whether a blood vessel will develop into an artery or vein depends on the nature of blood flowing within.

Circulatory System of Tadpole

Tadpole of frog is an aquatic fish-like animal and till it breathes by means of gills, its blood vascular system closely resembles to that of fish.

The Heart

The heart of tadpole, like fish, is a venous heart, exhibiting unicircuit circulation. It is a twisted, S-shaped tube consisting of a posterior receiving and anterior forwarding part. The receiving part consists of the sinuous venosus and atrium; while the forwarding part is formed of ventricle and bulbous aorta.

Afferent Branchial System

The bulbous aorta is continued forward as ventral aorta. It bifurcates into right and left branches. At the external gill stage each branch divides into two afferent vessels to the first and second branchial arches. These vessels carry deoxygenated blood to the external gills. There is an incipient afferent branchial to the third branchial arch, arising from the second afferent branchial. The fourth arch is with afferent vessel.

At the internal gill-stage each branch of ventral aorta divides into three branchials and the third bifurcates again into two. Thus at this stage the tadpole possesses four pairs of afferent vessels.

Efferent Branchial Vessels

From the gill the oxygenated blood is collected by two pairs of efferent branchial vessels. At their distal end these are connected to the efferent branchials through cross connections. Third and fourth pairs of efferent branchial vessels are also present. At the internal gill stage there are four pairs of efferent vessels. The efferent arteries of one side join to form the dorsal aorta of its side. The two dorsal aortae also unite mesially forming the median dorsal aorta.

In addition to these four pairs of branchials, the primordia of vessels to hyomandibular and hyoid arches are also present but they never attain full development.

Thus the tadpole possesses six sets of branchial vessels, of which first three are complete, the fourth one incomplete and the hyomandibular and hyoidean rudimentary.

Arterial System

The two dorsal aortae extend forward into the head as carotid arteries and supply the head and brain region. In its course behind, the median dorsal aorta issues pharyngeal arteries to the pharyngeal and oesophageal region, several lumbar arteries to the body wall, mesenteric arteries to the viscera, and iliac arteries to the hindlimbs. A pair of *subclavian arteries* emerge out from the second efferent vessel, and a pair of *pulmonary arteries* from the fourth efferent vessels.

Venous System

The venous system also develops on piscian pattern. The major veins are the anterior cardinals, posterior cardinals, cuvierian ducts, iliacs, and the caudals.

The anterior cardinals receive blood from the head region by external and internal jugular vein. The posterior cardinals develop at the region of pronephros and collect blood from the hinder part of the body. The anterior and posterior cardinals of each side unite to form the common cardinal vein or *ductus* Cuvieri or Cuvierian duct.

The blood from the caudal region is collected by a median *caudal vein* which breaks off in the kidney into a pair of *subcardinal veins.* These give off afferent veins in the substance of kidney and finally join the posterior cardinals. The afferent veins capillarize in the kidney and then reunite into efferent veins.

The vitelline veins form a network of sinusoids in liver and only the left vein exists as hepatic portal vein.

Changes in the Blood Vascular System at the Time of Metamorphosis

Heart : The auricle of the heart gets divided into two chambers by the downgrowth of a septum from its roof. The circulation of blood becomes bicircuit.

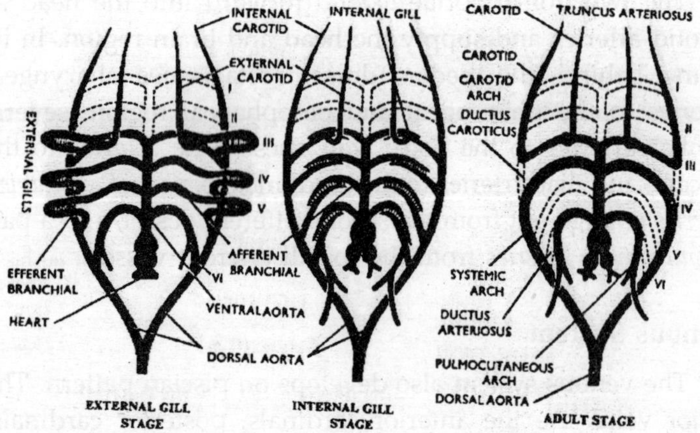

Changes in the blood vascular system of tadpole of frog.

Branchial Vessels : The vessels of hyomandibular and hyoid arches disappear. The first pair of branchial vessels form the *carotid arch.* The second becomes the *systemic arch.* The third pair disappears and the fourth pair forms the pulmocutaneous arch.

Arteries : A part of the mandibular arch forms the *lingual artery;* the anterior part of dorsal aorta forms the *internal carotid* and anterior part of the ventral aorta constitutes the *external carotid.* The systemic arch gives off various branches to forelimbs, vertebral column and oesophagus and ultimately units with its fellow to form the *dorsal aorta*. The dorsal aorta issues branches like *coeliacomesenteric, renals, gonadial*, etc. and finally divides to supply the hindlimbs.

Veins : The posterior vena cava is formed partly by subcardinals and partly by the right omphalomesenteric. The part of the left omphalomesenteric vein forms the hepatic vein. The lateral veins fuse to form the *anterior abdominal vein* which ramifies in the liver. The posterior cardinals and caudal veins disappear. The branches from the various parts of the alimentary canal unite to form the hepatic portal veins. The renal portal veins are formed by the union of sciatic and femoral veins.

Anteriorly, the ductus Cuvieri modifies into precaval veins receiving the external and internal jugular veins from head and a pair of subclavian veins from the forelimbs.

These total changes in the blood vascular system of tadpole lead to the circulatory system of the adult frog.

Embryology of Frog

In frog, sexes are separate and sexual dimorphism is evident during reproductive season.

(i) The male possesses a copulatory pad or amplexusory pad on the undersurface of the first digit of each forelimb. It is in the form of a darkly-coloured swelling, which enlarges during breeding season.

(ii) Male frogs possess vocal sacs and vocal cords. These produce croaking sound during reproductive season to attract the females for copulation.

(iii) The abdomen of mature male is comparatively narrow than in the mature female.

Sex Organs and Gametes

The Testes : Testes are a pair of whitish oval bodies attached to the upper end of kidneys. These are suspended by a double fold of peritoneum, known as mesorchium. Each testis is formed of numerous convoluted seminiferous tubules. In transverse section these appear as closely-packed, oval sacs embedded in the interstitial connective tissue. Each seminiferous tubule is lined with germinal epithelium.

The primordial germ cells of germinal epithelium give rise to spermatogonia or sperm mother cells. Spermatogonia undergo spermatogenesis and form spermatozoa. 20-40 spermatozoa are found together attached to the sertoli cells. Their heads lie embedded in the cytoplasm of sertoli cells which act as nurse cells and supply nourishment to the spermatozoa.

The Sperm

A mature spermatozoon averages about 0.03 mm in length. It has a typical structure of a chordate sperm. The head is elongated and it encloses a darkly-stained nucleus and a pointed acrosome at the anterior end. The middle piece is short and indistinct. The tail is a filamentous extension about four times longer than the sperm head.

Mature sperm are liberated from the testes under the influence of sex-stimulating hormones. These are carried down into the vasa efferentia by the ciliary movement of their lining. These pass through the urinogenital duct. Prior to mating, sperm are stored shortly in the seminal vesicles and are finally discharged on the ova at the time of copulation.

The Ovary

The ovaries are paired multi-lobular organs attached to the dorsal body wall by a double fold of peritoneum known as mesovarium. The size and colour of the ovary varies with season. During reproductive season ovaries have steel-gray colour and are very large in size. But after the discharge of ova ovary becomes very incipient.

The outermost covering of ovary is theca externa formed of connective tissue, followed by a layer of germinal epithelium. In a young ovary, small clusters of oogonial cells are visible. Each cluster develops into one ovarian follicle. The central oogonium of the duster develops into oocyte and the surrounding cells form a peripheral layer of follicle cells. The growing ovary has several hundreds of ovarian follicles (2,000-20,000).

Each ovarian follicle comprises of (i) centrally-placed-large rounded oocyte (ii) peripheral of small flattened follicular cells (iii) a thin covering or connective tissue, theca interna.

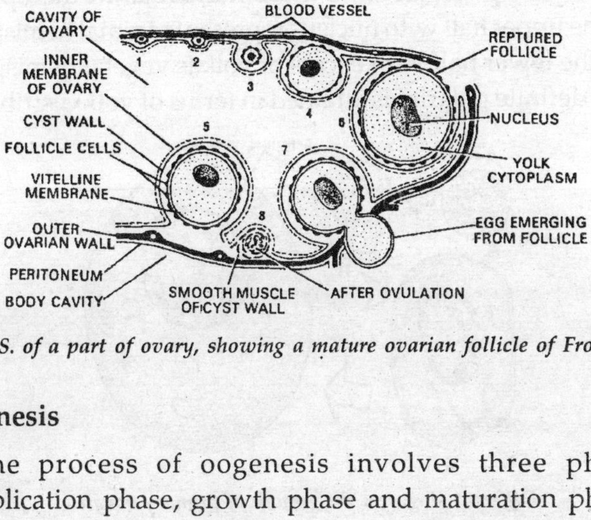

T.S. of a part of ovary, showing a mature ovarian follicle of Frog.

Oogenesis

The process of oogenesis involves three phases, multiplication phase, growth phase and maturation phase.

Multiplication Phase : The oogonia divide by mitosis and form clusters of oogonial cells. The multiplication of oogonia begins in the tadpole, when gonads are formed and occurs every year even in the older adult stages.

Growth Phase : One of the cells in each cluster of oogonial cells starts increasing in size and is known as primary oocyte. The increase in size (growth) is achieved by the accumulation of yolk. The chromosomes acquire loops and assume the appearance of lampbrush chromosomes.

At these loops RNA is synthesized in very large amount. This accumulates in the nucleolus, which divides into a large number of nucleoli, arranged on the periphery of the nucleus. Some of the nucleolar RNA or (nucleoli themselves) pass out into the cytoplasm through pores of nuclear membrane and form 'yolk nuclei.' Yolk accumulated around these yolk nuclei. In smaller oocytes, there is no yolk and their nucleus is centrally placed. Yolk starts accumulating around yolk nuclei and forms yolk plates. In the beginning yolk plates form a ring around the nucleus and then becomes evenly distributed. With increase in yolk mass, the nucleus is pushed towards one side and the yolk plates become more numerous in the opposite half. The upper half with nucleus represents animal hemisphere, while the lower half with excess of yolk is vegetal hemisphere. Thus a definite polarity is attained in terms of yolk distribution.

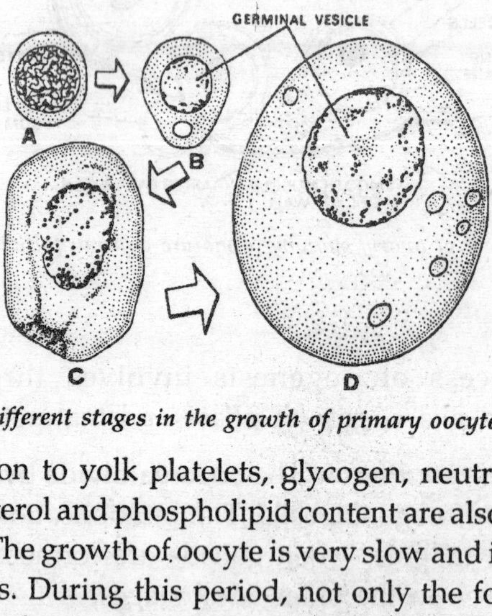

Different stages in the growth of primary oocyte.

In addition to yolk platelets, glycogen, neutral fats, fatty acids, cholesterol and phospholipid content are also distributed in ooplasm. The growth of oocyte is very slow and is completed in three years. During this period, not only the food contents but the cytoplasm also increases considerably, and black pigment (melanin) is deposited in the animal pole. Due to the unequal distribution of yolk, the egg is called telolecithal.

During growth phase the nucleus of primary oocyte enters into prophase of meiotic division and pairing of homologous chromosomes takes place. Subsequent stages of meiosis are postponed till the egg enters maturation phase. The nucleus or germinal vesicle increases in size by the formation of large amount of nuclear sap. Vitelline membrane is also formed around primary oocyte during the growth phase. It is secreted by the oocyte itself aided by the surrounding follicle cells.

Maturation Phase: First maturation division occurs at the time of ovulation. Prior to ovulation the nucleus of oocyte appears as a large, pale and irregularly shaped vesicle. Soon its nuclear wall dissolves and chromosomes (tetrads) are arranged on the equator of meiotic spindle. When egg enters the oviduct the first polar body is extruded out and the egg enters the secondary oocyte stage. Immediately after the first maturation division, second meiotic spindle is formed and chromosomes enter the metaphase of second maturation divison. The division is retarded at this stage and the remaining stages are completed after fertilization.

Ovulation

The ova are released into the body cavity by the rupture of theca externa and peritoneum of ovary and their emergence from their individual follicles. The process is initiated by the sex hormone FSH secreted by the anterior pituitary. The ovulated eggs are naked except for a thin transparent vitelline membrane.

Deposition of Tertiary Egg Membranes : Ciliary currents produced by cells of peritoneum force the eggs into the ostium and oviduct. The eggs at first accumulate in the anterior portion of the oviduct, and are pushed backward in a single file. During their passage down the narrow part of the oviduct, the eggs are enveloped by three distinct, thin and gelatinous membranes. These are known as tertiary membranes. These are formed of several coatings of albumen. The outermost of these is adhesive and tends to hold eggs together in a single mass. Two to four hours after ovulation eggs reach the uterus and retained for few hours, until these are laid down during amplexus.

Spawning

The eggs of frog are laid down in water in a single mass. The outermost albumen coat of all the eggs swells up on coming in contact with water and becomes jelly-like. With the help of jelly eggs stick together forming a spawn. Spawn is laid down during amplexus, when male clasps the female and deposits its semen over the eggs as they leave cloaca.

Utility of Jelly and Spawn

1. Jelly forms a protective covering and protects the eggs from heat, dust and atmospheric pressure.
2. Jelly swells upto many times its original volume and thus separates the eggs from one another. This provides a more favourable environment for each egg.
3. Air bubbles get entangled in the jelly and provide buoyancy to the spawn so that it can float on water surface.
4. Jelly is not tasty. Therefore, fishes, birds and worms do not eat the spawn.

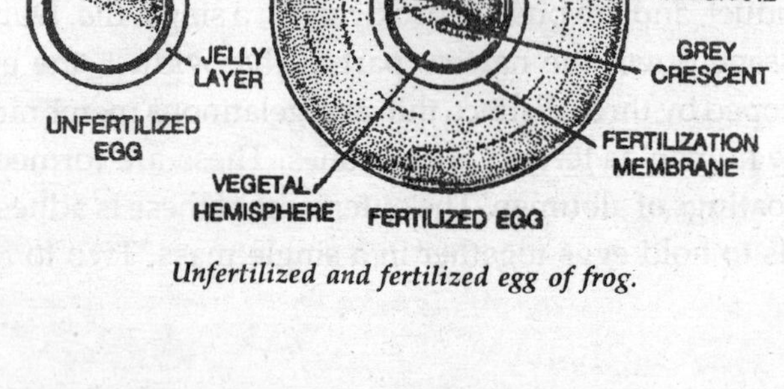

Unfertilized and fertilized egg of frog.

5. Ova and sperm are brought together in the jelly. Therefore, it facilitates fertilization.

Structure of Unfertilized Egg : Fully mature oocyte of frog measures about 400 to 500 μ in diameter. It is spherical in form and is invested with vitelline membrane and a thick jelly-coat, formed of three concentric layers of albuminous substance.

The ripe amphibian egg is differentiated into :

(i) vegetal half which is white in colour. It contains densely-packed mass of yolk and very little pigment, *(ii)* animal half which is dark brown or black. Its cytoplasm is rich in pigment granules but contains just few small yolk platelets. The egg nucleus or germinal vesicle lies in the animal half and forms a sort of inverted saucer. *(iii)* marginal zone is the transitional zone which includes the gradually fading area found between the animal and vegetal half. The ooplasm of the egg is differentiated into cortex and endoplasm :

Cortex : The superficial layer of ooplasm which underlies the plasma membrane of the egg is in roughly gelated state and is known as cortex. It is 2μ -3μ in thickness. It is thick around the animal pole and gradually thins out towards the vegetal pole. It is a colloidal complex of proteins, phosphatides, RNA and calcium ions.

Embedded in the cortex are found cortical granules. These are spherical bodies about 3μ in diameter and composed of acid mucopolysaccharides. These are secreted by Golgi complex and arranged in a layer close to plasma membrane. At the time of fertilization, the cortical granules break and their contents accumulate in the perivitelline space as vitelline fluid, contributing to the formation of fertilization membrane.

The cortex is very stable. It remains in the same position for entire period of growth and development. The large cytoplasmic inclusions are either embedded or attached to the cortical layer by cortical microfilaments. It is also considered to be the site of morphogenetic patterns relating to polar, bilateral and general organization of developing egg.

Endoplasm : It contains nucleus and melanin pigment in the animal half and yolk in the vegetal half. Because of uneven distribution of yolk, frog's eggs are called mesolecithal and telolecithal.

Yolk is in the form of a cup-shaped mass of yolk-platelets, and has been described as vitelline cupola. The yolk platelets are largest near the vegetal pole and smaller, less densely packed towards the animal pole. Thus, a polar axis is established with the egg constituents arranged radially around it and with a concentration gradient from vegetal to animal pole. This polar axis is known as vegetal axis.

Fertilization

Fertilization is external. The sperms are deposited on the eggs before these come in contact with water. The spermatozoon enters the ovum in animal hemisphere region. The point of entrance of sperm is predetermined. The entire sperm enters the ovum but only sperm head proceeds towards the female pronucleus. The entry of sperm causes following radical changes in the egg:

Formation of Fertilization Membrane : The penetration of sperm causes cortical reaction resulting in the lifting up of vitelline membrane from egg surface. This separated membrane is known as fertilization membrane and the space between it and the egg surface froms the perivitelline space. It gets filled with a fluid within which the egg is free to rotate.

Rotation of Egg : The vegetal hemisphere being yolky is heavier than the animal hemisphere. Therefore, the egg rotates slowly within its perivitelline space, brings the animal hemisphere above and vegetal hemisphere below.

Completion of Second Maturation Division : The sperm entry activates the nucleus of ovum, which had become quiescent at metaphase of second maturation division. The division is now completed and second polar body is given off.

Penetration and Copulation Path : In frog the complete spermatozoon enters the ovum. The tail then disintegrates and the head and middle piece move towards the female pronucleus along a cone-shaped path which corresponds to the egg radius. This is known as penetration path. Some of the pigment granules from the cortical layer of egg move along with sperm nucleus and get accumulated on the penetration path.

In some cases the sperm does not move straight and changes its course after penetration. This changed path is known as copulation path. Like penetration path it is also marked by a trail of pigment.

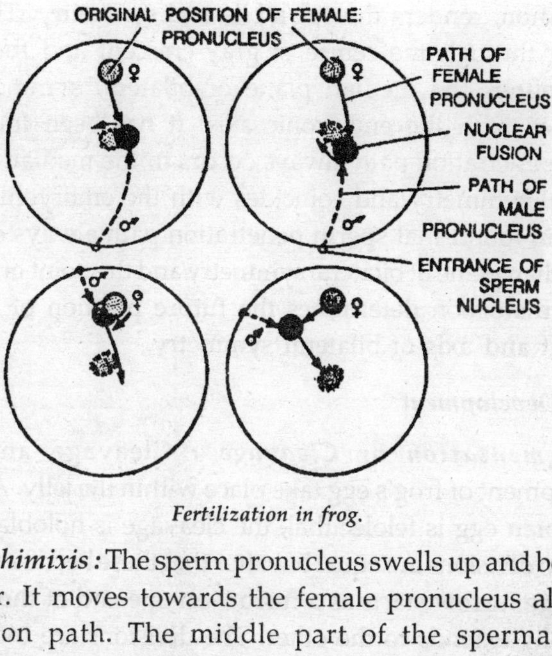

Fertilization in frog.

Amphimixis : The sperm pronucleus swells up and becomes vesicular. It moves towards the female pronucleus along its copulation path. The middle part of the spermatozoon contributes the centrosome. This divides and the resulting two centrosomes establish an axis at right angles to the direction of sperm movement.

Simultaneously, the female pronucleus moves towards the centre. Finally the male and female pronuclei fuse together to form the zygote nucleus.

Formation of Gray Crescent : About ten minutes after the penetration of sperm, the yellow cortical ooplasm of the egg starts flowing towards the sperm entrance. At the future dorsal side, the cytoplasm moves towards the animal pole, and at the opposite side (the future ventral side) it moves towards the vegetal pole. This exposes a lightly pigmented crescent-shaped area of marginal cytoplasm on the dorsal side, exactly opposite the point of sperm entrance. This is known as gray crescent.

Establishment of Bilateral Symmetry : Unfertilized egg is radially symmetrical, but the formation of gray-crescent after fertilization, renders the egg's bilateral symmetry. The plane passing through the centre of gray crescent and the animal pole defines the median plane of bilateral symmetry and coincides with the embryonic axis. It has been found that sperm penetration path always occurs in the median plane of bilateral symmetry and coincides with the embryonic axis. It has been found that sperm penetration path always occurs in the median plane of bilateral symmetry and the point of entrance of spermatozoon determines the future position of the gray crescent and axis of bilateral symmetry.

Early Development

Segmentation or Cleavage : Cleavage and early development of frog's egg take place within the jelly. Although amphibian egg is telolecithal, the cleavage is holoblastic. The first two divisions are equal but after that these become unequal. Cleavage furrow starts as a furrow on one end of the egg and gradually extends to the other. The divisions are more rapid in the animal hemisphere and pass slowly in the vegetal hemisphere because of the inert yolk mass. Thus, the succeeding cell divisions in the animal half start even before the first cleavage is completed in the vegetal half. The temperature and water effect the cleavage rate.

(1) First cleavage is meridional or vertical and bisects the egg into two indentical blastomeres. Its cleavage furrow appears at the animal pole about 2-1/2 hours after fertilization. After about 3 hours the egg is completely divided into two blastomeres. The plane of first cleavage furrow is determined by the direction of approach of sperm nucleus and includes the copulation path.

(2) Second cleavage is also meridional but at right angles to the first one.

(3) Third cleavage is horizontal or equatorial or latitudinal, but at right angles to the first two cleavage furrows. Its cleavage furrow is slightly above the equator towards the animal pole. Therefore, it divides the blastomeres unequally. The upper four blastomeres are smaller and are known as micromeres. The lower four blastomeres are large and are known as macromeres or megameres.

The deflection of third cleavage furrow towards the animal pole away from equator is due to the presence of more cytoplasm and less yolk in the animal half and more yolk in the vegetal half. The yolk puts resistance to the cleavage forces.

(4) Fourth cleavage is again vertical and comprises of two cleavage furrows laid down simultaneously. These furrows run into the first and second cleavage furrows. The egg attains 16-celled stage.

(5) Fifth cleavage also comprises of two cleavage furrows laid down horizontally—one in the animal hemisphere and other in the vegetal hemisphere. Therefore, 32 blastomeres are formed, arranged in four tiers. The

upper two tiers (16 cells) are formed of micromeres and lower two tiers are macromeres. The cleavage furrows in macromeres laid down slightly later than that in micromeres.

(4) From now onward the regularity in cleavages is lost and micromeres divide faster than macromeres. As a result a sphere of closely packed cells is formed. These cells vary in size. The more numerous small micromeres are present in the animal hemisphere and the macromeres many times the size of micromeres and very few in number are found in vegetal hemisphere.

This stage has been described as morula by some, but actually a morula is a solid ball of cells. In frog's embryo the blastocoel appears as early as eight-celled stage. It gradually increases corresponding to the increase in the number of blastomeres. Therefore, a morula stage is absent in frog.

Blastula

When embryo is at eight-celled stage, a cavity becomes apparent in its centre. It is formed by the roundening of the inner edges of blastomeres. This cavity is known as blastocoel.

The blastomeres in the early cleavage stages tend to acquire spherical form and independent cell boundaries. Their mutual pressure flattens the surfaces at which blastomeres lie in contact with each other, but the free surfaces of each blastomere remain spherical. Naturally a space develops in the form of narrow crevices in the centre of the embryo by the roundening of the inner margins. The blastocoel increases in size as the division proceeds further and at 32-celled stage it becomes very distinct. It is filled with an albuminous fluid, secreted by the surrounding blastomeres.

A blastula, therefore, appears as a hollow sphere enclosing blastocoel. The roof of blastocoel is formed of two or more layers of micromeres and its floor is formed of non-pigmented, large-sized macromeres, while the side walls are formed of several layers of micromeres. The floor of blastocoel is more or less flat and blastocoel is eccentric. It is situated in the animal hemisphere.

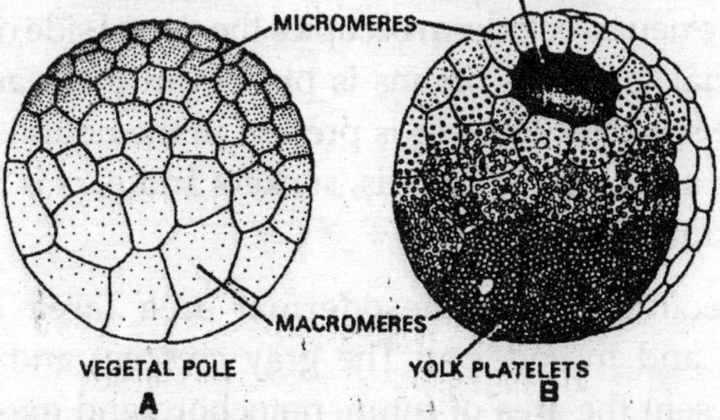

Blastula of frog. A-Early blastula B-V.S. blastula

After 32-celled stage a gradient of cleavage is established, the most active region being animal pole and least active vegetal pole. Due to active division of micromeres in the animal hemisphere, the cells start growing over the macromeres in the equatorial region and form a sort of pigmented girdle in the equatorial region. The band or girdle is known as germ ring or marginal zone or marginal belt Due to the migration of cells the roof of blastocoel becomes thin and double-layered. The outer layer of cells contains most of the pigment and represents the epidermal layer. The inner layer of blastula roof is less pigmented and is called nervous layer.

Fate Map of Blastula

By simple staining, amphibian blastula appears like a ball of cells of two types, but by using Vogt's vital staining method it is possible to identify the various prospective areas on its surface which will form different organs of the adult. A fate map of blastula of frog showing presumptive areas of future organs or structures had been given by Vogt. According to the fate map studies, the surface of the blastula has been divided into following three areas.

Presumptive Ectoderm Area : The pigemented area on and around the animal pole represents the presumptive ectoderm. It covers major portion of animal hemisphere.

The prospective epidermal ectoderm, which forms skin epidermis occupies the antero-ventral side of the blastula. The prospective neural ectoderm occupies the dorsal side of blastula. The material for sense organs is present in these areas only. The future sub-area for eyes is present in the neural ectoderm and future sub area for nostrils, suckers and ears is located in the epidermal ectoderm.

Prospective chorda-mesodermal area (area of future notochord and mesoderm): The gray crescent and marginal zone represent the area of future notochord and mesoderm of embryo. The major portion of gray crescent, present on the dorsal side develops into the notochord. On either side of the notochordal area is present future mesoderm area.

Prospective Endodermal Area : The cells in the vegetal hemisphere constitute the prospective endoderm.

Gastrulation

Gastrulation is a critical stage in the development which results in the differentiation of three prospective germ layers and the movement of prospective organ-forming-areas from the surface of blastula to their respective position in the embryo. During gastrulation the presumptive material of gut, notochord and mesoderm disappears from the surface of embryo into the interior and the ectodermal cells spread out on the entire outer surface. The mass migration of cells during gastrulation is described as formative movements. The process is much complicated in frog embryo due to the presence of yolk in the cells of vegetal hemisphere. It is brought about by the following processes occurring simultaneously. All these processes are self-determined and related to one another. But for convenience, these are described separately.

Epiboly (Spreading of Presumptive Ectoderm) : The micromeres of the animal hemisphere of blastula continue to divide rapidly and grow downward from all directions towards the vegetal pole. Simultaneously, the cells from deeper layers of marginal zone migrate from their original position and spread over the white macromeres from all sides except near the gray crescent, where dorsal lip of blastopore is to be formed. This spreading of micromeres over macromeres is described as epiboly. This spreading of micromeres over macromeres is described as epiboly. This spreading tendency is inherent in the cells of both the superficial and the inner layers of ectoderm. As a result of continued epiboly, the cells of presumptive ectoderm cover the entire surface of the embryo except in the region of blastopore, where some of the unpigmented macromeres could be seen projecting out of the blastopore.

Invagination : Continued epiboly of the marginal cell zone exerts an inward pressure on the yolk-endoderm cells (macromeres). The macromeres are, therefore, pushed inside into the blastocoel. The process is known as pseudo-invagination.

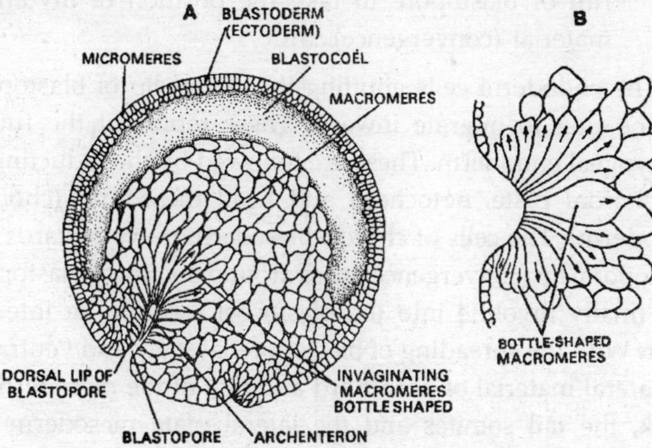

Alteration in the morphology of cells of endoderm during the formation of blastopore.

As a result of invagination a tiny crescent-shaped groove appears at the marginal zone where gray-crescent meets the vegetal macromeres. This groove marks the beginning of archenteron. Its opening is known as blastopore and the upper margin of the groove is referred as dorsal lip of blastopore.

The process of invagination is not a passive phenomenon. The cells of the outermost layer of sinking endoderm assume bottle-shaped or flask-shaped appearance. Their steadily elongated narrow necks remain attached to the surface of embryo, whereas the internal broad ends remain free. This appearance is regarded to be the result of intrinsic cellular contractibility, which causes them to thrust into the interior of the egg. It is regarded to be a form of amoeboid movement.

Involution of Pharyngeal Endoderm and Chorda-mesoderm : The onset of invagination is followed by two types of morphogenetic movements of the cells :

(i) the rolling of the superficial cells over the rim of blastopore into the interior (involution) and

(ii) the flow of new portions of blastoderm towards the rim of blastopore to take the position of involuted material (convergence).

The endoderm cells abutting the dorsal lip of blastopore are the first to migrate inward. These represent the future pharyngeal endoderm. These are followed by the inducting of pre-chordal plate, notochord and head mesoderm (chordo-mesoderm). The cells of chordo-mesoderm move towards the blastoporal lip (convergence), pass around the rim of blastopore and finally involute into the blastocoel forming an internal layer. With the spreading of blastopore laterally and ventrally, the lateral material of notochord and that of the mesoderm of trunk, the tail somites and the lateral plate mesoderm are tucked in progressively along the dorso-lateral, lateral and ventral rims of blastopore.

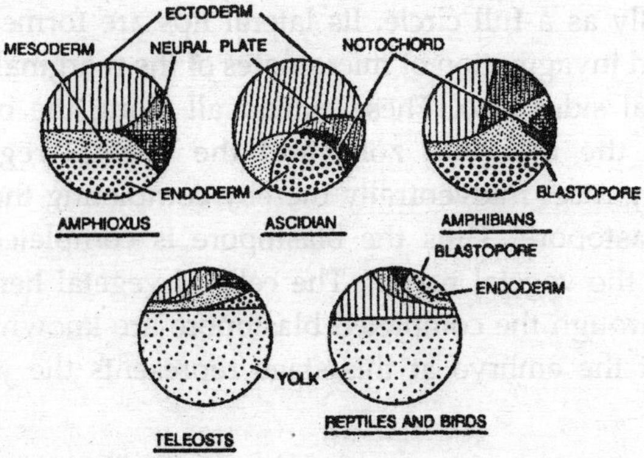

Demonstration of convergence and involution of areas during gastrulation by using vital stain.

If blastoderm above the rim of blastopore is marked with spots of vital stain, it can easily be seen that the stained areas stretch towards the lips of blastopore, approach its rim, roll over the edge and disappear inside.

Convergence : Once the above-mentioned materials of pre-chordal plate (= pharyngeal endoderm) and chordo-mesoderm have flown inward around the rim of blastopore, these do not come to rest but continue their movement in the interior of the embryo. But this time these move away from the blastopore and converge in the middle-line, forming a layer of future chorda-mesoderm between the ectoderm and endoderm. These form the roof of archenteron. This phenomenon of transference of particular cell type from the surface of embryo and their accumulation in the specific region is known as convergence. This was a described by VOGT.

Formation and Contraction of Blastoporal Lips : Blastopore appears in the beginning of gastrulation when invagination of macromeres starts at the lower margin of gray crescent. Its dorsal lip is formed by the involution of micromeres of the grey crescent (marginal zone). Gradually the invagination increases and spreads laterally, so that the crescent-shaped blastopore first appears as a half moon, then horse-shoe-shaped and finally as a full circle. Its lateral lips are formed by the continued invagination of micromeres of the marginal zone on the lateral sides also. These extend all along the boundary between the marginal zone and the vegetal region and ultimately meet midventrally thereby completing the ventral lip of blastopore. Thus the blastopore is completed and it encircles the vegetal region. The cells of vegetal hemisphere visible through the completed blastopore are known as yolk-plug and the embryo at this stage represents the yolk-plug stage.

When the lips of blastopore are being formed, the rim of blastopore gradually shifts over the macromeres of vegetal region. As a result of combined action of epiboly and convergence the blastopore which is a wide aperture gradually narrows until at the end of gastrulation the blastopore is recognizable only as a narrow slit and the protruding yolk-plug is drawn inside into the archenteron.

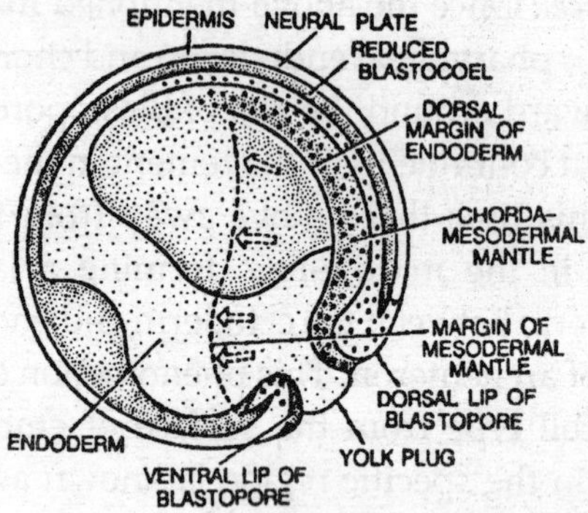

V.S. embryo at yolk plug stage

Other Changes during Gastrulation : As a result of above-mentioned changes, the following morphological changes also occur during gastrulation :

1. Archenteron gradually increases in size and in so doing encroaches the blastocoel. The blastocoel is ultimately completely obliterated.

2. The rearrangement of embryonic areas takes place. The chorda-mesoderm cells form the roof of archenteron. The chorda cells (future notochord) lie in the middle-line and are flanked on either side with the mesoderm of future somites and the lateral plates.
3. Reduction of blastocoel and the enlargement of archenteron change the gravitational axis of the embryonic mass, which is shifted at about 90° away from the blastopore.

Movement of Organ specific Areas during Gastrulation : The most important event of gastrulation is the mass movement of cells from the surface of blastula and their rearrangement in such a way that they come to lie in their definitive positions in the embryo. These movements are known as formative movements and are accomplished by several types of activities such as invagination, involution and epiboly. The displacement and movements of different areas of blastula can be discussed separately:

Ectoderm : The micromeres of animal hemisphere represent the presumptive ectoderm. It includes material of presumptive epidermis and presumptive nervous system. These cells proliferate and spread over the macromeres present in the vegetal half. By the end of gastrulation, when mesoderm and endoderm have involuted inside, the ectoderm covers the whole embryo.

The presumptive epidermis spreads in all directions. The area of presumptive nervous system expands in longitudinal direction in antero-posterior axis, but contracts in transverse direction and the cells of the lateral horns of crescentic area aie drawn towards the dorsal side of the embryo. The nervous area, therefore, becomes oval and elongated in antero-posterior direction.

Notochord : The cells of the presumptive notochord are located in the gray crescent. During gastrulation, these roll over the dorsal lip of blastopore and involute into the interior of the embryo. These form a strip in the mid-dorsal line in the roof of archenteron. This elongates in the antero-posterior axis but contracts in the transverse direction.

Pre-chordal Plate: The presumptive area of prechordal plate lies just below the presumptive notochord. It is a part of mesoderm and is the first part to involute along the dorsal lip of blastopore. It forms a part of the roof of archenteron just in front of the notochordal area.

Mesoderm : Most of the presumptive mesodermal tissue invaginates in the interior by rolling over the lateral and ventral lips of blastopore. Inside the embryo, it moves in anterior direction as a sheet of cells underneath the ectoderm. This mesodermal and the notochordal material together form a continuous sheet between the ectoderm and endoderm.

This is known as chorda-mesodermal mantle. In the interior of the embryo mesodermal mantle moves from the posterior to the anterior end. It is thickest in the roof of archenteron adjoining the notochord.

Endoderm : In the blastula stage the presumptive endoderm is located in the marginal zone and in the vegetal region. Both of them are drawn inside by invagination but in two different manners. The presumptive endoderm of marginal zone is absorbed into the blastopore, while that of the vegetal region is covered by the overgrowth of ectodermal cells of the animal half.

The blastopore appears as an invagination between the endoderm of marginal zone and vegetal region. The marginal zone endoderm invaginates as a part of the dorsal lip of blastopore and forms the endoderm of pharyngeal and oral regions. The endoderm of vegetal region forms the floor of archenteron. In later stages endoderm of pharyngeal and oral regions expands to form a spacious foregut.

Physiology of Gastrulation

Gastrulation involves two Important Events :

1. Movement of parts of embryo—Morphogenetic movements
2. Rearrangement of cells of the embryo.

Morphogenetic Movements

Gastrulation is essentially a process of movement of parts of the embryo. As a result of these movements, the structure of the embryo is changed and new structural elements are created in place of simple layer of cells found in blastula. These movements have been described as morphogenetic movements by VOGT (1925) and TRINKAUS (1969). The morphogenetic movements are represented by invagination and epiboly.

Ectoderm	*Mesoderm*	*Endoderm*
1. Epidermis and its glands	1. Dermis	1. Epithelium or internal lining of midgut.
2. Central nervous system epithelium (peritoneum)	2. Coelom and coelomic	2. Liver and pancreas
3. Receptor organs (i) Eye lens (ii) Retina and conjunctiva	3. Voluntary and involuntary	3. Gastric and intestine glands
(iii) Iris and its muscles (iv) Membranous labyrinth	4. Pericardium	4. Lungs and trachea
(v) Olfactory epithelium	5. Heart and Blood Vessels	5. Eustachian tube
4. Epithelium of stomodeum and proctodaeum (foregut	6. Endoskeleton	6. Urinary bladder
and hindgut) of aliment-ary canal.	7. Urinogenital ducts	7. Thyroid and thymus.
	8. Urinogenital organs	
	9. Medullary sheath of nerve fibres, neurilemma and neurogloea.	
	10. Spleen	
	11. Remaining parts of eye (except lens conjunctiva and cornea)	
	12. Eye muscle	
	13. Notochord	
	14. Dentine.	

The invagination of macromeres in the marginal zone just below the gray crescent results in the formation of blastopore. Invagination occurs on account of change in shape and movement of macromeres of the marginal zone. The cells undergoing invagination become bottle-shaped. Their outer ends which are firmly attached to the outer surface, become attenuated like the necks of bottles, whereas the distal free ends expand. This change in shape is presumed to be a form of amoeboid movement. This is an intrinsic phenomena and is performed by the cells themselves. The cells at the surface of the embryo are firmly held together and adhere to each other very closely at their distal ends. Most probably these are joined by some cementing substance. The collective inward movement of these are joined by some cementing substance. The collective inward movement of these cells in the marginal zone causes the surface of the embryo to be pulled inside with the formation of a pocket-like invagination, the rudiment of archenteron.

There exists a force in the region of invagination and the cells are pushed inside away from the rim of blastopore with force. The force can easily be measured by inserting a steel ball in the way of invaginating cells and measuring the force, which is necessary to keep the ball in position. Therefore, these migratory cells carry more and more cells inside and as a result the invagination deepens and increases in circumference.

Rearrangement of Cells

As a result of morphogenetic movements, the cells of different organ-forming-areas come to occupy their specific positions and get arranged in three primary embryonic layers of germinal layers.

Fate Map of Primary Germinal Layers : During gastrulation, the three embryonic membranes are established. The outer layer of micromeres forms the ectoderm of the embryo. The micromeres which invaginate along the dorsal lip of blastopore constitute the chordamesoderm. This further splits up to form the notochord and mesodermal layer. The large macromeres forming the floor and sides of archenteron form the endoderm. All the structures and organs of the adult are developed from these primary germ layers. The details are summarised in the table.

Post-gastrular Development

With the completion of gastrula, the various organ rudiments take their final positions in the embryo, where these develop into respective organs and organ systems. This is known as morphogenesis or organogenesis. It is concerned with the moulding of cells of the three primary germ layers of the embryo into organs and organ systems of the adult. In the early stages of organogeny, the following processes occur almost simultaneously.

1. Development of nerve cord — Neurulation.
2. Development of notochord —Chordogenesis.
3. Development of alimentary canal.

Neurulation (Development of Neural Tube) : The neural tube develops from the presumptive neuroectoderm, which occupies mid-dorsal position in the fully-formed gastrula. By the thickening of cells in this region, the neuroectoderm gets differentiated into an elongated pear-shaped area, the neural plate or the medullary plate. It extends as a median band of thickening from the dorsal lip of blastopore all along the antero-posterior axis of the embryo. Its formation is initiated (induction) by the chorda-mesoderm cells, which lie in the roof of archenteron. The cells of the neural plate become elongated and arranged into columnar epithelium.

During further development, the edges of the neural plate become more thickened and are raised above forming the neural folds or ridges. The neural plate between them gradually sinks due to progressive uprising and incurving of the neural folds. The depression or groove thus formed is known as neural groove. This marks the beginning of central nervous system and the embryo at this stage is known as neurula. The neural folds grow inward towards one another, meet in the middle-line and finally fuse together, thereby completing the formation of neural tube.

The closure of neural tube begins just in front of the middle region and proceeds both anteriorly and posteriorly. At the front end the neural folds remain unfused for some time leaving an aperture, the neuropore. The cavity of neural tube (neurocoele) for a short period communicates with the exterior through neuropore. At the posterior end, the neural folds merge into the sides of blastopore and their union encloses the blastopore. Therefore, the archenteron of the embryo communicates with the neurocoele. The original blastopore assumes the form of a temporary tubular connection between neurocoele and archenteron and is known as neurenteric canal.

Finally, the completed neural tube gets constricted off from the dorsal ectoderm. The two free edges of epidermal ectoderm grow over the neural tube and fuse forming a continuous sheet above. The ectoderm of neural tube, which lines the neurocoele is ciliated and pigmented.

The broad anterior part of the neural tube develops into the brain and the neural tube forms the spinal cord.

Neural Crests

When the neural tube separates from the presumptive epidermal ectoderm, a flattened mass of cells is left out as a semicircular peripheral band around the neural tube. It is known as neural crest. At first, it is continuous across the middle line above the neural tube, but soon it separates into two patches, lying dorsolaterally one on either side of the neural tube immediately below the ganglia of central and sympathetic nervous system.

Neural Induction

The development of neural tube is induced by the chorda-mesoderm cells, which come to lie in the roof of archenteron in the late gastrula. The chordomesoderm is therefore, known as neural inductor and has been named as primary organizer by SPEMANN (1983). The neural inductor imposes regional specificity on the neural tube. The anterior part of chorda-mesoderm tissue induces the formation of head organs i.e., the brain, eyes, ear and nose, etc., and is known as head organizer. The posterior part of neural inductor initiates the differentiation of trunk organs and tail buds. It is known as trunk or spinocaudal inductor. The head organizer (cephalic inductor) can be further differentiated into (i) archencephalic inductor, inducing the differentiation of forebrain, eyes and nose rudiments and (ii) deuterncephalic inductor inducing the differentiation of hind brain and ear ossicles (LEHMANN 1945)

Mechanism of Neurulation

Roux (1885) presumed that the events occurring during neurulation are caused by the changes in the shape of cells of neural plate. The cells of neural plate become taller and then flask-shaped. The free surfaces of these cells become narrower than the basal ends. Therefore, the layer of these cells tends to curve. Differential rate of cell division in the neural plate and lateral ectoderm is also considered responsible for neurulation.

C.O. Jacobson (1962) has drawn the following conclusions on neurulation in Axolote. 'The neural plate which gives rise to the brain and spinal nerves is not at all essential for nerural tube formation. Rather, the presence of chordo-mesodermal plate, which forms the roof of archenteron is essential. The lengthening of chordo-mesoderm cells causes the upward movement of the lateral ectoderm. Which in turn forms the neural folds or neural ridges. The drawing powers in the neural plate and underlying chordo-mesoderm cells brings the ridges close together.

Under electron microscope, the microtubules and microfilaments have been observed in the cells of neural groove and neural folds and in the elongated cells of blastopore region. These help in changing the cell shape and assist in neurulation.

Chordogenesis (Development of Notochord) : During gastrulation, the presumptive chorda cells along with the presumptive mesoderm involute, stream upward and stretch out along the longitudindal axis to form a narrow sheet in the mid-dorsal region of the roof of archenteron. This sheet of chordo-mesoderm cells is known as chordo-mesoderm mantle. By the time the blastopore closes, the chordo-mesoderm mantle separates from the adjoining endoderm and comes lying between endoderm and ectoderm in its definitive position. Later, the chordo-mesodermal mantle delaminates into the prechordal plate (presumptive notochord) in the middle and somatic mesoderm on the sides. The cells of prechordal plate organize themselves into a cyclindrical rod. Later, these assume vacuolated appearance and secrete a collagenous notochordal sheath. As a result the rod becomes turgid and represents the notochord. Its lengthening occurs by the swelling of notochordal cells which interdigitate in the long axis of the sheath.

Differentiation of Mesoderm

The mesoderm of the head of the pharyngeal region is in the form of mesenchyme which develops into visceral arches. Posterior to the pharynx in the remaining part of the body, the mesoderm occurs in inverted horse-shoe-shape around the archenteron and lateral to notochord. It thickens on either side of notochord and gets subdivided by transverse grooves into a series of somites. Each somite can be separated into three parts:

(i) Uppermost part that lies lateral to the nerve and notochord is the dorsal somite mass or vertebral plate or epimere.

(ii) Intermediate cell mass or mesomere or nephrotome.

(iii) Ventral and lateral part of mesoderm is the lateral plate mesoderm or hypomere.

Epimere—Subsequently, the epimere also delaminates into three parts:

(a) the outermost, narrow strip of mesoderm cells just inside the ectoderm is the dermatome, which contributes to the dermis of skin.

(b) the middle, thick sheet of mesoderm that represents the major portion of epimere is the myotome. It gives rise to the skeletal muscles. The space between dermatome and myotome is the myocoel,

(c) a group of scattered mesenchyme cells that lies between the myotome and notochord is the sclerotome or the skeleton-forming tissue. It forms vertebral coelum.

Mesomeres or nephrotomes give rise to the future kidney. Hypomere or lateral plate mesoderm on each side of archenteron splits into two layers, an outer somatic layers or parietal layer and an inner visceral layer or splanchnic layer of mesoderm. The somatic mesoderm lies along the inner surface of ectoderm and together form somatopleure. The somatopleure gives rise to the skin, its blood vessels, connective tissue and the coelomic epithelium. The splanchnic mesoderm lies along the outer surface of endoderm and collectively form splanchnopleure. The splanchnopleure gives rise to vesceral layer of coelomic epithelium (peritoneum), smooth muscles and blood vessels of mid and hind gut, the blood and the blood vessels.

The space between somatic and visceral layers of mesoderm is called splanchnocoel or coelom, that forms the primary body cavity.

The lateral plate mesoderm extends into the head ventral to pharynx as mesenchyme which gives rise to heart and pericardium.

Tabulation of Endoderm (Completion of Enteron) : At the end of gastrulation, the roof of archenteron is formed of chromesoderm cells. Once these delaminate from the endoderm of archenteron, the endoderm is left as an open through. As neurulation begins, the free margins of endoderm unite in the middle line beneath the notochord. This completes the formation of definite gut or enteron. The floor of enteron is thick and is occupied by large yolky macromeres.

The blastopore formed during gastrulation is first occluded by the yolk plug. Later on, with the withdrawal of yolk-plug in the floor of archenteron the blastopore becomes elongated and δ -shaped. The upper part of 8 forms the neurenteric canal and the lower part marks the position of future invagination of ectoderm to form the proctodeal invagination. It grows forward and becomes continuous with the archenteron. This completes the development of hindgut.

Similarly, stomodaeum appears as an invagination of ectoderm at the anterior end ventral of the neural tube in the middle of an elevated area of ectoderm. The opening of stomodaeum forms mouth, whereas the stomodeal imposing differentiates in buccal cavity. It grows behind to join the archenteron. The archenteron itself modifies into pharynx, oesophagus, stomach and intestine. Liver develops as a diverticulum from the floor of gut. The lumen of liver diverticulum forms the bile duct, whereas the cells of wall proliferate to form liver. The wall of the pharyngeal region proliferates into three pairs of visceral pouches. The remaining two pouches develop later on. The visceral pouches form the gills.

During neurulation, the embryo stretches antero-posteriorly and also flattens sideways so that it becomes narrow and distinct from the head and which is broad in comparison. The part above the blastopore grows out beyond the blastopore and forms the tail rudiment or tail bud. The embryo at this stage is called tail bud larva.

Post-neurular Development

During neurula stage the embryo starts elongating. Its dorsal convex surface becomes concave and anterior part of neural tube widens to form brain. Finally the cells just above the blastopore grow backward and form a tail-like projection. This is known as tail bud. The embryo at this stage is called tail bud larva. It takes about 84 hours.

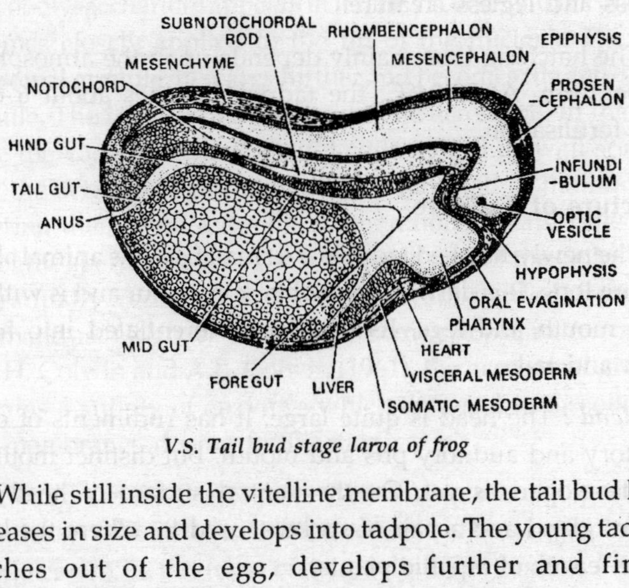

V.S. Tail bud stage larva of frog

While still inside the vitelline membrane, the tail bud larva increases in size and develops into tadpole. The young tadpole hatches out of the egg, develops further and finally metamorphoses into the' adult. The complete process can be studied under the following headings.

Formation of Tadpole

The tail bud larva is markedly different from the tadpole larva. It undergoes following changes while still inside the egg membranes *i.e.,* before hatching into the tadpole.

Hatching

At this stage, larva hatches out of the egg after about 6-15 days of embryonic life. The adhesive organ or sucker is used for fixing the larva to one point on the egg membrane. After fixing its anterior end, the larva to one point on the egg membrane. After fixing its anterior end, the larva performs movements around the fixed point.

The cilia present over the body help in such movement. The frontal gland situated anterior to adhesive organ is rubbed against the egg membrane, which ultimately soften and gives way. The tadpole larva hatches out of the egg as a mouthless, eyeless and legless creature.

The hatching time mainly depends upon the atmospheric temperature. At 30-34°C, the tadpole hatches about 6 days after fertilisation.

Structure of Tadpole

The newly-hatched tadpole is a small fish-like animal about 6-7 mm long. It is dark brown or black in colour and is without eyes, mouth and legs. Its body is differentiated into head, trunk and tail.

Head : The head is quite large. It has rudiments of eyes, olfactory and auditory pits and mouth. But distinct mouth is not developed as yet. On the ventral surface of head is a cement gland and a pair of suckers, used to adhere the larva to the leaves of aquatic plants.

Trunk : The trunk bears three pairs of visceral clefts at the junction of head and trunk. These develop into external gills. The rest of the trunk and tail has > > -shaped myotomes. A depression present at the junction of trunk and tail marks the beginning of proctodaeum.

Tail : The tail is very small. It has notochord, nerve cord, myotomes and blood vessels.

Habit and Habitat of Tadpole

The tadpole is totally different from frog in habit, habitate and structure. It is fishlike in appearance and swims with its tail fin. It breathes with gills and has a soft vascular skin. Its vascular system also resembles that of fish.

Tadpole is purely herbivorous. It lives on or near the bottom of pond, pool or lake, with the help of rasping papillae of the lips and horny jaws it scraps moss algae and chew floating vegetation. It also feeds on bottom mud rich in organic matter.

Adaptation to Aquatic Mode of Life : Tadpoles exhibit following structural modifications which make them adapted to live in water:

1. Fish-like body-form.
2. Presence of external or internal gills.
3. Two-chambered heart like that of fish and circulatory system.
4. A long broad tail with a tail fin that assists in swimming.
5. Presence of a lateral-line system.
6. Excretion of nitrogenous wastes in the form of ammonia.

Late Larval Period

24 hours after hatching, changes begin in the external as well as internal structure of tadpole. The larval life can be separated into following stages:

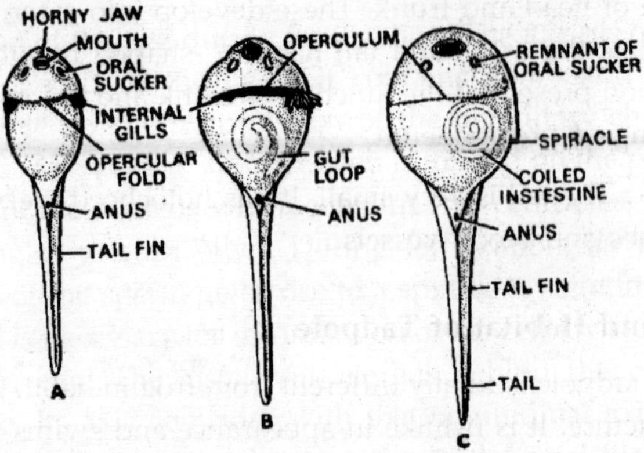

Diagram showing development of operculum in tadpole.

External Gill-stage : During external gill stage following changes occur almost simultaneously.

(i) Proctodaeum is formed by invagination at the junction of trunk and tail. The invagination grows inside and finally joins the archenteron. Its opening to the exterior forms anus.

(ii) The stomodaeum begins as an invagination on the ventral surface of head just in front of suckers. The stomodaeum also gets connected with the archenteron, completing the formation of alimentary canal. Its opening forms mouth.

(iii) Mouth develops horny jaws bearing strong rasping papillae or teeth in several rows. The larva is now able to scrap vegetable matter and chew leaves.

(iv) External gills grow out as feathery outgrowths just behind the head. In the beginning, these are two but become three on each side after some time.

These correspond to 3rd-4th and 5th visceral arches. In this stage larva is called external gill stage.

(v) Tail bud elongates and forms a full-fledged tail. The

skin along its dorsal and ventral sides form a tail fin. The tail functions as a powerful swimming organ.

(vi) Olfactory pit becomes more prominent and eyes become fully-developed.

(vii) The gut becomes much elongated and coiled, like a watch spring. This causes bloating of abdomen. It gets differentiated into pharynx, oesophagus, stomach intestine, etc.

(viii) Liver and urinary bladder are also formed.

(ix) Pronephric kidneys becomes fully developed and functional.

The larva at this stage swims actively by its tail, feeds on aquatic vegetation and increases in size.

Internal Gill Stage : The external gills are of short duration, these are soon replaced by internal gills.

(i) About 28 hours after the formation of external gills, the skin between the external gills starts invaginating and finally joins the pharyngeal wall. Thus 4 branchial clefts are formed on either side. The gill-filaments develop along the anterior and posterior edges of each branchial cleft. These filaments are highly vascular and form internal gills.

(ii) The opercular fold appears from the sides of the head just behind the hyoid arches and in front of gills as double fold of skin. It grows backward over the gills completely enclosing them inside opercular chamber. The opercular chamber projects out as a siphon on the left side and opens outside by a spiracle. Simultaneously, the external gills disappear.

At this stage tadpole respires like a fish. It takes water in through mouth, bathes the gills in pharynx and opercular chamber and comes out of it through spiracle. Simultaneously, the external gills disappear.

At this stage tadpole respires like a fish. It takes water in through mouth, bathes the gills in pharynx and opercular chamber and comes out of it through spiracle.

(iii) The suckers are lost and cement gland appears no more.

(iv) Lateral-line as present on the fish-body develops on the larval body also.

(v) The tail is laterally flattened with dorsal, ventral and caudal fins.

(vi) The tadpole is about 10-15mm long and fish-like in appearance having laterally compressed body, tail-fin and lateral-line sense organs. It swims and breathes like a fish.

Limb Stage : After two-three weeks of free larval life, the limb-buds appear in the tadpole. The hindlimb buds are formed first as small stumps one on each side of cloaca. The forelimb buds are seen later, because these remain hidden under the opercular fold.

Metamorphosis

Tadpole stage lasts for about 15 days or more under normal conditions of temperature and food supply. After this, the fish-like aquatic herbivorous tadpole undergoes drastic changes in habitat, way of life and its structure and metamorphoses or changes into a terrestrial, carnivorous and tailless frog.

Metamorphosis is initiated by the functional development of *thyroid gland,* the hormonal secretion of which is carried to the various body organs through the blood stream, and enhances the changes.

To start with, larva loses its appetite and stops feeding. It now relies upon the reserve food of larval tissue. The further changes can be discussed under three headings.

Changes in Habit and Habitat (Ecological Changes)

1. The herbivorous tadpole larva changes to an insectivorous adult.
2. The preying habits develop and the adult frog becomes more active and swift moving.
3. It leaves water and comes to the land, although it prefers damp places and jumps often and on into the water.
4. In addition to the swimming in water it also jumps on land.

Morphological Changes

The structural or morphological changes occurring during metamorphosis are of two types :

Regressive Changes : These include destructive morphological changes. The organs or structures during larval life but no longer required in the adult are either lost or modified. These include:

1. The internal gills are reabsorbed. The gill clefts are closed.
2. Operculum and spiracle disappear.
3. The tail along with its fin-folds is reabsorbed and at the end of metamorphosis it disappears completely.
4. The horny jaws with rasping teeth are shed. These are replaced by true jaws, which are cartilaginous in the beginning and bony later on.
5. Shape and size of mouth changes. The small subterminal and rounded mouth of tadpole changes into a wide, terminal and crescentric opening.
6. Lateral line system and its sense organs present in the tadpole skin disappears.

7. Aortic arches become reduced and modified in the adult frog.
8. The long and highly-coiled tadpole intestine is replaced by a comparatively short and almost straight tube.
9. Coccal tube becomes short and reduced.

Progressive Changes : The progressive changes are constructive and are as follows :

(i) Both forelimbs and hindlimbs enlarge in size and differentiate with the development of joints and toes. The forelimbs develop under the operculum and come out by breaking it.

(ii) The eyes protrude out on the dorsal side of head and develop eyelids and nictitating membrane.

(iii) The middle ear develops in connection with the first pharyngeal pouch. It is followed by the development of tympanic membrane and circular tympanic cartilage.

(iv) Tongue develops from the floor of buccal cavity and quardrate cartilage rotates backwards increasing the mouth gap.

(v) External nostrils communicate with the buccal cavity through internal nostrils.

(vi) Lung and asspcoated structures become fully developed.

Remodelling of Existing Larval Structure : These include changes in the internal anatomy and are as follows :

(i) The double-layered epidermis of tadpole during metamorphosis increases the number of layers of cells and the surface layers become cornified adapted to live on land. Multicellular mucous and serous glands develop as pockets and sink from the surface into the subcutaneous connective tissue layer. Pigmentation of the skin is changed, characteristic pattern of pigmentation appear.

(ii) Due to insectivorous habit the alimentary canal reduces much in length.

(iii) The stomach and liver become more prominent.

(iv) The two-chambered heart becomes three-chambered due to the septum being laid in the auricle.

(v) Drastic changes occur in the blood vascular system.

(vi) The pronephros of the larva is replaced by the mesonephros.

(vii) Brain becomes more highly differentiated.

(viii) Cartilaginous endoskeleton of larva is replaced in part or as a whole by bones. At the cellular level, cell modifications are evident in eyelids, limb, lungs, tongue, eardrum, operculum, skin, liver pancreas and intestine. Probably no cell or tissue or organ remains entirely unaffected.

Physiological Changes during Metamorphosis

Physiological changes occur simultaneously with the morphological changes. These are of adaptive value for transition to terrestrial habit.

(i) Aquatic larva metamorphoses into the terrestrial adults and, therefore aquatic respiration is modified into terrestrial one.

(ii) There is a change from ammonotelism to ureotelism *i.e.* the kidney starts excreting urea instead of ammonia.

(iii) Liver starts converting ammonia into urea.

(iv) There is an increase in the serum albumin and other serum proteins.

(v) Larval haemoglobin is changed to adult haemoglobin.

(vi) Certain additional digestive enzymes are also produced.

(vii) Endocrine functioning of pancreas starts at metamorphosis for glycogenesis and is associated with increased turn over of carbohydrates.

(viii) There are changes in the metabolism of carbohydrate, lipid, nucleic acids and nitrogen.

(ix) Auto dissolution of tail and reduction in the general size of the body.

(x) Larval visual pigment porphyropsin is replaced by rhodopsin or retinine-I.

(xi) Synthesis of new enzymes, pigmentation of skin, etc. are other physiological changes.

Since the destructive processes play a considerable role in metamorphosis, the body weight and size at the end of metamorphosis is smaller than at the beginning. This is due to de-growth process. The reduction of the body mass is not only due to loss of some parts like gills, tail, etc. but other larval parts except a few, appear to shrink during metamorphosis. As a visible the head and trunk of metamorphosed frog are smaller than in larva.

Causes of Metamorphosis

Metamorphosis in amphibians is an excellent example of the control of morphogenetic processes by *hormones*. The initial signal for metamorphosis in frog is given by the anterior lobe of pituitary gland when it reaches a certain degree of differentiation and become capable of producing the *thyrotropic* hormone. This hormone activates the thyroid gland which builds up and releases the *thyroxine* hormone; now this hormone affects the tissue directly, causing the degeneration and necrosis of some cells and stimulating the growth and differentiation of others (GUDERNATSCH, 1912 and ALLEN, 1918).

Another pituitary hormone, the prolactin is also found to be involved in metamorphosis (ETKIN, 1968). Fresh thyroid tissue contains protein, *thyroglobulin,* having iodine in its molecules. Iodine is not only essential for the working of thyroxine hormone, it has been found that iodine alone can cause metamorphosis even in *thyroidectomized* axolotles.

Endocrine Control of Metamorphosis

Metamorphosis is initiated by the functional development of thyroid gland, its secretion, the thyroid hormone, is carried by blood to different parts of the body and enhances the changes. Thyroid is essential for initiating metamorphosis has been proved by following experiments:

1. The thyroidless tadpoles remain in the larval stage only and continue to grow to attain much larger size than the normal tadpole.
2. Feeding the young tadpoles with thyroid gland or injecting thyroid extract, can induce the metamorphosis to occur in young larvae.
3. Addition of traces of iodine to water causes metamorphosis to occur at an early stage, while eliminating iodine from diet postpones the process.
4. During later part of tadpole stage, the amount of thyroid hormone gradually increases so that initially the metamorphic changes are slow. Towards the end of tadpole life, there is great increase in this hormone and so the metamorphic changes are also rapid.

It is presumed that at a critical point of development the genetic mechanism of tadpole stimulates its neurosecretory apparatus of hypothalamus to release thyrotropin releasing factor (TRF) which in turn stimulates the anterior pituitary to secrete thyroid stimulating hormone (TSH). This causes an orderly increase in thyroid secretion raising its level in blood of tadpole, which initiates metamorphic changes in tadpole.

Bibliography

Alcock, John : *Exploring Animal Behavior : Readings from American Scientist*, Sinauer, London, 1992.

Arbel, T. : *Annual Review of Genetics*, Oxford, New York, 1993.

Arey, L.B. : *Developmental Anatomy*, W.B. Saunders Company, London, 1954.

Austin, C.R. : *Ultra Structure of Fertilization*, Rinehart and Winston International, New York, 1968.

Balinsky, B.I. : *An Introduction to Embryology*, W.B. Saunders Company, London, 1920.

Benson, G. John and Bernard, E. : *The Well-Being of Farm Animals : Challenges and Solutions*, Blackwell, London, 2004.

Berill, N.J. : *Developmental Biology*, McGraw Hill Book Company, New York, 1971.

Black, Jonathan : *Biological Performance of Materials : Fundamentals of Biocompatibility*, Dekker, London, 1999.

Bodemer, C.W. : *Modern Embryology*, Rinehart and Winston International, New York, 1968.

Bolhuis, J.J. and Hogan, J.A. : *The Development of Animal Behaviour : A Reader*, Blackwell, London, 1999.

Bonner, J.T. : *Morphogenesis*, Oxford and IBH Publishing Company, Calcutta, 1965.

Bos, Cees J. : *Fungal Genetics : Principles and Practice*, Dekker, London, 1996.

Campbell, N.A. : *Biology : Concepts and Connections*, Oxford, New York, 1997.

Chaudhry, G. Rasul : *Biological Degradation and Bioremediation of Toxic Chemicals*, Dioscorides P., London, 1994.

Cooper, R. : *The Biology-Chemistry Interface : A Tribute to Koji Nakanishi*, Dekker, London, 1999.

Deen, Roger T. and Kelly, T. : *Atherosclerosis : Gene Expression, Cell Interactions and Oxidation*, Oxford, New York, 2000.

Dick, Stevan J. : *The Biological Universe : The Twentieth-Century Extraterrestrial Life Debate*, Cambridge, New York, 1999.

Dudley, Elizabeth C. : *The Unity of Evolutionary Biology : Proceedings of the Fourth International Congress*, Dioscorides Pub., London, 1991.

Ebert, J.D. and Sussex, I.M. : *Interacting Systems in Development*, Rinehart and Winston International, New York, 1970.

Ewen, R.S. : *Vertebrate Embryology*, Oxford and IBH Publishing Company, New Delhi, 1980.

Ferl, Robert J. : *Biology : The Realm of Life*, Harper Collins, London, 1996.

Fosberg, Dombois : *Vegetation of the Tropical Pacific Islands*, Springer, London, 1998.

Gould, Dr. E. : *Encyclopaedia of Mammals : A Comprehensive Illustrated Guide*, Academic Pub., London, 1998.

Gould, Laura : *Cats Are Not Peas : A Calico History of Genetics*, Copernicus, London, 1996.

Green, Ronald M. : *The Human Embryo Research Debates : Bioethics in the Vortex of Controversy*, Oxford, New York, 2001.

Gutmann, F. : *Charge Transfer Complexes in Biological Systems*, Dekker, London, 1997.

Helms, Doris R. : *Biology in the Laboratory*, Worth Pub., London, 1994.

Hunter, M.L. : *Fundamentals of Conservation Biology*, Blackwell, London, 1996.

Kardong : *Vertebrates*, McGraw-Hill, London, 2001.

Larket C.L., and A. Usprung : *Developmental Genetics*, Prentice-Hall of India Pvt. Ltd., New Delhi, 1974.

Linzey, Donald : *Vertebrate Biology : Biological Sciences*, McGraw-Hill, London, 2001.

Luettner, A.F. : *Fundamentals of Comparative Embryology*, The MacMillan Company, New York, 1949.

Martin, E.H. : *Developmental Behavior Genetics : Natural, Biometrical and Evolutionary Approaches*, Oxford, New York, 1990.

McGleenan, T. : *Genetics and Insurance*, BIOS, London, 1999.

Minkoff, Eli C. : *Biology Today : An Issues Approach*, McGraw-Hill, London, 1996.

Moody, Sally A. : *Cell Lineage and Fate Determination*, Academic Pub., London, 1999.

Nalbandov, A.V. : *Reproductive Physiology*, W.H. Freeman and Company, London, 1985.

Nelson, O.E. : *Comparative Embryology of the Vertebrates*, The Balkiston Company, New York, 1953.

Newell, Grove and Carthy : *Animal Biology*, University Tutorial Press Ltd., London, 1966.

Odell, W.D. and Moyer, D.L. : *Physiology of Reproduction*, St. Louis, Mosby, 1971.

Patten, B.M. : *Early Embryology of the Chick*, Tata McGraw-Hill Publishing Company Ltd., New Delhi, 1971.

Pedigo, Larry P. : *Entomology and Pest Management*, Prentice Hall, London, 1999.

Roodrich, E.S. : *Studies on the Structure and Development of Vertebrates,* The MacMillan Company, New York, 1958.

Rugh, Roberts : *A Laboratory Manual of Vertebrate Embryology,* Burgess Publishing Company, Bombay, 1962.

———: *The Frog : Its Reproduction and Development,* Tata McGraw-Hill Publishing Company, New Delhi, 1972.

Russo, V.E.A. : *Development : Genetics, Epigenetics and Environmental Regulation,* Springer, London, 1999.

——— : *Development : The Molecular Genetic Approach,* Springer, London, 1992.

Samuel, S. : *Biological Control of Crop Diseases,* Dekker, London, 2002.

Saunders, J.W. : *Pattern and Principles of Animal Development,* MacMillon Company, London, 1970.

Scheuer, P.J. : *Bio-Organic Marine Chemistry,* Springer, London, 1988.

———: *Biotechnology and Genetics in Fisheries and Aquaculture,* Blackwell, London, 2003.

Segel, Lee A. : *Biological Kinetics : Cambridge Studies in Mathematical Biology,* Cambridge, New York, 1991.

Shair, H.N. : *Developmental Psychobiology : New Methods and Changing Concepts,* Oxford, New York, 1991.

Singh, Bijay K. : *Plant Amino Acids : Biochemistry and Biotechnology,* Dekker, London, 1999.

———: *Practical Genetics for Aquaculture,* Blackwell, London, 2001.

Slafer, Gustavo A. : *Genetic Improvement of Field Crops,* Dekker, London, 1994.

Slater, P.J.B. : *Essentials of Animal Behaviour,* Oxford, New York, 1999.

Slickinger, R.A. : *Developmental Biology Dubuque,* MacMillan, London, 1966.

Spencer, J.F.T. : *Yeasts : Natural and Artificial Habitats*, Springer, London, 1997.

Spratt, N.T. : *Introduction to Cell Differentiation*, Van Nostrand Reinhold, New York, 1964.

Sreeman, W.H. and B. Bracegirdle : *An Atlas of Embryology*, Heinemann Educational Books, London, 1977.

Starr, C. : *Biology : The Unity and Diversity of Life*, Wadsworth, London, 1998.

Sussman, M. : *Animal Growth and Development*, Prentice Hall, New Delhi, 1958.

Taylor, D.J. : *Biological Science*, Oxford, New York, 1997.

Torrey, T.W. : *Morphogenesis of the Vertebrates*, John Wiley & Sons, London, 1971.

Townsend, R.R. : *Techniques in Glycobiology*, Dekker, London, 1997.

Trempy, J. : *Fundamental bacterial Genetics*, Blackwell, London, 2003.

Waddington, C.H. : *Principle of Development and Differentiation*, MacMillan, New York, 1966.

Walker, P.M.B. : *Chambers Biology Dictionary*, Chambers, London, 1989.

Wang, T.L. and Cuming, A. : *Embryogenesis : The Generation of a Plant-EPBS*, BIOS, London, 1996.

Weisz, Paul B. : *The Science of Biology*, McGraw-Hill Book Company, New York, 1971.

[illegible] London, 1957.

[illegible] Reinhold, New York, [illegible]

[illegible] Blackwell Books, London, [illegible]

[illegible] Wadsworth, London, [illegible]

[illegible] Prentice Hall, New Delhi, [illegible]

Taylor, D.J.: [illegible] Oxford, New York, 1997.

[illegible] John Wiley & Sons, London, 1971.

[illegible] Dekker, London, [illegible]

[illegible] Blackwell, London, [illegible]

[illegible] New York, [illegible]

[illegible] London, [illegible]

[illegible] BIOS, London, [illegible]

[illegible] Book Company, New York, 1971.